T0263544

Emerging Pathogens

Guest Editors

A. WILLIAM PASCULLE, ScD
JIM SNYDER, PhD, D(ABMM), F(AAM)

CLINICS IN LABORATORY MEDICINE

www.labmed.theclinics.com

Consulting Editor
ALAN WELLS, MD, DMSc

March 2010 • Volume 30 • Number 1

SAUNDERS an imprint of ELSEVIER, Inc.

W.B. SAUNDERS COMPANY
A Division of Elsevier Inc.

1600 John F. Kennedy Boulevard • Suite 1800 • Philadelphia, Pennsylvania 19103-2899

http://www.theclinics.com

CLINICS IN LABORATORY MEDICINE Volume 30, Number 1

March 2010 ISSN 0272-2712, ISBN-13: 978-1-4377-1235-3

Editor: Katie Hartner
Developmental Editor: Donald Mumford

Reprints. For copies of 100 or more, of articles in this publication, please contact the Commercial Reprints Department, Elsevier Inc., 360 Park Avenue South, New York, New York 10010-1710. Tel. (212) 633-3813, Fax: (212) 462-1935, E-mail: reprints@elsevier.com.

Clinics in Laboratory Medicine (ISSN 0272-2712) is published quarterly by Elsevier Inc., 360 Park Avenue South, New York, NY 10010-1710. Months of issue are March, June, September, and December. Business and Editorial offices: 1600 John F. Kennedy Blvd., Suite 1800, Philadelphia, PA 19103-2899. Periodicals postage paid at New York, NY and additional mailing offices. Subscription prices are $220.00 per year (US individuals), $347.00 per year (US institutions), $114.00 (US students), $253.00 per year (Canadian individuals), $438.00 per year (foreign institutions), $157.00 (foreign students). Foreign air speed delivery is included in all *Clinics* subscription prices. All prices are subject to change without notice. POSTMASTER: Send address changes to *Clinics in Laboratory Medicine*, Elsevier Health Sciences Division, Subscription Customer Service, 3251 Riverport Lane, Maryland Heights, MO 63043. **Customer Service: 1-800-654-2452 (US). From outside of the US and Canada, call 1-314-447-8871. Fax: 1-314-447-8029. E-mail: journalscustomerservice-usa@elsevier.com (for print support) or journalsonlinesupport-usa@elsevier.com (for online support).**

Clinics in Laboratory Medicine is covered in *EMBASE/Exerpta Medica, MEDLINE/PubMed (Index Medicus), Cinahl, Current Contents/Clinical Medicine, BIOSIS* and *ISI/BIOMED.*

Printed and bound by CPI Group (UK) Ltd, Croydon, CR0 4YY

Transferred to Digital Print 2012

Contributors

GUEST EDITORS

A. WILLIAM PASCULLE, ScD
University of Pittsburgh Medical Center, Pittsburgh, Pennsylvania

JIM SNYDER, PhD, D(ABMM), F(AAM)
Department of Pathology and Laboratory Medicine, University of Louisville Hospital, Louisville, Kentucky

AUTHORS

KAREN C. BLOCH, MD, MPH
Infectious Disease Department, Vanderbilt University School of Medicine, Nashville, Tennessee

SCOTT CURRY, MD
Assistant Professor of Medicine, Division of Infectious Diseases, University of Pittsburgh School of Medicine, Pittsburgh, Pennsylvania

JARED D. EVANS, PhD
Member, Center for Vaccine Research, Assistant Professor, Department of Microbiology and Molecular Genetics, University of Pittsburgh, Pittsburgh, Pennsylvania

LYNNE S. GARCIA, MS, MT, CLS, FAAM
LSG and Associates, Santa Monica, California

CHRISTINA L. GARDNER, PhD
Post-doctoral Fellow, Center for Vaccine Research, Department of Microbiology and Molecular Genetics, University of Pittsburgh, Pittsburgh, Pennsylvania

AMY L. HARTMAN, PhD
Research Manager, University of Pittsburgh, Regional Biocontainment Laboratory, Center for Vaccine Research; Research Instructor, Department of Infectious Diseases and Microbiology, University of Pittsburgh Graduate School of Public Health, Pittsburgh, Pennsylvania

CHRISTINA R. HERMOS, MD
Clinical Fellow, Division of Infectious Diseases, Department of Medicine, Children's Hospital Boston, Boston, Massachusetts

MICHAEL HOLBROOK, PhD
Associate Professor, Department of Pathology, West Virginia University, West Virginia; Director, Robert Shope BSL-4 Laboratory; Director, Emerging and High Risk Pathogens, University of Texas Medical Branch, Galveston, Texas; NIAID Integrated Research Facility, Frederick, Maryland

JOHN M. HUNT, PhD
Independent Consultant, Clinical and Public Health Microbiology, St Paul; Instructor, School of Ophthalmic Medical Technology, Regions Hospital, Minneapolis, Minnesota

NAHED ISMAIL, MD, PhD
Department of Pathology and Department of Microbiology and Immunology, Meharry Medical College, Nashville, Tennessee

P. ROCCO LASALA, MD
Director, Clinical Microbiology Laboratory, Assistant Professor, Department of Pathology, West Virginia University, Morgantown, West Virginia

MICHAEL J. LOEFFELHOLZ, PhD
Associate Professor, Director, Clinical Microbiology Division, Department of Pathology, University of Texas Medical Branch, Galveston, Texas

ALEXANDER J. MCADAM, MD, PhD
Assistant Professor of Pathology, Department of Pathology, Harvard Medical School; Medical Director, Infectious Diseases Diagnostic Division, Department of Laboratory Medicine, Children's Hospital Boston, Boston, Massachusetts

JERE W. MCBRIDE, PhD
Department of Pathology, Center for Biodefense and Emerging Infectious Diseases, University of Texas Medical Branch, Galveston, Texas

MOHAMMED A. MIR, PhD
Assistant Professor, Department of Microbiology, Molecular Genetics and Immunology, Kansas University Medical Center, Kansas

THOMAS S. MURRAY, MD, PhD
Associate Research Scientist, Departments of Pediatrics and Laboratory Medicine, School of Medicine, Yale University, New Haven, Connecticut

STUART T. NICHOL, PhD
Chief, Molecular Biology Activity, Special Pathogens Branch, Division of Viral and Rickettsial Diseases, Centers for Disease Control and Prevention, Atlanta, Georgia

ANN M. POWERS, PhD
Chief, Alphavirus Laboratory, Centers for Disease Control and Prevention, Division of Vector-Borne Infectious Diseases, Fort Collins, Colorado

SHANNAN L. ROSSI, PhD
Postdoctoral Scholar, Center for Vaccine Research, Department of Microbiology and Molecular Genetics, University of Pittsburgh, Pittsburgh, Pennsylvania

TED M. ROSS, PhD
Member, Center for Vaccine Research; Associate Professor, Department of Microbiology and Molecular Genetics, University of Pittsburgh, Pittsburgh, Pennsylvania

KATE D. RYMAN, PhD
Associate Professor, Center for Vaccine Research, Department of Microbiology and Molecular Genetics, University of Pittsburgh, Pittsburgh, Pennsylvania

EUGENE D. SHAPIRO, MD
Professor of Pediatrics, Epidemiology and Public Health and Investigative Medicine, Department of Pediatrics, School of Medicine, Yale University, New Haven, Connecticut

CHARLES W. STRATTON, MD
Associate Professor of Pathology and Medicine, Vanderbilt University Medical Center, Nashville, Tennessee

YI-WEI TANG, MD, PhD
Associate Professor of Pathology and Medicine, Vanderbilt University Medical Center; Molecular Infectious Disease Laboratory, Vanderbilt University Hospital, Nashville, Tennessee

JONATHAN S. TOWNER, PhD
Microbiologist, Molecular Biology Activity, Special Pathogens Branch, Division of Viral and Rickettsial Diseases, Centers for Disease Control and Prevention, Atlanta, Georgia

SARA O. VARGAS, MD
Associate Professor of Pathology, Department of Pathology, Harvard Medical School; Department of Pathology, Children's Hospital Boston, Boston, Massachusetts

SRIRAM VENNETI, MD, PhD
Division of Neuropathology, Department of Pathology and Laboratory Medicine, Hospital of the University of Pennsylvania, Philadelphia, Pennsylvania

Contents

> Malaria has had a greater impact on world history than any other infectious disease. More than 300 to 500 million individuals worldwide are infected with *Plasmodium* spp, and 1.5 to 2.7 million people a year, most of whom are children, die from the infection. Malaria is endemic in over 90 countries in which 2400 million people live; this represents 40% of the world's population. Approximately 90% of malaria deaths occur in Africa. Despite continuing efforts in vaccine development, malaria prevention is difficult, and no drug is universally effective. This article examines malaria caused by the 4 most common *Plasmodium* spp that infect humans, *P vivax*, *P ovale*, *P malariae*, and *P falciparum*, as well as mixed infections and the simian parasite *P knowlesi*. A comprehensive review of the microbiology, clinical presentation, pathogenesis, diagnosis, and treatment of these forms of malaria is given.

> Respiratory tract infections (RTI) are the leading cause of death in low-income countries and the second leading cause of death worldwide in children less than 5 years old. Most RTI are viral. Human metapneumovirus (hMPV) was discovered in 2001 in routine viral cultures of respiratory specimens from children with RTI and has been implicated as a common cause of RTI in children and adults and a cause of severe disease in immunocompromised hosts. This article describes the microbiology, epidemiology, clinical presentation, pathogenesis, diagnosis, treatment, prognosis, long-term outcome, immunity and reinfection of hMPV.

> Dengue is the most prevalent arthropod-borne virus affecting humans today. The virus group consists of 4 serotypes that manifest with similar symptoms. Dengue causes a spectrum of disease, ranging from a mild febrile illness to a life-threatening dengue hemorrhagic fever. Breeding sites for the mosquitoes that transmit dengue virus have proliferated, partly because of population growth and uncontrolled urbanization in tropical and subtropical countries. Successful vector control programs have also been eliminated, often because of lack of governmental funding. Dengue viruses have evolved rapidly as they have spread worldwide, and genotypes associated with increased virulence have spread across Asia and the Americas. This article describes the virology, epidemiology, clinical manifestations and outcomes, and treatments/vaccines associated with dengue infection.

> Ebola and Marburg viruses cause a severe viral hemorrhagic fever disease mainly in Sub-Saharan Africa. Although outbreaks are sporadic, there is

the potential for filoviruses to spread to other continents unintentionally because of air travel or intentionally because of bioterrorism. This article discusses the natural history, epidemiology, and clinical presentation of patients infected with Ebola and Marburg viruses. Clinicians in the United States should be aware of the symptoms of these viral infections in humans and know the appropriate procedures for contacting local, state, and national reference laboratories in the event of a suspected case of filoviral hemorrhagic fever.

Staphylococcus aureus has been recognized as an important human pathogen for more than 100 years. *S aureus* has been able to adapt and evolve in terms of its resistance traits and virulence factors; it is among the most important causes of human infections in the twenty-first century. Rapid molecular identification in the clinical microbiology laboratory of these resistance and virulence factors expressed by *S aureus* will play an important role in the future in decreasing the morbidity and mortality of infections. This article addresses the emerging aspects of infections caused by *S aureus*, including microbiology, epidemiology, clinical presentation, pathogenesis, diagnosis, treatment and prognosis, and immunity.

Chikungunya virus is a zoonotic, vector-borne pathogen that has been responsible for numerous outbreaks of febrile arthralgia since its discovery in the early 1950s. In the past decade, the virus has re-emerged more frequently, causing massive epidemics that have moved from Africa throughout the Indian Ocean to India and Southeast Asia. A discussion of the virus, its epidemiology, diagnostic criteria, and immunity are presented in this article.

There has been a remarkable increase in tick-borne flaviviral disease incidence throughout the past 2 decades. Transmission of tick-borne viruses, like other vector-borne agents, is impacted by a very broad set of factors, both natural (eg, climate and ecology) and man-made (eg, human mobility and agricultural patterns). As our encroachment into areas of virus endemicity intensifies, and as changes in global economic and environmental conditions continue to promote the expansion of tick populations, we will undoubtedly continue to observe attendant increases in rates of disease attributable to these vector-borne pathogens. This article focuses on a some of the major tick-borne flaviviral diseases, caused in particular by tick-borne encephalitis virus, louping ill virus, Powassan virus, Kyasanur Forest disease virus, and Omsk hemorrhagic fever virus, as well as their subtypes.

erthyma migrans, early disseminated disease includes multiple erythema migrans, meningitis, cranial nerve palsies, and carditis; late disease is primarily arthritis. The symptoms and signs of infection resolve in most patients after treatment with appropriate antimicrobials for 2 to 4 weeks. Serologic testing should be used judiciously as it often results in misdiagnosis when performed on blood from patients with a low prior probability of disease and those with only nonspecific symptoms such as fatigue or arthralgia without objective signs of infection.

Clostridium difficile has re-emerged as a major hospital-acquired infection since 2001. Despite development of polymerase chain reaction–based testing, no single clinical diagnostic test has emerged with sufficient sensitivity, specificity, and turnaround time to be entirely reliable for disease diagnosis. The importance of *C difficile* acquired outside the hospital environment remains an unknown factor and awaits further epidemiologic investigation. This article discusses the changing epidemiology, clinical presentation, and pathogenesis of *C difficile* infection and highlights the ongoing challenges of laboratory diagnosis, treatment, and disease relapse.

THE CLINICS ARE NOW AVAILABLE ONLINE!

Access your subscription at:
www.theclinics.com

Avian Influenza A H5N1 Virus

Michael J. Loeffelholz, PhD

KEYWORDS

• Influenza • Avian influenza A H5N1 virus
• Diagnosis • Epidemiology

OVERVIEW

Although influenza A viruses of avian origin have long been responsible for influenza pandemics, including the "Spanish flu" pandemic of 1918, human infections caused by avian subtypes of influenza A virus, most notably H5N1, have emerged since the 1990s (H5N1 in 1997,[1] H9N2 in 1999,[2] and H7N7 in 2003[3]). The wide geographic distribution of influenza A H5N1 in avian species, and the number and severity of human infections are unprecedented. Together with the ongoing genetic evolution of this virus, these features make influenza A H5N1 a likely candidate for a future influenza pandemic. This article discusses the epidemiology, pathogenesis, and diagnosis of human infections caused by influenza A H5N1 virus.

MICROBIOLOGY

Influenza A virus is a member of the family Orthomyxoviridae. This family also consists of influenza B and C viruses. These 3 influenza virus types are separated taxonomically by differences in the matrix and nucleoproteins. Influenza viruses are enveloped, with a single-stranded, negative-sense RNA genome. The genome consists of 8 (influenza A and B viruses) or 7 (influenza C virus) segments approximately 800 to 2500 nucleotides in length. Prominent proteins in the lipid envelop are hemagglutinin (H) and neuraminidase (N). Point mutations in H, referred to as antigenic drift, result in the emergence of new strains of influenza A and B viruses and the resultant annual outbreaks and epidemics. New influenza A virus subtypes emerge as the result of reassortment of genes between 2 distinct strains, referred to as antigenic shift. These new subtypes of influenza A virus are responsible for influenza pandemics. During the twentieth century, influenza pandemics occurred in 1918, 1957, and 1968. The subtypes causing these pandemics all had avian origins, and adapted to high transmissibility among humans. Subtyping of influenza A virus is based on antigenic

Clinical Microbiology Division, Department of Pathology, University of Texas Medical Branch, 301 University Boulevard, Galveston, TX 77555-0740, USA
E-mail address: mjloeffe@utmb.edu

Clin Lab Med 30 (2010) 1–20
doi:10.1016/j.cll.2009.10.005   labmed.theclinics.com
0272-2712/10/$ – see front matter © 2010 Elsevier Inc. All rights reserved.

characteristics of H and N. There are currently 16 recognized H subtypes and 9 recognized N subtypes. Although virtually all combinations of influenza A subtypes naturally infect waterfowl and shorebirds, certain subtypes infect poultry and mammalian species. Subtypes H1N1, H3N2, H2N2, and H1N2 have circulated, or are currently circulating widely, among humans. Subtype H5N1, causing highly pathogenic avian influenza, was identified in humans in 1997 in Hong Kong.[1] Studies on the evolutionary dynamics of influenza A H5N1 indicate that the prototype virus (A/goose/Guangdong/1/96) was derived from a low pathogenic H5 subtype carried by migratory waterfowl, and introduced into poultry in 1996. This was followed by the evolution of novel genotypes locally in poultry through reassortment events, and the rapid increase in genetic diversity (**Table 1**).[4,5] Influenza A virus H5N1 continues to evolve rapidly in avian species,[6] and is significant, although not unique, in its ability to cross normal species barriers and directly infect humans. Although avian subtypes H9N2[2] and H7N7[3] have also recently caused infection in humans, the wide geographic distribution of H5N1 in avian species, and the number and severity of human infections, are unprecedented.

EPIDEMIOLOGY

The classic epidemiologic cycle of influenza A virus includes wild waterfowl and shorebirds, which are naturally infected; domestic waterfowl and poultry, which acquire virus from wild birds; pigs, which serve as "mixing vessels" for avian- and mammalian-adapted strains; and humans, who are susceptible to the reassorted viruses. Reassortment can also occur during human to human transmission. Influenza A virus also infects marine mammals, including seals and whales, dogs, and horses. The H5N1 virus has bypassed this epidemiologic cycle, crossed normal species barriers, and is capable of being transmitted directly from poultry to humans. First identified as a cause of highly pathogenic avian influenza in southern China in 1997, the virus has since spread and caused human infections in Asia, Southeast Asia, the Middle East, and Africa (**Fig. 1**). H5N1 has been found in domestic fowl and a variety of migratory and resident wild bird species. The presence of H5N1 in several migratory bird species has resulted in its rapid spread among continents. The virus has caused outbreaks among poultry in numerous countries across Asia, Southeast Asia, the Middle East, Europe, and Africa (**Fig. 2**). In avian species, influenza A H5N1 infects the intestinal tract and is shed at high titers in feces. Transmission rates are high among birds

Table 1	
Emergence and geographic spread of H5N1 clades causing human disease	
Clade	**Characteristic**
0	China (1997[a])[29]
1	China and Southeast Asia (predominant in Vietnam, Thailand, Cambodia 2004–2005)[29,30]
2.1	Indonesia (2005)[31]
2.2	China (2005), followed by spread to Southeast Asia, Middle East, Europe, Africa[29,32]
2.3	China (predominant in southern China since late 2005), followed by spread to Southeast Asia[13,29,33]
7	China (2003)[6]

[a] Year represents first detection of human disease.

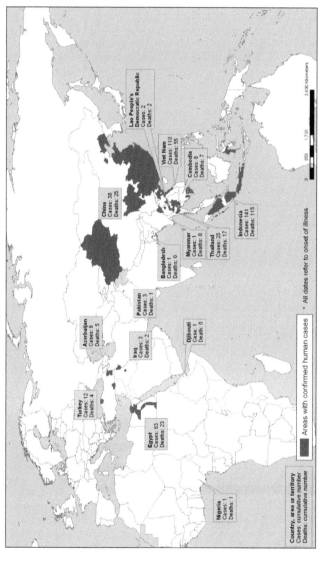

Fig. 1. Worldwide distribution of human influenza H5N1 cases, 8 April 2009. (*Courtesy of World Health Organization; with permission.*)

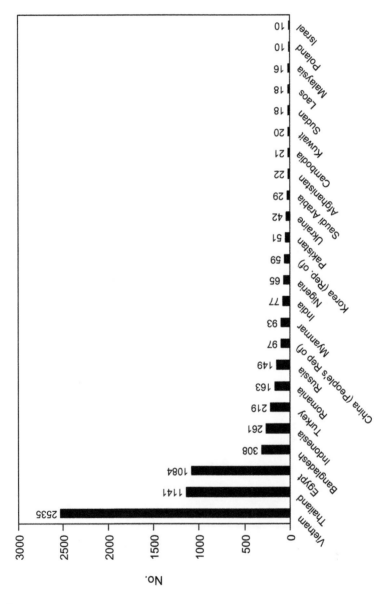

Fig. 2. Outbreaks of influenza H5N1 in poultry, late 2003 to March 2009. (*Courtesy of World Organization for Animal Health; with permission.*)

congregating at bodies of water. In addition to birds, the virus has also been found in several mammalian species. Felines have become infected via the oral route, and probably the respiratory route as a result of consumption of infected dead birds. Cats and ferrets transmit influenza A H5N1 within their own populations, and could possibly infect humans.[7]

Human H5N1 infections are the result of exposure to high viral titers in infected birds or feces. Wet poultry markets, where live poultry is sold and butchered fresh, are sources of transmission to humans (**Table 2**).[8,9] The route of exposure in poultry markets may be contact or droplet, and this risk factor is most commonly reported among adults. Among children, playing with diseased poultry is a more common risk factor.[10] Transmission from diseased poultry to humans is inefficient, as indicated by the absence of neutralizing antibodies in persons who had frequent, direct contact with poultry.[11] The occurrence of cases in persons with indirect or no known contact with diseased poultry suggests that other factors may be involved in transmission and disease. There is evidence of human to human transmission of influenza A H5N1, yet secondary cases are limited due to avian host specificity of H5N1.[8,12] Causes for the emergence and spread of influenza A H5N1 include:

1) Vaccination of poultry using a narrow-range vaccine.
   a) The emergence and spread of a new clade, 2.3, in China and Southeast Asia since late 2005 may have been facilitated by the vaccination of poultry with a vaccine that generated low neutralizing antibodies to clade 2.3 viruses. This selection allowed the rapid spread and predominance of clade 2.3 over a large region, and was associated with an increased incidence of human disease.[13]

Table 2
Epidemiologic features of H5N1 patients: countries with the highest number of reported human cases

Characteristic	China[28]	Vietnam[34]	Indonesia[35]	Egypt[29]
No. of cases investigated	24	28	54	38
Year in which onset occurred	NR[a]	2004	2005–2006	2006–2007
Age (y)				
Median	25	15	18.5	12.5
Range	6–44	1–31	1.5–45	1–75
Male sex, no. (%)	6 (25)	14 (50)	33 (61)	12 (32)
Rural residence, no. (%)	24 (100)	NR	33 (61)	NR
Contact with poultry during previous 2 weeks, no. (%)	24 (100) 16 (67) exposed to sick or dead poultry, and 8 (33) exposed to wet poultry market	28 (100)[b]. 15 (54) exposed to sick or dead poultry in household	41 (76). 23 (43) with direct contact	31 (82)

[a] NR, not reported.
[b] Contact with poultry during previous 7 days.

2) Movement of poultry and wild bird migration.
   a) The movement of poultry and migration of wild birds are associated with the spread of influenza A H5N1. Poultry trade is likely responsible for introduction of H5N1 clades into new areas of Southeast Asia,[6,14] whereas introduction into Europe was most likely through migratory birds.[15]
   b) Multiple lineages have been introduced independently into Africa, consistent with wild bird migration.[16,17,18] Phylogenetic analysis also suggests that influenza A H5N1 was introduced into Egypt through a migratory bird (common teal).[19] A central Asian cold spell in 2006 may have altered bird migration patterns, resulting in the introduction of influenza A H5N1 clade 2.2 from Eurasia to Africa.[20]
   c) Wild birds are not likely hosts for introduction of influenza A H5N1 into North America for 2 reasons: (1) limited migration between eastern and western hemispheres; and (2) newly infected birds that were able to cross hemispheres would likely die before being able to spread the virus.[15,21] However, phylogenetic studies showed evidence of movement of low pathogenic avian influenza viruses between Asia and Alaska via a species of duck.[22]
3) Within a defined geographic area, new virus reassortments may gradually replace established strains.[18,20]

There is evidence for winter seasonal patterns of influenza A H5N1. Although outbreaks in poultry and human cases occur year-round, most outbreaks among poultry in Southeast Asia occur during the winter months.[23] As of June 2, 2009 more than 400 confirmed human cases of avian influenza H5N1 have been reported to the World Health Organization (WHO),[24] and the mortality rate has exceeded 60%. Human cases have been reported from Azerbaijan, Bangladesh, Cambodia, China, Djibouti, Egypt, Indonesia, Iraq, Laos People's Democratic Republic, Myanmar, Nigeria, Pakistan, Thailand, Turkey, and Vietnam (see **Fig. 1**). Cases from Indonesia and Vietnam represent more than 58% of the total reported cases.

CLINICAL PRESENTATION

Influenza caused by H5N1 shares features with those caused by the Spanish influenza pandemic of 1918. Morbidity and mortality are severe in previously healthy, young, and middle-aged persons. Although an aggressive course with severe pneumonia and high mortality rates are the norm, atypical infections such as encephalitis and diarrhea without respiratory symptoms occur.[25,26] Evidence indicates that mild disease and asymptomatic infections occur but are rare.[27] The incubation period is generally 2 to 7 days for all routes of exposure (visiting a wet poultry market, handling sick or dead poultry, and human to human).[8,9,28] One study showed a significantly shorter incubation period after handling sick or dead poultry (median, 4.3 days) compared with visiting a wet poultry market (median, 7 days).[28] The incubation period after exposure to a human case can be as long as 8 to 9 days.[29] Symptomatic cases are characterized by high fever, cough, and lower respiratory tract symptoms (shortness of breath, pulmonary infiltrates) in virtually all patients (**Fig. 3**). At hospital admission the presence of symptoms varies (**Table 3**), likely related to the duration of symptoms before hospitalization. Gastrointestinal symptoms occur more frequently than with influenza caused by human-adapted subtypes. The presence of vomiting or diarrhea ranged from 5% to 50% of cases at hospitalization (see **Table 3**). The frequency of pneumonia and gastrointestinal symptoms distinguish avian from seasonal influenza. Lymphopenia and thrombocytopenia were common among hospitalized cases in several countries, with the exception of Egypt (**Table 4**). Elevated liver function

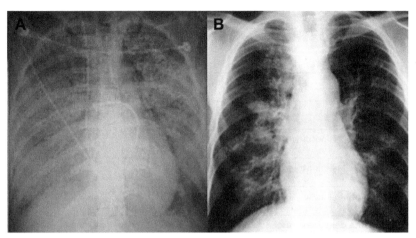

Fig. 3. Chest radiographs of (*A*). Influenza H5N1 pneumonia showing bilateral interstitial infiltration. (*B*) Pneumococcal pneumonia showing multifocal bronchopneumonia in para-hilar regions of both lungs. (*From* Apisarnthanarak A, Kitphati R, Thongphubeth K, et al. Atypical avian influenza (H5N1). Emerg Infect Dis 2004;10(7):1321–4; Shah RM, Gupta S, Angeid-Backman E, et al. Pneumococcal pneumonia in patients requiring hospitalization: effects of bacteremia and HIV seropositivity on radiographic appearance. Am J Roentgenology 2000;175:1533–6.)

enzymes, creatinine kinase, and lactate dehydrogenase were frequently reported (see **Table 4**). The WHO has developed a case definition and risk assessment for human influenza caused by influenza A H5N1 (**Table 5**). The case definition is based on signs and symptoms, results of laboratory testing, and a relevant exposure, which includes close contact with poultry in an H5N1-endemic region, a human H5N1 case, a known infected wild animal, or a laboratory exposure. When there is a suspect case, clinicians

Table 3
Reported signs and symptoms of influenza A H5N1 cases at hospital admission

Sign or Symptom, no./total no. (%)	China[36] Year: 2005–2008 Clade: 2.2, 2.3	Vietnam[33] Year: 2007 Clade: 2.3	Indonesia[35] Year: 2005–2006 Clade: 2.1	Turkey[10] Year: 2005–2006 Clade: ND[a]	Egypt[29] Year: 2006–2007 Clade: 2.2
Fever	18/26 (69)	8/8 (100)	54/54 (100)	8/8 (100)	34/38 (89)
Headache	4/26 (15)	NR[b]	7/54 (13)	1/8 (12)	19/38 (50)
Sore throat	4/26 (15)	2/3 (67)	NR	6/8 (75)	26/38 (68)
Cough	20/26 (77)	8/8 (100)	50/54 (93)	7/8 (88)	27/38 (71)
Dyspnea	6/26 (23)	8/8 (100)	51/54 (94)	NR	14/38 (37)
Pneumonia	26/26 (100)	8/8 (100)	54/54 (100)	7/8 (88)	23/38 (61)
Vomiting	3/26 (12)	2/6 (33)	6/54 (11)	NR	3/38 (8)
Diarrhea	2/26 (8)	3/6 (50)	6/54 (11)	3/8 (38)	2/38 (5)
Myalgia	8/26 (31)	NR	7/54 (13)	4/8 (50)	17/38 (45)

[a] ND, not determined.
[b] NR, not reported.

Table 4
Reported laboratory findings of influenza A H5N1 cases at hospital admission

Variable [no./total no. (%)]	China[36]	Vietnam[33]	Indonesia[35]	Turkey[10]	Egypt[29]
Lymphopenia (<1000 cells/μL)	16/26 (62)	5/8 (63)	16/29 (55)	5/8 (63)	4/25 (16)
Thrombocytopenia (<150,000 cells/μl)	13/26 (50)	6/8 (75)	29/45 (64)	6/8 (75)	8/26 (31)
Elevated alanine aminotransferase (>45 U/L)	13/24 (54)	7/8 (88)	NR[a]	2/8 (25)	15/27 (56)[b]
Elevated aspartate aminotransferase (>45 U/L)	23/24 (89)	8/8 (100)	NR	7/8 (88)	[b]
Elevated creatinine kinase (>130 IU/L)	15/20 (75)	NR	NR	5/8 (63)	NR
Elevated lactate dehydrogenase (>250 U/L)	20/21 (95)	3/3 (100)	NR	7/8 (88)	NR

[a] NR, not reported.
[b] Reported as increased aminotransferase levels.

and infection control practitioners should work closely with public health department epidemiologists to perform a case risk assessment.

PATHOGENESIS

Infection of cells of the human airway epithelium is crucial for the replication and transmission of influenza viruses. Influenza viruses bind to host cells via a specific interaction between the viral hemagglutinin protein and sialic acid residues of cell surface glycoproteins or glycolipids. Whereas human-adapted influenza viruses preferentially infect cells expressing α2,6-linked sialic acid receptors, avian influenza viruses infect cells expressing α2,3-linked sialic acid receptors. α2,6-Linked sialic acids are predominant in the upper respiratory tract, but cells expressing α2,3-linked sialic acids do occur and likely serve as the target cells for human cases of avian influenza.[37] Alternatively, there may be other binding sites on the upper respiratory epithelium that mediate virus entry.[38] Alveolar cells of the lower respiratory tract (macrophages, pneumocytes) express α2,3-linked sialic acid receptors and may also be a site of initial infection.[39] The absence of an influenza A H5N1 pandemic to date is due to the receptor specificity of the H5N1 hemagglutinin protein, and likely to suboptimal virus replication within cells of the upper respiratory tract[37] and the relative inaccessibility of alveolar cells of the lower respiratory tract to casual exposures.

High levels of viral replication and disseminated infection are essential to the pathogenesis of influenza A H5N1 infection.[40] Unlike human-adapted influenza virus subytpes, H5N1 is found in high titers in lower respiratory tract specimens, throat swabs, and stool. In severe cases, H5N1 virus has been detected from blood.[29,40] Death is primarily due to fulminant viral pneumonia followed by respiratory or multiorgan failure. The host immune response is in large part responsible for the severe disease and mortality associated with influenza caused by H5N1. A strong cytokine response, associated with high levels of viral replication, causes fluid accumulation and tissue damage to the lungs.[40] Pathologic findings in the lungs include alveolar damage with hyaline membrane formation, interstitial infiltrates, and pulmonary congestion with hemorrhage.[29]

Table 5		
WHO influenza A H5N1 case definition		
Suspect	**Probable**	**Confirmed**
Acute lower respiratory illness with fever (>38°C) and cough, shortness of breath or difficulty breathing AND One or more of the following exposures in the 7 d before symptom onset: a. Close contact (within 1 m) with a suspected, probable, or confirmed H5N1 case b. Exposure (eg, handling, slaughtering, defeat hering, preparation for consumption) to poultry or wild birds or their remains or to environ ments contaminated by their feces in an area in which H5N1 infections in animals or humans have been suspected or confirmed in the last month c. Consumption of raw or undercooked poultry products in an area in which H5N1 infections in animals or humans have been suspected or confirmed in the last month d. Close contact with a confirmed H5N1 in fected animal other than poultry or wild birds e. Handling samples (animal or human) sus pected of containing H5N1 virus in a labora tory or other setting	Probable definition 1: Criteria for a suspected case AND One of the following additional criteria: a. infiltrates or evidence of acute pneumonia on chest radiograph plus evidence of respi ratory failure (hypox emia, severe tachypnea) OR b. positive laboratory confirmation of an influenza A infection but insufficient labora tory evidence for H5N1 infection Probable definition 2: A person dying of an unexplained acute respiratory illness who is considered to be epidemiologically linked by time, place, and exposure to a probable or confirmed H5N1 case	Criteria for a suspected or probable case AND One of the following positive results conducted in a WHO-designated national, regional or international influenza laboratory: a. Isolation of an H5N1 virus; b. Positive H5 PCR results from tests using 2 different PCR targets c. A fourfold or greater increase in neutraliza tion antibody titer for H5N1 based on testing of an acute serum spec imen (collected 7 d or less after symptom onset) and a convales cent serum specimen. The convalescent anti body titer must be 1:80 or higher d. A microneutralization antibody titer for H5N1 of ≥1:80 in a single serum specimen collected at day 14 or later after symptom onset and a positive result using a different serologic assay, for example, a horse red blood cell HI titer of ≥1:160 or an H5-specific Western blot positive result

Adapted from World Health Organization. WHO case definitions for human infections with influenza A(H5N1) virus. http://www.who.int/csr/disease/avian_influenza/guidelines/case_defini tion2006_08_29/en/index.html (accessed June 1, 2009); with permission.

DIAGNOSIS

The Centers for Disease Control (CDC) has provided guidance on when to perform influenza H5N1 laboratory testing on persons in the United States.[41] These recom-mendations are appropriate for the current stage in which human infections worldwide are rare, limited to certain countries, and absent in the United States. They are intended to prevent testing of persons in whom disease due to influenza A H5N1 virus is highly unlikely, as positive test results in this setting are more likely to be false than they are to be true. These recommendations are based on a combination of clinical and epidemiologic criteria (**Table 6**).

Specimen Collection and Handling

Detection of influenza A H5N1 virus is more likely from specimens collected within the first 3 days of illness onset. Specimens should generally be stored at refrigerated temperatures, unless specified otherwise by test procedures. For virus isolation, specimens should be stored at refrigerated temperatures no longer than 2 to 3 days, or frozen at −70° or less, and shipped on dry ice.

Respiratory specimens

Throat swabs and lower respiratory samples such as bronchoalveolar lavages and tracheal aspirates are the preferred specimens for detection of influenza A H5N1 virus. Nasal swabs and aspirates may contain lower titers than throat swabs.[29,40] This is an

Table 6
Conditions warranting influenza A virus H5N1 testing in the United States

Clinical Criteria	Epidemiologic Criteria
Illness that requires hospitalization or is fatal AND Documented temperature of ≥38°C OR history of fever during past 24 h AND Radiographically confirmed pneumonia or other severe respiratory evidence AND (see epidemiologic criteria)	Has at least 1 of the following exposures during 7 d before symptom onset: 1. Travel to country with documented influenza H5N1 infections in poultry, wild birds, or humans, AND at least 1 of the following during travel: a. Direct contact with well-appearing, sick, or dead poultry or wild birds b. Direct contact with surfaces contaminated with poultry feces or parts c. Visiting a market where live poultry are sold d. Consumption of undercooked poultry products e. Close contact (within 1 m) with a confirmed influenza H5N1 virus-infected animal other than birds (eg, cat), or a person hospitalized or who died due to a severe respiratory illness f. Handling animal or human samples suspected of containing influenza H5N1 virus 2. Close contact (within 1 m) with an ill person with confirmed influenza H5N1 virus infection 3. Close contact (with 1 m) with an ill person under investigation for influenza H5N1 virus infection 4. Laboratory work with infectious influenza H5N1 virus

Courtesy of Centers for Disease Control and Prevention. Updated interim guidance for laboratory testing of persons with suspected infection with highly pathogenic avian influenza (H5N1) virus in the United States. Available at: http://www.cdc.gov/flu/avian/professional/guidance-labtesting.htm. Accessed June 1, 2009.

important distinction between H5N1 and seasonal influenza A subtypes. Collection of combined nasopharyngeal and throat swabs from the same patient would provide an optimal specimen for detection of seasonal and avian influenza strains. Dacron or rayon tipped swabs should be used for specimen collection, as other materials may inhibit reverse transcription polymerase chain reaction (RT-PCR) or virus isolation. Swabs placed in viral transport medium are generally suitable for RT-PCR testing. The collection of lower respiratory specimens generates aerosols, and requires infection control precautions for influenza A H5N1, including the use of gloves, gown, eye protection, and a respirator rated at least N-95.

Rectal specimens
In contrast to seasonal human influenza, diarrhea is a common symptom of H5N1 infections.[29] Influenza A H5N1 viral RNA has been detected in rectal swabs by RT-PCR.[40] However, current CDC testing recommendations do not include rectal specimens,[42] and rectal specimens are inappropriate for detection of seasonal influenza strains.

Serum
Influenza A H5N1–specific antibody can be detected in serum, most accurately by microneutralization and hemagglutination inhibition (HI) assays. Paired serum specimens, the first collected during acute illness and the second collected 2 to 4 weeks later, are required for definitive diagnosis.

Laboratory Tests
As other novel strains of influenza A virus could result in an epidemic or pandemic, such as the recent H1N1 strain of swine origin,[43] testing for the H5N1 virus alone is not recommended. Any influenza A viruses that cannot be subtyped should be referred to the CDC or a local public health laboratory for identification (**Table 7**).

Rapid antigen tests
Because rapid influenza antigen tests provide a result in 30 minutes or less, they can significantly affect patient treatment and management.[44,45] These tests are widely used for diagnosis of influenza in point-of-care locations such as physicians' offices. Several rapid antigen tests are commercially available, and most are able to distinguish between influenza A and B types. Some of these tests are "waived" under the Clinical Laboratory Improvement Amendment (CLIA) regulations. Rapid antigen tests are substantially less sensitive than culture or RT-PCR; reported sensitivities of 27% to 53% relative to RT-PCR[46,47] are typical for seasonal influenza. Although the specificity of rapid antigen tests is often high,[47] the positive predictive value is, as with all laboratory tests, reduced when disease prevalence is low. Therefore, positive rapid antigen test results outside of the influenza "season" should be interpreted with caution, and confirmed by additional tests. Although rapid antigen-capture assays may detect avian influenza subtypes, including H5N1, most commercially available tests are not capable of distinguishing specific influenza A subtypes. Recent evidence indicates that rapid antigen tests designed to detect seasonal strains of influenza are extremely insensitive for H5N1[29,48] and should not be used alone to rule out avian influenza in a suspect case, especially during the prepandemic phase. Since 2004 the overall sensitivity of rapid antigen testing performed on respiratory specimens in 4 countries has been 17%.[29] A study that evaluated the analytical sensitivities of several rapid antigen tests showed that they were at least as good for influenza A subtype H5N1 as they were for seasonal subtypes H1N1 and H3N2, although the detection limits of all kits were at least 1000-fold less than virus isolation.[49] A rapid

Table 7
Advantages and disadvantages of laboratory diagnostic tests for influenza A H5N1

Method	Advantages	Disadvantages
Rapid antigen	Simple Fast Can be performed at point of care	Poor sensitivity Poor positive predictive value in setting of low disease prevalence Most kits do not identify influenza A subtypes
Direct fluorescent antibody	Fast	Moderate sensitivity Subjective interpretation of fluorescent staining Commercially available antibodies do not identify influenza A subtypes
Virus isolation	Sensitive (requires infectious virus) High specificity Provides isolates for further characterization	Propagation of H5N1 requires BSL 3e[a] conditions Slow turnaround time Methods to confirm influenza A subtype (eg, HI, RT-PCR) are not widely available
Nucleic acid amplification	Excellent sensitivity Purified nucleic acids can serve as template for sequencing (genotyping, antiviral resistance mutations)	Food and Drug Administration (FDA)-cleared influenza A H5 tests not available in United States
Serology	Excellent sensitivity Can provide a retrospective diagnosis when other methods are negative	May require paired specimens for accurate diagnosis H5-specific reagents not widely available Labor-intensive Standard methods require infectious virus (BSL 3e conditions)

[a] BSL 3e: biosafety level 3 with enhancements. Refer to text for definition of BSL 3e conditions.

antigen test that detects the nonstructural protein of influenza A H5N1 was recently cleared by the US Food and Drug Administration (FDA) (AVantage A/H5N1 Flu Test; Arbor Vita Corp, Sunnyvale, CA, USA). Rapid antigen testing can be performed on respiratory specimens from suspected avian influenza cases under standard BSL 2 conditions in a class II biologic safety cabinet.[50]

Fluorescent antibody staining of antigens
The specific staining of antigens with fluorescent antibodies is an additional rapid test for the direct detection of influenza viruses in patient specimens (**Fig. 4**). When performed directly on cells from respiratory specimens, this method can provide results in less than an hour. Availability of fluorescent antibody staining is restricted to laboratories with immunofluorescent microscopes and trained technologists able to accurately interpret fluorescent staining patterns. Because this test is performed in a central microbiology laboratory, the factors that affect turnaround time of test results are specimen transport to the testing laboratory, and batching of specimens.

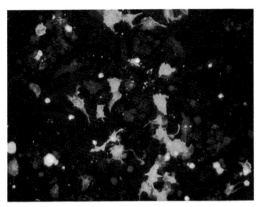

Fig. 4. Immunofluorescent stain of influenza A virus antigens in mixed mink lung and A549 cells (R-Mix™, Diagnostic Hybrids, Inc, Athens, OH). Cell monolayer infected with Influenza A 2009 H1N1; stained with pool of 2009 H1N1-specific monoclonal antibodies 18 hours post infection. Magnification ×200. (*Courtesy of* Diagnostic Hybrids, Inc.)

Fluorescently labeled antibodies specific for influenza A and B viruses are available. Some commercially available influenza antibodies are provided in pools with antibodies to other common respiratory viruses. Fluorescent antibody staining is more sensitive than rapid antigen tests.[46] Specificity is high, but depends on well-trained, experienced technologists. Fluorescent antibody staining reagents specific for influenza A virus will detect avian influenza A H5N1.[48] Currently there are no H5N1-specific fluorescent antibody reagents commercially available. Fluorescent antibody staining can be performed on respiratory specimens from suspected avian influenza cases under BSL 2 conditions in a class II biologic safety cabinet.

Virus isolation
Virus isolation in cell cultures provides highly specific laboratory diagnosis of influenza, but requires fresh, refrigerated specimens for optimal sensitivity. Specimens in viral transport medium must be kept at 2 to 8°C and processed within 2 to 3 days to avoid excessive decrease in viral titer. With proper specimen handling, virus isolation is significantly more sensitive than antigen detection methods.[49] Historically, isolation methods have been considered too slow to affect patient management. Incubation for at least 5 days is generally required to detect influenza virus in tube cultures. Tubes are generally held for 14 days before reporting a negative result. Influenza virus is detected in tube cultures by the presence of cytopathic effect (CPE), adsorption or agglutination of red blood cells, and fluorescently labeled antibodies specific for influenza A and B viruses. Spin-amplified shell vial cultures have reduced the time to detection to 1 to 3 days. In addition to its diagnostic role, virus isolation is important to obtain isolates for strain characterization, surveillance, and vaccine production. Influenza A H5N1 will grow in primary cells and cell lines commonly used for isolation of human-adapted influenza virus, including primary monkey kidney, Madin Darby canine kidney, A549, and others. Microbiology laboratories should be aware that H5N1 and other highly pathogenic novel subtypes can be cultivated unknowingly from unrecognized human cases. Virus isolation of suspected avian influenza A H5N1 requires enhanced BSL 3 laboratory conditions.[50] Enhancements include use of respirators, decontamination of all waste (solid and liquid), and showering of personnel before exiting. Highly pathogenic avian influenza viruses, including H5N1,

are select agents regulated by the Animal and Plant Health Inspection Service (APHIS) of the US Department of Agriculture (USDA). If live H5N1 virus is isolated from a clinical specimen, the CDC or APHIS must be notified, and the agent must be transferred or destroyed.

Serology

Serologic test methods to detect influenza virus–specific antibodies include HI, micro-neutralization, immunofluorescence assay (IFA), enzyme immunoassay (EIA), and complement fixation (CF).[51,52,53,54] Of these methods, only HI and microneutralization are adequately sensitive and specific, and are considered the gold standards for detection of anti-H5–specific antibodies in humans.[52,53] A drawback of HI and micro-neutralization methods is the requirement for enhanced BSL 3 conditions. In response, pseudotype reporter viruses expressing H5 have been engineered and incorporated into microneutralization assays.[55,56] The diagnostic usefulness of serology is limited by the need, generally, to collect acute and convalescent sera to identify seroconver-sion or a fourfold increase in antibody titer. As such, serologic methods that detect IgG responses have a limited effect on patient management, but play a significant role in epidemiologic studies and vaccine development. IFA and other methodologies that detect IgM antibodies can detect acute infection, but sensitivity is reduced because serum IgM levels are usually low due to repeated exposure to vaccine or circulating virus.

Nucleic acid amplification

Nucleic acid amplification methods such as RT-PCR and nucleic acid sequence-based amplification (NASBA) are becoming more commonly used for detection of seasonal and novel influenza viruses and other respiratory viruses.[46,47,57,58,59,60,61] Indeed, testing has become sufficiently established in human and animal diagnostic laboratories such that quality assurance programs have been established.[60] Using real-time fluorescent detection of amplified product, laboratories are able to perform molecular tests in less than 3 hours. These are consistently the most sensitive methods for detection of influenza virus, including H5N1. Molecular diagnostic tests should target conserved sequences of the matrix or nucleoprotein genes to avoid false negatives due to genetic mutations in the more variable hemagglutinin gene.[29] High specificity requires judicious selection of primers and probes, optimization of amplifi-cation conditions, and interpretation of results. Continuous adherence to laboratory protocol is essential to avoid false positives due to carry-over contamination. Currently, there are 3 commercially available FDA-cleared tests that detect influenza viruses by nucleic acid amplification. ProFlu+ (Prodesse, Waukesha, WI) identifies influenza A and B viruses and human respiratory syncytial (RSV) virus. RVP ID-Tag (Lu-minex, Austin, TX) identifies influenza A and B viruses, H1, H3 (seasonal subtypes), and 7 additional respiratory viruses. A CDC-developed assay detects and differenti-ates influenza A, B, H1, H3, (seasonal subtypes) and H5. This test is distributed only to Laboratory Response Network (LRN) reference laboratories. In addition to the CDC influenza subtyping RT-PCR test, some commercial and hospital laboratories may offer laboratory developed ("home-brewed") nucleic acid amplification testing for influenza A H5N1. Unlike FDA-cleared tests, these assays are developed and vali-dated in house by each laboratory. As such, the performance characteristics of the tests may vary between laboratories. The limited availability of influenza A H5N1 refer-ence materials restricts the ability of most laboratories to robustly develop and thor-oughly validate home-brewed H5N1 tests.

Initial processing of specimens for amplified molecular testing can be performed within a biologic safety cabinet under BSL 2 conditions. If the specimen lysis buffer is known to inactivate influenza viruses, further processing and testing can be performed outside of the biologic safety cabinet.

Recent developments in laboratory diagnosis

Recent developments in the laboratory diagnosis of H5N1 infections include the use of monoclonal antibodies for antigen-capture EIA, IFA, and immunohistochemical staining,[62,63,64] H5 epitope–specific EIAs for detection of antibodies,[65] and the use of microarrays[66] and PCR-mass spectrometry[67] for subtyping and strain characterization.

DIFFERENTIAL DIAGNOSIS

Patients with avian influenza typically present with an influenzalike illness with or without severe pneumonia. The differential diagnosis of community-acquired pneumonia includes bacteria (*Streptococcus pneumoniae*, *Mycoplasma pneumoniae*, *Chlamydophila pneumoniae*, *Legionella* species) and viruses (seasonal strains of influenza viruses, RSV, human metapneumovirus, and adenoviruses). In the absence of pneumonia, the common manifestations of fever, cough, myalgia, and malaise can be indistinguishable from those caused by seasonal strains of influenza viruses and other respiratory viruses including RSV, human metapneumovirus, rhinovirus, parainfluenza viruses, and adenovirus.

TREATMENT, PROGNOSIS, AND LONG-TERM OUTCOME

The worldwide case fatality rate for avian influenza is more than 60%, and ranges between 33% and 88% in countries with at least 8 confirmed human cases.[24] Among these countries, Egypt and Turkey have experienced the lowest case fatality rates, 37% and 33%, respectively. Influenza A H5N1 clade 2.2 is the cause of disease in these countries, but multiple variables in health care practices, access to health care, and epidemiology make it difficult to make associations between prognosis and virus clade.[29] Factors likely affecting prognosis the most are receiving antivirals early in disease and supportive care (hospitalization).[10,29,36] Because there are so many other variables, differences in proportions are not always significant.[68]

Recent isolates of influenza A H5N1 show varying resistance to the adamantanes (amantadine and rimantadine). Clade 1 viruses are resistant, whereas the susceptibility of clade 2 viruses varies by lineage and geographic region.[29] The neuraminidase inhibitors, oseltamivir and zanamivir, are active against influenza A H5N1. However, the emergence of high-level resistance to oseltamivir during oseltamivir treatment has been demonstrated in some patients with influenza A H5N1 infections.[69] Quantitatively, the susceptibility of influenza A H5N1 clades to oseltamivir varies, with clade 1 viruses being 15 to 30 times more sensitive than clade 2 viruses.[29] Resistance of influenza A H5N1 to oseltamivir has been associated with H274Y and N292S neuraminidase mutations.[29,70] Additional neuraminidase inhibitors and other antiviral agents are under investigation.[71]

Corticosteroids are not recommended in current WHO treatment guidelines,[72] and may be associated with adverse outcomes.[29] Randomized controlled studies are not practical or ethical, and the presence of multiple variables makes it difficult to observe a statistically significant relationship between corticosteroid therapy and outcome.[68] Yu and colleagues[36] showed that the length of treatment with corticosteroids was directly related to the rate of survival among avian influenza cases.

IMMUNITY AND REINFECTION

Following influenza A H5N1 infection, neutralizing antibodies are detectable 10 to 14 days after the onset of illness.[73] Natural infection with, or immunization against, seasonal strains of influenza viruses does not provide protection against influenza A H5N1. H5 vaccines that are safe and offer cross-clade immunogenicity have been developed.[29,74,75,76,77] Adjuvants varied in their ability to improve (immunogenicity or cross-clade protection) the immune response. Cell culture–derived vaccines have been developed.[77,78] Potential advantages over egg-based vaccines include a faster production schedule and increased production capacity. An adenovirus vector–based vaccine has been shown to be cross-clade immunogenic in mice.[79]

REFERENCES

1. Class EC, de Jong JC, van Beek R, et al. Human influenza virus A/Hong Kong/156/97 (H5N1) infection. Vaccine 1998;16:977–8.
2. Peiris M, Yuen KY, Leung CW, et al. Human infection with influenza H9N2. Lancet 1999;354:916–7.
3. Fouchier RAM, Schneeberger PM, Rozendaal FW, et al. Avian influenza A virus (H7N7) associated with human conjunctivitis and a fatal case of acute respiratory distress syndrome. Proc Natl Acad Sci U S A 2004;101(5):1356–61.
4. Vijaykrishna D, Bahl J, Riley S, et al. Evolutionary dynamics and emergence of panzootic H5N1 influenza viruses. PLoS Pathog 2008;4(9):e1000161.
5. Duan L, Bahl J, Smith GJD, et al. The development and genetic diversity of H5N1 influenza virus in China, 1996–2006. Virology 2008;380:243–54.
6. Nguyen T, Davis CT, Stembridge W, et al. Characterization of a highly pathogenic avian influenza H5N1 virus sublineage in poultry seized at ports of entry into Vietnam. Virology 2009. DOI:10.1016/j.virol.2009.03.006.
7. Thiry E, Zicola A, Addie D, et al. Highly pathogenic avian influenza H5N1 virus in cats and other carnivores. Vet Microbiol 2007;122:25–31.
8. Wang H, Feng Z, Shu Y, et al. Probable limited person-to-person transmission of highly pathogenic avian influenza A (H5N1) virus in China. Lancet 2008;371:1427–34.
9. Yu H, Feng Z, Zhang X, et al. Human influenza A (H5N1) cases, urban areas of People's Republic of China, 2005–2006. Emerg Infect Dis 2007;13(7):1061–4.
10. Oner AF, Bay A, Arslan S, et al. Avian influenza A (H5N1) infection in eastern Turkey in 2006. N Engl J Med 2006;355(21):2179–85.
11. Vong S, Coghlan B, Mardy S, et al. Low frequency of poultry-to-human H5N1 transmission, southern Cambodia, 2005. Emerg Infect Dis 2006;12(10):1542–7.
12. Ungchusak K, Auewarakul P, Dowell SF, et al. Probable person-to-person transmission of avian influenza A (H5N1). N Engl J Med 2005;352(4):333–40.
13. Smith GJD, Fan XH, Wang J, et al. Emergence and predominance of an H5N1 influenza variant in China. Proc Natl Acad Sci U S A 2006;103(45):16936–41.
14. Wang J, Vijaykrishna D, Duan L, et al. Identification of the progenitors of Indonesian and Vietnamese avian influenza A (H5N1) viruses from southern China. J Virol 2008;82(7):3405–14.
15. Kilpatrick AM, Chmura AA, Gibbons DW, et al. Predicting the global spread of H5N1 avian influenza. Proc Natl Acad Sci U S A 2006;103(51):19368–73.
16. Ducatez MF, Olinger CM, Owoade AA, et al. Multiple introductions of H5N1 in Nigeria. Nature 2006;442:37.

17. Ducatez MF, Olinger CM, Owoade AA, et al. Molecular and antigenic evolution and geographical spread of H5N1 highly pathogenic avian influenza viruses in western Africa. J Gen Virol 2007;88:2297–306.

18. Salzberg SL, Kingsford C, Cattoli G, et al. Genome analysis linking recent European and African influenza (H5N1) viruses. Emerg Infect Dis 2007;13(5):713–8.

19. Saad MD, Ahmed LS, Gamal-Eldein MA, et al. Possible avian influenza (H5N1) from migratory bird, Egypt. Emerg Infect Dis 2007;13(7):1120–1.

20. Owoade AA, Gerloff NA, Ducatez MF, et al. Replacement of sublineages of avian influenza (H5N1) by reassortments, sub-Saharan Africa. Emerg Infect Dis 2008; 14(11):1731–5.

21. Rappole JH, Hubalek Z. Birds and influenza H5N1 virus movement to and within North America. Emerg Infect Dis 2006;12(10):1486–92.

22. Koehler AV, Pearce JM, Flint PL, et al. Genetic evidence of intercontinental movement of avian influenza in a migratory bird: the northern pintail (*Anas acuta*). Mol Ecol 2008;17(21):4754–62.

23. Park AW, Glass K. Dynamic patterns of avian and human influenza in east and southeast Asia. Lancet Infect Dis 2007;7:543–8.

24. World Health Organization. Cumulative number of confirmed human cases of avian influenza A/(H5N1) reported to WHO. Available at: http://www.who.int/csr/disease/avian_influenza/country/cases_table_2009_06_02/en/index.html. Accessed June 7, 2009.

25. Apisarnthanarak A, Kitphati R, Thongphubeth K, et al. Atypical avian influenza (H5N1). Emerg Infect Dis 2004;10(7):1321–4.

26. de Jong MD, Cam BV, Qui PT, et al. Fatal avian influenza A (H5N1) in a child presenting with diarrhea followed by coma. N Engl J Med 2005;352:686–91.

27. Uyeki TM. Global epidemiology of human infections with highly pathogenic avian influenza A (H5N1) viruses. Respirology 2008;13:S2–9.

28. Huai Y, Xiang N, Zhou L, et al. Incubation period for human cases of avian influenza A (H5N1) infection, China. Emerg Infect Dis 2008;14(11):1819–21.

29. Writing Committee of the Second World Health Organization (WHO) Consultation on Clinical Aspects of Human Infection with Avian Influenza A (H5N1) Virus. Update on avian influenza A (H5N1) virus infection in humans. N Engl J Med 2008;358(3):261–73.

30. Buchy P, Mardy S, Vong S, et al. Influenza A/H5N1 virus infection in humans in Cambodia. J Clin Virol 2007;39:164–8.

31. Kandun IN, Wibisono H, Sedyaningsih ER, et al. Three Indonesian clusters of H5N1 virus infection in 2005. N Engl J Med 2006;355(21):2186–94 [Erratum N Engl J Med 2007;356:1375].

32. Editorial team. Seven human cases of H5N1 infection confirmed in Azerbaijan, and one case in Egypt. Euro Surveill 2006;11(12). pii=2927. Available at: http://www.eurosurveillance.org/ViewArticle.aspx?ArticleId=2927. Accessed June 1, 2009.

33. Le MTQ, Wertheim HFL, Nguyen HD, et al. Influenza A H5N1 clade 2.3.4 virus with a different antiviral susceptibility profile replaced clade 1 virus in humans in northern Vietnam. PLoS One 2008;3(10):e3339.

34. Dinh PN, Long HT, Tien NTK, et al. Risk factors for human infection with avian influenza A H5N1, Vietnam, 2004. Emerg Infect Dis 2006;12(12):1841–7.

35. Sedyaningsih ER, Isfandari S, Setiawaty V, et al. Epidemiology of cases of H5N1 virus infection in Indonesia, July 2005-June 2006. J Infect Dis 2007;196(15):522–7.

36. Yu H, Gao Z, Feng Z, et al. Clinical characteristics of 26 human cases of highly pathogenic avian influenza A (H5N1) virus infection in China. PLoS One 2008; 3(8):e2985.

37. Matrosovich MN, Matrosovich TY, Gray T, et al. Human and avian influenza viruses target different cell types in cultures of human airway epithelium. Proc Natl Acad Sci U S A 2004;101(13):4620–4.
38. Nicholls JM, Chan MCW, Chan WY, et al. Tropism of avian influenza A (H5N1) in the upper and lower respiratory tract. Nat Med 2007;13(2):147–9.
39. Shinya K, Ebina M, Yamada S, et al. Influenza virus receptors in the human airway. Nature 2006;440(23):435–6.
40. de Jong M, Simmons CP, Thanh TT, et al. Fatal outcome of human influenza A (H5N1) is associated with high viral load and hypercytokinemia. Nat Med 2006;12:1203–7.
41. Centers for Disease Control and Prevention. Updated interim guidance for laboratory testing of persons with suspected infection with highly pathogenic avian influenza (H5N1) virus in the United States. Available at: http://www.cdc.gov/flu/avian/professional/guidance-labtesting.htm. Accessed June 1, 2009.
42. U.S. Department of Health & Human Services. HHS pandemic influenza plan. Available at: http://www.hhs.gov/pandemicflu/plan/. Accessed June 1, 2009.
43. Centers for Disease Control and Prevention. Swine influenza A (H1N1) infection in two children—Southern California, March-April 2009. Morb Mortal Wkly Rep 2009;58(15):400–2.
44. Falsey AR, Murata Y, Walsh EE. Impact of rapid diagnosis on management of adults hospitalized with influenza. Arch Intern Med 2007;167(4):354–60.
45. Abanses JC, Dowd MD, Simon SD, et al. Impact of rapid influenza testing at triage on management of febrile infants and young children. Pediatr Emerg Care 2006;22(3):145–9.
46. Landry ML, Cohen S, Ferguson D. Real-time PCR compared to Binax NOW and cytospin-immunofluorescence for detection of influenza in hospitalized patients. J Clin Virol 2008;43(2):148–51.
47. Uyeki TM, Prasad R, Vukotich C, et al. Low sensitivity of rapid diagnostic test for influenza. Clin Infect Dis 2009;48(9):e89–92.
48. Fedorko DP, Nelson NA, McAuliffe JM, et al. Performance of rapid tests for detection of avian influenza A virus types H5N1 and H9N2. J Clin Microbiol 2006;44(4):1596–7.
49. Chan KH, Lam SY, Puthavathana P, et al. Comparative analytical sensitivities of six rapid influenza A antigen detection test kits for detection of influenza A subtypes H1N1, H3N2 and H5N1. J Clin Virol 2007;38:169–71.
50. Centers for Disease Control and Prevention. Outbreaks of avian influenza A (H5N1) in Asia and interim recommendations for evaluation and reporting of suspected cases—United States, 2004. Morb Mortal Wkly Rep 2004;53(5):97–100.
51. Jia N, Wang SX, Liu YX, et al. Increased sensitivity for detecting avian influenza-specific antibodies by a modified hemagglutination inhibition assay using horse erythrocytes. J Virol Methods 2008;153(1):43–8.
52. Rowe T, Abernathy RA, Hu-Primmer J, et al. Detection of antibody to avian influenza A (H5N1) virus in human serum by using a combination of serologic assays. J Clin Microbiol 1999;37(4):937–43.
53. Noah DL, Hill H, Hines D, et al. Qualification of the hemagglutination inhibition assay in support of pandemic influenza vaccine licensure. Clin Vaccine Immunol 2009;16(4):558–66.
54. Stelzer-Braid S, Wong B, Robertson P, et al. A commercial ELISA detects high levels of human H5 antibody but cross-reacts with influenza A antibodies. J Clin Virol 2008;43(2):241–3.
55. Wang W, Butler EN, Veguilla V, et al. Establishment of retroviral pseudotypes with influenza hemagglutinins from H1, H3, and H5 subtypes for sensitive and specific detection of neutralizing antibodies. J Virol Methods 2008;153(2):111–9.

56. Nefkens I, Garcia J-M, Ling CS, et al. Hemagglutinin pseudotyped lentiviral particles: characterization of a new method for avian H5N1 influenza sero-diagnosis. J Clin Virol 2007;39:27–33.
57. Mahony JS, Chong F, Merante S, et al. Development of a respiratory virus panel test for detection of twenty human respiratory viruses by use of multiplex PCR and a fluid microbead-based assay. J Clin Microbiol 2007;45:2965–70.
58. Wang W, Ren P, Mardi S, et al. Design of multiplexed detection assays for identification of avian influenza A virus subtypes pathogenic to humans by SmartCycler real-time reverse transcription-PCR. J Clin Microbiol 2009;47(1):86–92.
59. Chantratita W, Sukasem C, Kaewpongsri S, et al. Qualitative detection of avian influenza A (H5N1) viruses: a comparative evaluation of four real-time nucleic acid amplification methods. Mol Cell Probes 2008;22(5–6):287–93.
60. Stelzer-Braid S, Escott R, Baleriola C, et al. Proficiency of nucleic acid tests for avian influenza viruses, Australasia. Emerg Infect Dis 2008;14(7):1126–8.
61. Yuen KY, Chan PKS, Peiris M, et al. Clinical features and rapid viral diagnosis of human disease associated with avian influenza A H5N1 virus. Lancet 1998;351: 467–71.
62. Ho HT, Qian HL, He F, et al. Rapid detection of H5N1 subtype influenza viruses by antigen capture enzyme-linked immunosorbent assay using H5- and H1-specific monoclonal antibodies. Clin Vaccine Immunol 2009;16(5):726–32.
63. Du A, Daidoji T, Koma T, et al. Detection of circulating Asian H5N1 viruses by a newly established monoclonal antibody. Biochem Biophys Res Commun 2009;378(2):197–202.
64. He F, Du Q, Ho Y, et al. Immunohistochemical detection of influenza virus infection in formalin-fixed tissues with anti-H5 monoclonal antibody recognizing FFWTILKP. J Virol Methods 2009;155(1):25–33.
65. Prabakaran M, Ho HT, Prabhu N, et al. Development of epitope-blocking ELISA for universal detection of antibodies to human H5N1 influenza viruses. PLoS One 2009;4(2):e4566.
66. Gall A, Hoffmann B, Harder T, et al. Design and validation of a microarray for detection, hemagglutinin subtyping, and pathotyping of avian influenza viruses. J Clin Microbiol 2009;47(2):327–34.
67. Michael K, Harder TC, Mettenleiter TC, et al. Diagnosis and strain differentiation of avian influenza viruses by restriction fragment mass analysis. J Virol Methods 2009;158(1–2):63–9.
68. Hien ND, Ha NH, Van NT, et al. Human infection with highly pathogenic avian influenza virus (H5N1) in Northern Vietnam, 2004–2005. Emerg Infect Dis 2009; 15(1):19–23.
69. de Jong MD, Thanh TT, Khanh TH, et al. Oseltamivir resistance during treatment of influenza A (H5N1) infection. N Engl J Med 2005;353:2667–72.
70. Malaisree M, Rungrotmongkol T, Nunthaboot N, et al. Source of oseltamivir resistance in avian influenza H5N1 virus with the H274Y mutation. Amino Acids 2008. DOI:10.1007/s00726-008-0201-z.
71. Hayden F. Developing new antiviral agents for influenza management: what does the future hold? Clin Infect Dis 2009;48:S3–13.
72. World Health Organization. Clinical management of human infection with avian influenza A (H5N1) virus. Available at: http://www.who.int/csr/disease/avian_influenza/guidelines/clinicalmanage07/en/. Accessed June 1, 2009.
73. Writing Committee of the World Health Organization (WHO) Consultation on Human Influenza A/H5. Avian influenza A (H5N1) infection in humans. N Engl J Med 2005;353(13):1374–85.

74. Nolan TM, Richmond PC, Skeljo MV, et al. Phase I and II randomized trials of the safety and immunogenicity of a prototype adjuvanted inactivated split-virus influenza A (H5N1) vaccine in healthy adults. Vaccine 2008;26(33):4160–7.
75. Levie K, Leroux-Roels I, Hoppenbrouwers K, et al. An adjuvanted, low-dose, pandemic influenza A (H5N1) vaccine candidate is safe, immunogenic, and induces cross-reactive immune responses in healthy adults. J Infect Dis 2008; 198(5):642–9.
76. Fazekas G, Martosne-Mendi R, Jankovics I, et al. Cross-reactive immunity to clade 2 strains of influenza virus A subtype H5N1 induced in adults and elderly patients by Fluval, a prototype pandemic influenza virus vaccine derived by reverse genetics, formulated with a phosphate adjuvant, and directed to clade 1 strains. Clin Vaccine Immunol 2009;16(4):437–43.
77. Ehrlich HJ, Muller M, Oh HML, et al. A clinical trial of a whole-virus H5N1 vaccine derived from cell culture. N Engl J Med 2008;358:2573–84.
78. Hu AY, Weng TC, Tseng YF, et al. Microcarrier-based MDCK cell culture system for the production of influenza H5N1 vaccines. Vaccine 2008;26(45):5736–40.
79. Hoelscher MA, Singh N, Garg S, et al. A broadly protective vaccine against globally dispersed clade 1 and clade 2 H5N1 influenza viruses. J Infect Dis 2008; 197(8):1185–8.

Shiga Toxin–Producing *Escherichia coli* (STEC)

John M. Hunt, PhD[a,b,*]

KEYWORDS

• Escherichia coli • STEC • Enterohemorrhagic • Verotoxigenic
• Diarrhea • Hemolytic uremic syndrome

Shiga toxin–producing *Escherichia coli* (STEC) comprise one of four generally recognized groups of *E coli* causing diarrhea in humans who acquire infections by ingestion of contaminated food or water or another fecal-oral route. The natural reservoir for STEC is ruminant animals, notably cattle, in which STEC can occur as normal intestinal flora (**Fig. 1**).[1,2] STEC is unique among these *E coli* by virtue of harboring and expressing the genes for Shiga toxins type 1 (Stx1) and 2 (Stx2). Shiga toxin is named for the Japanese microbiologist Kiyoshi Shiga (1870–1957), for whom the genus *Shigella* is named, inasmuch as the toxin produced by *Shigella dysenteriae* type 1 is very similar to the Stx1 and Stx2 produced by STEC. **Table 1** provides a brief summary of these four well-characterized diarrheogenic *E coli*. They are distinct from the commensal *E coli* strains that inhabit the human gut and cause urinary tract infections, bacteremia, meningitis, and pneumonia in susceptible patients.[3]

Transmission of STEC to humans occurs through consumption of undercooked ground (minced) beef, foods eaten raw (eg, lettuce, sprouts, or spinach from manured gardens), water, or unpasteurized milk or juices, contaminated with STEC originating from cattle feces.[4] Direct animal-to-human and human-to-human transmission have occurred.[4,5] Worldwide, STEC are often referred to as "verotoxin-producing" or "verocytotoxin-producing" *E coli* (VTEC), making reference to their cytotoxic effect on the Vero monkey kidney cell line (**Fig. 2**).[6] In older literature, STEC was referred to as "enterohemorrhagic *E coli*" (EHEC), referring to bloody stools that are often a part of the clinical presentation,[4,7] and use of the EHEC acronym continues.

The author is employed as an independent contractor by Children's Hospitals and Clinics of Minnesota to provide consulting for laboratory test development.
[a] Clinical and Public Health Microbiology, 441 Desnoyer Avenue, St Paul, MN 55104, USA
[b] School of Ophthalmic Medical Technology, Regions Hospital, PO Box 1309, Minneapolis, MN 55440–1309, USA
* Clinical and Public Health Microbiology, 441 Desnoyer Avenue, St Paul, MN 55104.
E-mail address: jmhuntjr@comcast.net

Clin Lab Med 30 (2010) 21–45
doi:10.1016/j.cll.2009.11.001
0272-2712/10/$ – see front matter © 2010 Elsevier Inc. All rights reserved.

labmed.theclinics.com

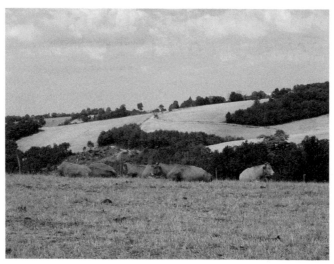

Fig. 1. Cattle and other ruminants are natural reservoirs of STEC. (*Courtesy of* Sarah Hunt, St Paul, MN.)

HISTORICAL EMERGENCE OF STEC AS A DIARRHEAL PATHOGEN

Reported as *E coli* strains having distinct O-antigenic serotypes associated with bloody diarrhea and postdiarrheal hemorrhagic colitis in children in Canada[6] and in the United States,[8] STEC has emerged as a frequent cause of food-borne gastroenteritis, both sporadically and in outbreaks, creating substantial risk of hemolytic uremic syndrome (HUS) and life-threatening renal failure in children.[9] Over the past 25 years, most attention has been focused on one particular STEC O-antigen serotype, O157, of flagellar serotype H7 (*E coli* O157:H7, or STEC O157), which predominates in reported outbreaks and sporadic cases in the United States and elsewhere worldwide, although not universally.[4] In Germany, for example, STEC O91 is the predominant serotype isolated from adult patients.[10] STEC O157 is notable for having caused an outbreak of diarrhea in the United States in 1982 traced to contaminated beef served by a fast-food restaurant chain that resulted in four deaths[8]; and a 1996 Japanese outbreak affecting an estimated 6000 children, three of whom died.[11]

The two toxins that can be produced by STEC have been referred to historically as "Shiga-like toxins," and "verotoxins" or "verocytotoxins." The acronyms STEC, EHEC, and VTEC are used interchangeably. Stx1 differs in one amino acid from Shiga toxin of *Shigella dysenteriae* serotype 1, whereas Stx2 shares only about 60% amino acid similarity with Stx1. Sequence variants of both Stx1 and Stx2 are known, and multiple variants may be produced by one STEC bacterium.[12]

With heightened awareness of the importance of STEC O157, and improvements in its laboratory detection in stool specimens,[3] sporadic infections and outbreaks of varying magnitude continue to be documented. Laboratory testing has improved to the point that a standard of care is to always suspect and test for this particular pathogen in stool specimens from patients with diarrhea. Importantly, it is the clinician's responsibility to communicate with the clinical microbiology laboratory to ensure that appropriate specimen collection and transport occurs, and that cultures are ordered and performed to recover and isolate STEC O157 from stool specimens submitted for bacterial cultures.[3,13] Isolation of a pure culture of STEC from patients

Table 1
Four major groups of diarrheogenic *E coli*

Diarrheogenic *E coli*	Toxins	Other Virulence Factors	Worldwide Disease Burden	Clinical and Public Health Aspects
STEC (EHEC, VTEC)	Produces Shiga toxins Stx1, Stx2 (Verotoxins)	Survival in undercooked beef, on raw vegetables, in milk, and in water and fruit juices; adhesins for adherence to intestinal epithelium	Significant cause of HUS following bloody or nonbloody diarrhea; O157:H7 most prevalent, but STEC non-O157 important	A zoonotic disease acquired from foods and water contaminated with feces of cattle and other ruminants; secondary cases likely; low infectious dose
EIEC	None	Low infectious dose; invades intestinal epithelium	Rare; endemic in some countries; localized outbreaks in nurseries	Similar to Shigella, with fever, pain, dysentery; food-borne and person-to-person transmission
EPEC	None	Protein factors for attachment to and effacement of enterocyte microvilli; distinct pili for attachment to enterocytes	Significant cause of infant (<1 y) diarrhea; associated with weaning in infants; dehydration may be severe and fatal	Watery diarrhea with mucus, fever, with nausea and vomiting; foodborne transmission
ETEC	Heat-labile toxin (LT), heat-stable toxin (ST)	Colonization factors (proteins) expressed in intestinal lumen	Many fatal cases in children <5 y; associated with weaning in infants; dehydration may be severe	Profuse watery diarrhea; usually self-limiting as a common complaint of adult travelers

Abbreviations: STEC (EHEC, VTEC), Shiga toxin–producing *E coli* (enterohemorrhagic *E coli*, verocytotoxin- or verotoxin-producing *E coli*); EIEC, enteroinvasive *E coli*; EPEC, enteropathogenic *E coli*; ETEC, enterotoxigenic *E coli*; HUS, hemolytic-uremic syndrome.

Data from Nataro JP, Bopp CS, Fields PI, et al. *Escherichia, Shigella,* and *Salmonella.* In: Murray PR, Baron EJ, Jorgensen JH, et al. editors. Manual of clinical microbiology. 9th edition. Washington, DC: American Society for Microbiology; 2007. p. 670–87; Fontaine O, Griffin P, Henao O, et al. Diarrhea, acute. In: Heymann DL, editor. Control of communicable diseases manual. 19th edition. Washington, DC: American Public Health Association; 2008. p. 179–95; Centers for Disease Control and Prevention. Diagnosis and management of foodborne illnesses: a primer for physicians and other health care professionals. MMWR Morb Mortal Wkly Res 2004;53:1–33.

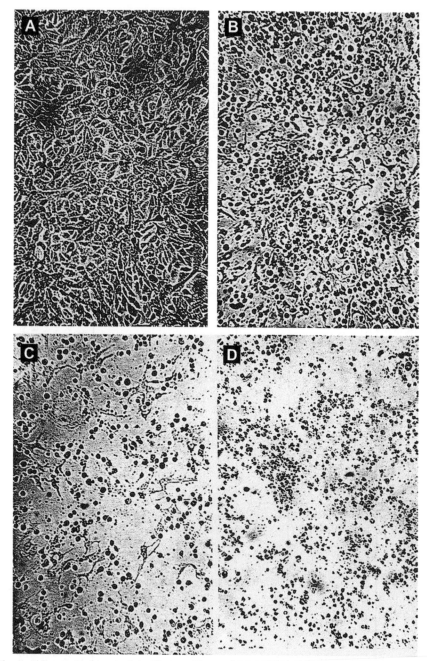

Fig. 2. Shiga toxin (Verotoxin) effect on Vero cell monolayers. (*A*) Medium control, 1 day, cells in continuous monolayer. With STEC filtrate, (*B*) 1 day, (*C*) 2 days, (*D*) 5 days; monolayer being destroyed. Phase-contrast microscopy. Magnification ×237. (*From* Konowalchuk J, Speirs JI, Stavrik S. Vero response to a cytotoxin of *Escherichia coli*. Infect Immun 1977;18:775–9; with permission.)

is the gold standard for confirming the diagnosis. In addition, pure cultures provide organisms for molecular epidemiology and outbreak investigations by public health laboratories working to prevent transmission in the community.[14,15] With the emerging awareness of STEC non-O157 as diarrheal pathogens, many clinical laboratories now offer immunoassay tests for Shiga toxins or for several non-O157 STEC O-antigens in parallel with stool cultures.[3,7] Immunoassay results can often be provided to the clinician before a final culture result is available. Culture confirmation of STEC should always be attempted by the clinical laboratory, however, or by a reference laboratory to which suspected STEC isolates are sent.[16]

EMERGENCE OF STEC NON-O157 DISEASE

Early recognition that STEC serotypes other than O157 were associated with diarrhea and hemorrhagic colitis prompted development of laboratory testing methods for the detection of now over 150 known STEC non-O157 strains.[3,6] In North America, STEC serotypes O26, O45, O103, O111, and O121 are the most common[3,4]; and in Europe, these serotypes, and O91 and O145, are most frequently isolated from ill patients.[3,4,10] Serotypes of STEC isolated from ruminant reservoir animals and from infected patients vary in prevalence worldwide, indicating a need for clinical laboratories to determine common endemic serotypes while being on the alert for less common or "imported" serotypes in sporadic infections.[1,2,4,17,18] The non-O157 STEC also harbor and express one or both of the Shiga toxin *Stx* genes present on temperate bacteriophages in the STEC genome and, like STEC O157, have caused diarrhea, hemorrhagic colitis, and HUS.[3,4,6,10] Detection of non-O157 STEC in stool cultures is problematic because unlike most O157 STEC, they do ferment sorbitol, and do not grow as sorbitol-negative (nonfermenting) colonies on sorbitol-MacConkey (SMAC) agar that has been so useful for recovery of sorbitol-nonfermenting STEC O157.[3,9]

EMERGING TRENDS IN STEC DISEASE

The severity and long-term sequelae associated with STEC disease warrant a careful consideration of how to improve patient outcome.[17,19] Awareness that STEC non-O157 serotypes are capable of causing postdiarrheal HUS is well established,[3,4,7] but the recovery of diverse serotypes by most clinical laboratories is difficult and can result in delays in providing useful information to clinicians. DNA amplification methods can be used to identify STEC independent of serotype, if genes encoding Stx1 or Stx2 are present.[20] This can be done from isolated colonies, from mixed growth on agar plates, or directly from stool specimens. Commercial kits for real-time amplification tests for Shiga toxin genes, using instrument platforms currently in use in clinical laboratories, may eventually be available.[21]

Sorbitol-fermenting STEC O157, the so-called "SF STEC," are typically nonmotile (H-) STEC O157 first identified in a 1988 outbreak of HUS in Germany.[22] These pathogens present identification challenges analogous to those of non-O157 STEC. The epidemiology of SF STEC O157:H- is interesting because of its geographic clustering in Europe.[20,22]

Loss of the genes that encode Shiga toxins during infection has recently been observed for patients with HUS following STEC diarrhea. Strains of *E coli* having typical STEC serotypes (eg, O26, O111, O103, O121, O145, and O157) but which lack genes for Stx1 and Stx2 have been isolated from stool specimens of HUS patients.[23] Assuming that these strains of *E coli* were the cause of HUS for these patients, the Shiga toxin genes were apparently lost during the course of the infection. This situation potentially renders ineffectual current Shiga toxin immunoassays and

Stx gene amplification testing of bacterial isolates from diarrheal stool specimens in search of STEC. Culturing early in the course of clinical illness,[13] and successive culturing, may allow recovery of toxin-producing STEC before the Shiga toxin genes are lost.[13]

MICROBIOLOGY
Bacterial Physiology and Genetics of STEC

Escherichia coli is the predominant gram-negative facultative anaerobe found as usual intestinal flora in warm-blooded animals, including humans, although it is outnumbered in the intestine by obligate anaerobes, such as *Bacteroides* spp.[24] *E coli* is typically motile by peritrichous flagella, the location of the *E coli* H-antigen, of which over 50 serotypes are known. Some commensal *E coli* may possess a capsule, the site of the *E coli* K-antigen, which serves as a virulence factor for extraintestinal colonization, urinary tract infections, and invasive disease. Over 80 serologically distinct K-antigen specificities are known.[24]

Enterobacteriaceae, the taxonomic family to which *E coli* belongs, includes opportunistic commensal genera, such as *Citrobacter, Enterobacter, Klebsiella,* and *Proteus,* and noncommensal human pathogens, such as *Salmonella, Shigella,* and *Yersinia.*[3,24] The gram-negative cell wall of the Enterobacteriaceae is characterized by the presence of a lipopolysaccharide that is the location of the O-antigen. The O-antigen is a polysaccharide composed of repeating monosaccharide trimers in diverse combinations and sequences. The O-antigen is anchored in the cell wall's outer membrane by a lipid moiety, Lipid A, by an oligosaccharide core (**Fig. 3**). The complex structure of these lipopolysaccharide polysaccharides generates the 100 to 200 distinct *E coli* O-antigen serotypes. Diarrheogenic *E coli* (STEC, ETEC, EIEC, and EPEC) (see **Table 1**) have a relatively restricted number of O-antigen serotypes,[3] and STEC is unique among these in its ability to produce Shiga toxins.

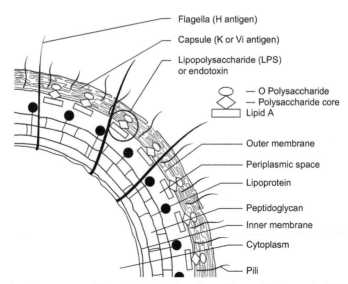

Fig. 3. Antigenic structure of Enterobacteriaceae. (*From* Murray PR, Rosenthal KS, Kabayashi S, et al. Enterobacteriaceae. In: Medical microbiology. 4th edition. Philadelphia: Elsevier Mosby; 2002. p. 267; with permission.)

The STEC O157 chromosome is a closed circular, double-stranded DNA molecule about 5.5 megabases in size.[11,25] **Fig. 4** provides a graphic representation of the STEC O157 chromosome from the strain responsible for the 1996 outbreak in Sakai City, Japan, derived from genome sequencing. The fourth circle of the figure indicates in black the locations of the temperate bacteriophage genomes integrated into the *E coli* chromosome that harbor the genes encoding Stx1 and Stx2. These bacteriophages account for some of the differences evident between the Sakai STEC O157 genome and the genome of a nonpathogenic laboratory strain of *E coli*. Other areas of difference illustrated in **Fig. 4** reflect virulence genes present in STEC O157 but not in a nonpathogenic *E coli*.[11,25]

The integrated, temperate bacteriophage genomes carrying the Shiga toxin genes can be induced to replicate lytically and generate bacteriophage progeny by exposure of STEC to chemical agents or ultraviolet light. These bacteriophages are lambdoid in morphology, with hexagonal heads and long tails.[26] They may be responsible for transmission of Shiga toxin genes between different strains of *E coli* in the gastrointestinal tract, and even toxin gene transfer to other genera and species of bacteria, such as *Citrobacter* spp, *Aeromonas* spp, and *Enterobacter* spp, in which Shiga toxin genes have been reported to occur.[12]

Diagnostic Microbiology of STEC

In the clinical microbiology laboratory, recovery of STEC O157 from stool specimens has been facilitated by the inability of most STEC O157 to ferment sorbitol.[3,9] Because of the worldwide occurrence of this pathogen and its well-documented ability to cause

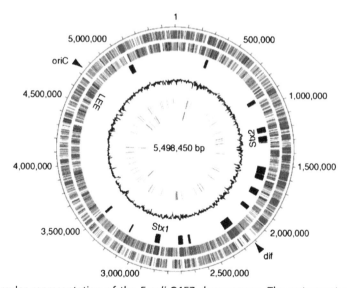

Fig. 4. Circular representation of the *E coli* O157 chromosome. The outermost circle indicates locations on the 5.5-MB genome. The second and third circles show in red the predicted genes in O157 that differ from those of a nonpathogenic laboratory strain of *E coli*. The fourth circle indicates in black the locations of the integrated temperate bacteriophage genomes encoding Stx1 and Stx2 in the O157 chromosome. (*From* Hayashi T, Makino K, Ohnishi M, et al. Complete genome sequence of enterohemorrhagic *Escherichia coli* O157:H7 and genomic comparison with a laboratory strain K-12. DNA Res 2001;8:13; with permission.)

serious disease, media chosen for bacterial cultures of all stools from patients with diarrhea or HUS should include SMAC agar for recovery and isolation of STEC O157. SMAC agar containing cefixime and potassium tellurite has been used to suppress interfering gram-negative bacterial growth when isolating STEC O157, but these agents prevent growth of some STEC and are not recommended for routine stool cultures.[3]

Chromogenic agars (eg, CHROMAgar, Becton Dickinson, Sparks, MD, USA) are selective differential media for the visual identification of specific pathogens based on their biochemical phenotypes. Chromogenic O157 agar, like SMAC agar, can provide the laboratory with isolated colonies after overnight incubation for presumptive visual identification as STEC O157, and facilitate prompt confirmation of suspect colonies as STEC O157:H7 by subculture and latex agglutination for O157 and H7 antigens, or for Shiga toxins.[3] Alternatively, "sweeps" of confluent growth from a plate with suspect STEC colonies can be tested for Shiga toxin or O-antigens using a commercial immunoassay for which this specimen source is approved according to the package insert.

Recovery of STEC non-O157 from stool specimens of patients with diarrhea is challenging. These pathogens ferment sorbitol and are not detected on SMAC or current chromogenic agars. The importance of testing for non-O157 STEC cannot be overemphasized, however, because at least one third of STEC isolated from ill patients are non-O157 serotypes.[3,4,27,28] Immunoassays from several manufacturers are available to test patient specimens or cultures for STEC.[29]

Direct testing of fresh stool specimens for Shiga toxins by immunoassay before culture can provide the clinician with a qualitative result in 20 minutes to 2 hours, depending on the type of test used. Only immunoassays specifying fresh stool as an acceptable specimen in the package insert should be used for direct "point-of-care" Shiga toxin testing. An optical immunoassay (eg, Biostar OIA SHIGATOX, Inverness Medical Professional Diagnostics, Princeton, NJ, USA) is available for direct testing of stool specimens, providing a toxin result in 20 minutes, without differentiation of Stx1 and Stx2.[28] A microwell plate immunoassay (eg, Premier EHEC, Meridian Bioscience, Cincinnati, OH, USA) for direct testing of stool specimens provides toxin results in about 2 hours. The sensitivity of these direct tests is good, between 80% and 100%, and specificity is 99%.[28] A greater variety of immunoassays is available for detection of Shiga toxins and O-antigens in growth from overnight (18–24 hours) cultures, either in broth or on agar media. If no toxins are detected in direct testing of stool specimen, a Shiga toxin immunoassay can be repeated from overnight growth, usually with greater sensitivity than can be obtained from direct testing of stool specimens.[27,28]

One approach is to sample "sweeps" of mixed colonial growth from SMAC or other agar media after overnight incubation. Individual colonies of potential STEC growing on SMAC or other enteric culture plates may be picked for identification by serotyping or for Shiga toxin immunoassay.[3]

Suspensions of the sweeps or colonies can be tested for Shiga toxins using an optical immunoassay (eg, Biostar OIA SHIGATOX),[28] a lateral flow immunoassay (eg, Meridian Immunocard STAT!EHEC, Meridian Bioscience, Cincinnati, OH, USA) (Fig. 5), or an enzyme immunoassay (eg, ProSpect Shiga toxin *Escherichia coli* Microplate Assay, Alexon-Trend, Ramsey, MI, USA).[27] Rapid tests (optical and lateral flow immunoassays) provide a qualitative Shiga toxin result in 10 to 15 minutes and microplate assays in about 2 hours. The sensitivity and specificity of immunoassays should not be assumed to be 100%, so results must be interpreted cautiously until STEC colonies are isolated and identified. Real-time polymerase chain reaction testing of stool specimens directly, or of overnight cultures, can also provide Stx1 or Stx2

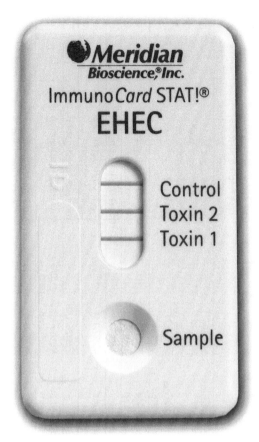

Fig. 5. Shiga toxin lateral-flow immunoassay device for testing broth and agar cultures. This device distinguishes Stx1 from Stx2. (*Courtesy of* Meridian Bioscience, Cincinnati, OH.)

gene results to clinicians in 30 to 60 minutes when available for clinical laboratories.[20,21] As with immunoassay results, molecular testing results must be confirmed by isolation of STEC from stool and culture.

Many STEC express a distinctive hemolytic phenotype on enterohemolysin (Ehly) agar (eg, Sifin, Berlin, Germany).[3,10,30] If this agar is available, individual colonies from Ehly agar can be picked and tested by latex agglutination for common STEC O-antigen serotypes, such as O157, O26, and O111, or for Shiga toxins by immunoassay.[3,6]

Immunomagnetic separation is used in the food industry for enhancing the recovery of diverse STEC serotypes.[3] It could be used on a research use only basis for the enrichment of stool specimens or broth cultures for STEC by incubation with sterile magnetic beads to which selected STEC O-antigen–specific antibody molecules have been attached. Following incubation the beads are aseptically rinsed and cultured, and colonies or mixed growth tested as described previously. Reagents for immunomagnetic separation are commercially available for several STEC (eg, O157, O111, O26, from Denka Seiken, Japan; O157, from Invitrogen Dynal, Oslo, Norway). Beads for immunomagnetic separation could be custom-requested from manufacturers by laboratories based on local STEC serotype prevalence in patients and animal reservoirs.[1–4]

Table 2
Recent STEC outbreaks, 2006–2009

Country and Year of Outbreak	STEC Serotype	Transmission Source or Vehicle	Cases/Hosp/HUS/Deaths[a]	Action Taken	Text References
United Kingdom, Wales, 2009	O157:H7	Fast food outlet	4/2/2/0	Analysis of isolates by PT, PFGE, VNTR; active case finding by local practitioners	33
United Kingdom, Wales, 2009	O157:H7	Dance camp; campsites on farms with animals; unchlorinated water being investigated	2/–/–/–	Contacts sought by social network Web sites, telephone, e-mail	34
United States, 2009	O157:H7	Refrigerated cookie dough, uncooked	72/34/10/0	Recall of product by manufacturer	35
Netherlands, 2008–2009	O157:H- (nonmotile)	Raw minced beef	20/7/0/0	Traceback investigation	36
United States, 2008	O157:H7	Commercial ground (minced) beef	49/27/1/0	Beef product recall (5.3 million pounds)	37
Canada, 2008	O157:H7	Raw onions	235/26/1/0	Traceback investigation	38
Netherlands and Iceland, 2007	O157:H-	Lettuce processed at Dutch plant	Netherlands: 41/0/0/0 Iceland: 9/0/0/0	Traceback investigation	39
Scotland, 2007	O157:H7	Cold meat salad	9/2/0/0	Public notified; hotel kitchen closed and cleaned; disinfectant washing procedure instituted	40
United States, 2007	O157:H-	Petting zoo (goats, sheep, llama)	7/2/0/0	Case finding among staff, visitors; zoo closed; animals tested for colonization	5

United States, 2006	O157:H7	Spinach	199/102/31/3	Public warning; product recall; PFGE analysis of outbreak strains	[41]
Norway, 2006	O103:H25 (notable for loss of Stx2 gene during infection)	Cured mutton sausage	17/–/10/1	Public warning; product recall; sheep slaughter changes implemented	[42]
Japan, 2006	O26	Nursery school; person-to-person spread from index patient inferred	26/0/0/0	Case finding; PFGE analysis of isolates	[43]
Japan, 2006	O103	Nursery school; person-to-person spread from index patient inferred	8/0/0/0	Case finding; PFGE analysis of isolates	[44]

Abbreviations: HUS, hemolytic uremic syndrome; PFGE, pulsed-field gel electrophoresis; PT, phage typing; VNTR, variable number of tandem repeats.

[a] Numbers of: No. of Cases/No. hospitalized/No. with HUS/No. deaths.

Data from Refs. [5,33–44]

EPIDEMIOLOGY

STEC infection is a zoonotic disease, for which small and large ruminant animals, notably cattle, are the natural reservoir, harboring STEC as normal gastrointestinal flora.[1,2] Transmission to humans commonly occurs through consumption of STEC-contaminated raw or undercooked meat, or of produce contaminated with cattle feces through farming or production practices. The infectious dose of STEC is low, about 100 bacteria,[3] so person-to-person transmission can occur, leading to secondary cases in contacts of infected persons. Clinically recognized STEC diarrhea, and probably many subclinical STEC infections, occurs through direct animal-to-human contact.[5] Risk of transmission to humans from food sources can be substantially reduced by careful washing of produce; pasteurization of juices and milk; and cooking to allow the internal temperature of meat, especially ground (minced) beef, to reach 70°C (160°F).[4]

Approximately 75% of cases of HUS occur in children, following diarrhea caused by an STEC infection. HUS is a significant cause of acute renal failure in children.[9,19] In the United States, approximately 90% of HUS cases are caused by STEC O157:H7, but only 50% or less in other countries.[3,4,9,13] Children under 10 years of age are at greatest risk for serious STEC infections. Approximately 15% of children with STEC diarrhea develop HUS.[9,31] Half of these require dialysis for renal failure, and the HUS case-fatality rate is approximately 5%.[4,9,19] The incidence of HUS worldwide varies widely. In Argentina, the incidence is 12 per 100,000 children under 5 years of age,[32] but can be 10-fold lower elsewhere in the world.[9]

The worldwide distribution and diversity of STEC serotypes in recent outbreaks is evident from **Table 2**. Several interactive sources for tracking STEC disease and serotypes worldwide are accessible electronically. Data for STEC from 36 reporting countries are available from Enter-Net, funded by the European Center for Disease Control (http://ecdpc.europa.eu/documents/ENTER_NET/vtec07q2.pdf; accessed August 5, 2009).

Similar data, both in tabular and map format, are available for the United States in publications from the Centers for Disease Control and Prevention.[45] The World Health Organization Weekly Epidemiologic Record indexes "VTEC," with fewer entries for "STEC," at www.who.int/wer/en (accessed June 10, 2009). The World Health Organization provides interactive map building capability for the World Health Organization European Region through its Computerized Information System for Infectious Disease, accessible through www.who.int. For STEC, the Computerized Information System for Infectious Disease map query-builder uses "6080" as the reference number for generating distribution maps of "enterohemorrhagic E coli" (accessed June 10, 2009).

International interactive maps of disease occurrence are generated by ProMED, a global reporting system of emerging infectious diseases, at http://www.promedmail.org/. The maps are accessible at www.healthmap.org. A healthmap.org map locating current STEC outbreaks in the United Kingdom and Wales[33,34] is shown in **Fig. 6**.

Statutory reporting of STEC infections has evolved with the increasing recognition of serious disease from non-O157 STEC infections. Currently in the United States, STEC infections of all serotypes are reportable to the National Notifiable Diseases Surveillance System of the Centers for Disease Control and Prevention.[45] Molecular techniques, such as phage typing and pulsed-field gel electrophoresis, are useful for comparing STEC isolates from outbreaks to link ill patients with contacts and with potential sources of infection. Databases are available for using these techniques to compare newly isolated outbreak strains for tracking the sources of outbreaks.[14,15]

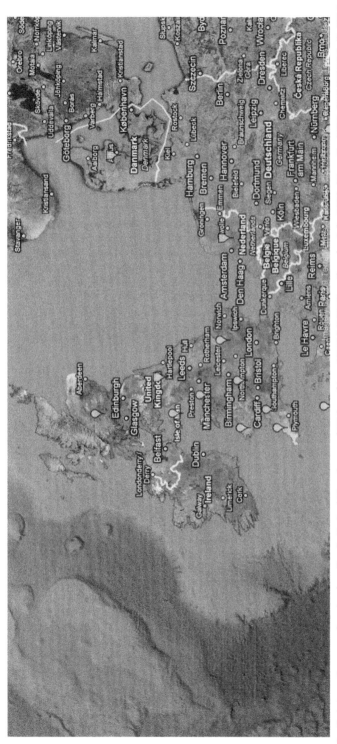

Fig. 6. Interactive map showing location in United Kingdom and Wales of two STEC O157:H7 outbreaks, July, 2009. (*From* ProMED. PRO/AH/EDR>E. COLI O157-UK: Wales dance camp, alert 17-Aug-2009. Archive Number 20090817.2915. Available at: http://www.promedmail.org and www.healthmap. org. Accessed August 18, 2009; Brownstein JS, Freifeld CC, Reis BY, et al. Surveillance sans frontières: internet-based emerging infectious disease intelligence and the healthmap project. PLoS Med 2008;5:e151; with permission.)

CLINICAL PRESENTATION

The clinical presentation of STEC infection is diarrhea, consisting of more than three unformed stools in a 24-hour period with or without blood.[5] The diarrhea may be intermittent, watery, or nonwatery, and may be associated with dehydration consistent with the fluid loss. Other symptoms often associated with STEC diarrhea include abdominal cramping, nausea, headache, vomiting, and fever.[3,4,7,9,19]

Based on experience with STEC O157 in children, diarrhea, abdominal pain, painful defecation, vomiting, and fever occur about 3 days after ingestion of an infectious dose of bacteria. Bloody diarrhea develops in 90% of children after another 3 days. The diarrhea symptoms abate about 7 days after onset. About 85% of children recover spontaneously, with 15% developing HUS and at risk of death (5% mortality).[9]

The clinical presentation of HUS in a patient with prior gastrointestinal or influenza-like symptoms is usually evidence of bleeding, either in vomitus or stool; severe oliguria; hematuria; microangiopathic hemolytic anemia; hypotension; and perhaps neurologic changes. Because of the risk of HUS, renal failure, and death in patients with intestinal STEC infections, especially in children, it is extremely important to assess renal function of the patient at presentation, which along with dehydration, may necessitate emergent care. The question of whether or not to treat a diarrheal infection caused by STEC must be considered promptly because of the generally accepted risk of increasing the severity of diarrhea and HUS caused by STEC if antimicrobial agents are given to STEC-infected patients.[4,9,19,31]

PATHOGENESIS

Ingested STEC reach the small intestine and the colon and multiply there in competition with the normal bacterial flora. A number of bacterial structures (fimbriae, pili) and adhesion molecules (adhesins) are thought to mediate adherence of STEC to the intestinal epithelial cells, allowing the Shiga toxins secreted by STEC to interact with the enterocyte plasma membrane surface.[23,46–48]

The STEC secrete Shiga toxins Stx 1 and Stx2, which bind to the enterocytes, the absorptive epithelial cells present on the luminal surface of the small and large intestines (**Fig. 7**). Stx1 and Stx2 are exotoxins of the AB5 class of toxins.[12] **Fig. 8** is a "ribbon diagram" illustrating the three-dimensional structure of the A and B polypeptides of Stx2 based on radiograph crystallography.[49,50] The pentameric B portion of the toxin, consisting of five identical B polypeptides, binds to the cellular glycolipid receptor globotriaosylceramide (Gb3) present on the plasma membrane of enterocytes and other cells. The monomeric A subunit of the Shiga toxin then enters the enterocyte by endocytosis and is transported to the rough endoplasmic reticulum by the Golgi apparatus.[12] The A subunit is proteolytically cleaved in the cell cytoplasm, liberating the N-terminal (A1) portion, a glycosidase that hydrolyzes a specific adenine-ribose bond in the ribosomal 28S RNA. This cleavage prevents aminoacyl-tRNA binding, and irreversibly inhibits protein synthesis, resulting in cell death (see **Fig. 2**).[48]

Once the Shiga toxins enter the bloodstream by the damaged intestinal epithelium, the precise mechanism of which is still unclear, capillary endothelial cells are exposed to the Shiga toxin and killed by the same mechanism. The endothelial cell lysis is accompanied by platelet activation and aggregation, leukocyte adherence, cytokine secretion, and vasoconstriction, contributing to fibrin deposition and clot formation within the capillary lumen and in the subendothelial tissue.[17,46,47] This thrombotic microangiopathy then occurs distally as the Shiga toxins are carried by the bloodstream

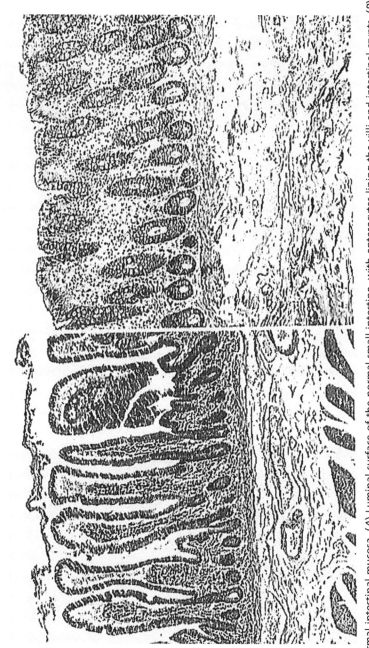

Fig. 7. Normal intestinal mucosa. (*A*) Luminal surface of the normal small intestine, with enterocytes lining the villi and intestinal crypts. (*B*) Normal colon histology showing colonic crypts and a flat mucosal surface lined with enterocytes. The enterocytes are the target of STEC Shiga toxins. H&E staining. Magnification ×70 approximately. (*From* Chen L, Crawford JM. The gastrointestinal tract. In: Kumar V, Abbas AK, Fausto N, editors. Robbins and Cotran pathologic basis of disease. 7th edition. Philadelphia: Elsevier Saunders; 2005. p. 828; with permission.)

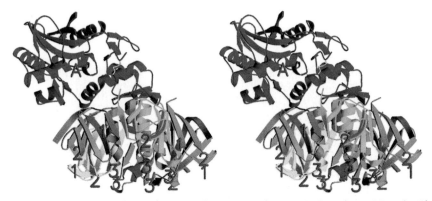

Fig. 8. Ribbon diagram of Stx2 from *E coli* O157:H7. Shiga toxin is a class AB5 toxin. The monomeric A polypeptide is red. The five B polypeptides are orange, cyan, green, yellow, and blue. Binding of the pentameric B portion of the toxin to the cell surface allows entry of the A subunit into the cell, where it functions enzymatically to stop protein synthesis and kill enterocytes and other cells to which the Shiga toxin binds. (*From* Fraser ME, Fujinaga M, Cherney MM, et al. Structure of Shiga toxin type 2 (Stx2) from *Escherichia coli* O157:H7. J Biol Chem 2004;279:27513; with permission.)

to the kidneys, resulting in fibrin deposition in glomerular capillaries, hematuria, and renal failure (**Fig. 9**).[9,31,47]

DIAGNOSIS

The clinical presentation of STEC infection is diarrhea, with or without blood present, which may be intermittent, watery, or nonwatery, often accompanied with abdominal cramping, nausea, headache, vomiting, and fever.[4,7,9,51]

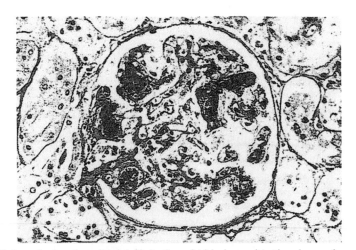

Fig. 9. Fibrin stain showing platelet-fibrin thrombi (*dark areas*) in the glomerular capillaries. Glomerular injury is characteristic of microangiopathic disorders, such as hemolytic uremic syndrome (HUS). Fibrin stain. Magnification ×240 approximately. (*From* Alpers CE. The kidney. In: Kumar V, Abbas AK, Fausto N, editors. Robbins and Cotran pathologic basis of disease. 7th edition. Philadelphia: Elsevier Saunders; 2005. p. 1010; with permission.)

Laboratory diagnosis of STEC infection in a patient with diarrhea is based on microscopic examination of stool when appropriate (eg, to exclude parasites and to visualize *Vibrio* and *Campylobacter* spp)[7]; bacterial stool cultures; detection of Shiga toxin by immunoassay; and detection of genes encoding Shiga toxin by DNA amplification. Confirmation of STEC as the etiologic agent of diarrhea requires the recovery and isolation in pure culture of STEC from a patient's stool specimen.[3]

Stool specimens should be obtained for culture as early as possible from the patient presenting with diarrhea, and specimens for culture collected successively if no pathogen is initially identified. In patients who develop HUS, STEC may be unrecoverable by the time HUS develops.[13] Ideally, specimens for toxin or O-antigen immunoassay, or DNA amplification, should be the same ones collected for cultures. These tests may provide preliminary information useful to clinicians in advance of a confirmatory culture result that requires 1 or more days to obtain. Any report from the laboratory stating that STEC O157 specifically was not recovered or detected should include a comment that STEC non-O157, such as STEC O26 and O111, can also cause diarrhea and HUS and should be considered as potential etiologies.[3,4] This reporting by the laboratory allows the clinician to request additional testing if it seems indicated.

STEC isolates recovered by the clinical laboratory, and cultures of any presumptive STEC identified by toxin immunoassay or other test, should be submitted to a local or national laboratory for confirmatory testing and outbreak investigation if appropriate.[3,14,15,45]

DIFFERENTIAL DIAGNOSIS

A patient presenting with diarrhea must be assessed not only for infection with gastrointestinal pathogens, but also for other illnesses and conditions with associated diarrhea, such as Legionnaire's disease, severe acute respiratory syndrome, influenza, and chemical and physical injury.[7,51]

Table 3 summarizes 23 causes of diarrhea, including STEC, and provides information useful in formulating a broad differential diagnosis, which can then be refined based on the patient's current illness course and exposure history (food consumption, contact with other ill persons, animals, fomites, social settings). An appreciation of this broad differential is essential to identify the most immediately life-threatening etiologies in a patient and begin a treatment plan without delay.

TREATMENT, PROGNOSIS, AND LONG-TERM OUTCOME

The treatment of patients with STEC diarrhea consists of fluid replacement, supportive care, and careful monitoring of kidney function, without antibiotic therapy.[4,31] Close attention must be given to the possible development of HUS or other associated thrombotic microangiopathy-associated conditions, such as hemorrhagic colitis or thrombotic thrombocytopenic purpura.[9,13,47] HUS can develop in patients of all ages, so vigilance must extend across the age spectrum.[13,47] Renal failure can usually be managed by dialysis and patients usually recover in several weeks.[13,31] Treatment of STEC infections with antimicrobial agents is not recommended because of studies demonstrating ineffectiveness and even potential harm to patients who receive antibiotics for STEC diarrhea.[19,31] Long-term follow-up studies to determine the outcome of patients who have experienced STEC diarrhea-associated HUS indicate that there is some increase in risk of renal impairment and hypertension in these patients.[19,31,47,48,52]

Table 3
Differential diagnosis of diarrhea in patients with suspected STEC

Pathogen	Incubation Period	Blood in Stool	Abdominal Cramping and Pain	Nausea or Vomiting	Fever	Other Signs and Diagnostic Aids	Diagnostic Laboratory Testing
Bacillus anthracis (gastrointestinal anthrax)	2 d to wk	+	+	+	+	Patient history: exposure may be accidental from consumption of infected meat	Culture of food, any lesions, blood; CDC select agent; culture hazard
Brucella spp	7–21 d	+	–	–	+	Patient history: bacteremia and fever; unpasteurized dairy product consumption; travel to endemic area; muscle and joint pain; headache	Blood cultures with special incubation request; CDC select agent; culture hazard
Campylobacter spp	2–5 d	+/–	+	+	+	Consumption of or contact with raw or undercooked poultry	Stool culture (special request)
Clostridium difficile (*C difficile* associated disease); Community-associated *C difficile* associated disease	Variable (d to mo)	+/–	+	+/–	+	May occur in patients with or without prior antibiotic use	Stool toxin EIA; anaerobic stool culture and toxin EIA of isolates
Cryptosporidium spp	2–28 d	–	+	+	+	May be chronic in ICH	Microscopic stool examination; DFA; EIA

Organism	Incubation				Clinical features	Diagnosis
Cyclospora spp	1–11 d	—	+	—	Fatigue; may be chronic if unrecognized	Microscopic stool examination
EIEC	10–18 h	— early; <10% + late	—	+	Fecal leukocytes late, as seen with Shigella spp	Stool culture for other pathogens
Entamoeba histolytica	2 d–4 wk	+	—	+	Invasive; liver abscess if chronic; may be confused with STEC; patient food and exposure history very important	Microscopic stool examination; serology for chronic or invasive disease; stool EIA or PCR
EPEC	9–12 h	+/–	+	+	Infant diarrhea; mucus in stool; dehydration severe; prolonged infections	Stool culture for other pathogens
ETEC	1–3 d	—	—	—	Patient history useful (travel, infant weaning)	Stool culture for other pathogens
Giardia spp	1–4 wk	—	—	—	Flatulence, bloating; may be chronic if unrecognized	O&P stool examination; stool DFA or EIA
Norovirus	24–48 h	—	+	+	Outbreak settings common; most common viral cause of gastroenteritis	PCR testing of stool
Rotavirus	1–3 d	—	+	+/–	Common in children; outbreak settings	Stool EIA for rotavirus

(continued on next page)

Table 3
(continued)

Pathogen	Incubation Period	Blood in Stool	Abdominal Cramping and Pain	Nausea or Vomiting	Fever	Other Signs and Diagnostic Aids	Diagnostic Laboratory Testing
Salmonella enterica subsp. enterica; 2500 serovars; nontyphoidal	1–3 d	−	+/−	+	+	May be chronic if not recognized or untreated	Stool culture
Shigella spp	1–2 d	+	+	+	+	*S dysenteriae* serotype 1 especially severe due to Shiga toxin; all *Shigella* are invasive of intestinal epithelium	Stool culture (special request for *S dysenteriae* serotype 1)
STEC, O157 or non-O157 (EHEC, VTEC)	1–8 d	+/−	+	+	+/−	Nonbloody diarrhea may precede blood in stool; oliguria, renal failure, hemolytic uremic syndrome; history of undercooked beef consumption	Stool culture to include SMAC agar for O157 STEC (special request); Shiga toxin EIA; O157 EIA; PCR testing of stool for Stx genes
Toxins, bacterial, preformed: *Bacillus cereus*, *Clostridium botulinum*, *Clostridium perfringens*, *Staphylococcus aureus*	1–16 h Bc; 12–72 h Cb; 8–16 h Cp; 1–6 h Sa	−	+	+	−/+	Sudden onset vomiting with Sa; diplopia and muscle paralysis with Cb; Cb is life-threatening	Toxin testing of food

Etiologic agent	Incubation period				Signs and symptoms	Laboratory testing
Toxins: fish, shellfish, and mushrooms	<30 min to 8 h	–	+	+/–	Visual disturbance, confusion, numbness, altered sensations; may be life-threatening	Toxin testing of food
Toxins, chemical: organic compounds, metals (As, Sn, Tl, Zn), nitrite, fluoride	5 min to 8 h	–	+	–	Headache, nervousness, twitching movements, visual disturbance	Toxin testing of food
Trichinella spp	1 d–8 wk	–	+	+	Myalgias, periorbital edema; cardiac and neurological involvement possible	Larval cysts detectable in muscle tissue by microscopy
Vibrio cholerae, serogroup 01 or 0139	1–3 d	–	+	–	Profuse watery diarrhea; dehydration life-threatening	Stool culture (special request)
Vibrio parahemolyticus, V mimicus, V fluvialis, V furnissii, V hollisae	2–48 h	+/–	+	+	Patient history of seafood consumption	Stool culture (special request)
Yersinia enterocolitica and pseudotuberculosis	24–48 h	+/–	+	+/–	Mesenteric lymphadenitis mimicking appendicitis	Stool culture (special request)

Symbols used: + usually present; +/– may be present; – rarely present.
Abbreviations: DFA, direct fluorescent antibody staining; EIA, enzyme immunoassay; ICH, immunocompromised host; Bc Cb Cp Sa (for toxins, bacterial, pre-formed) are *Bacillus cereus, Clostridium botulinum, Clostridium perfringens,* and *Staphylococcus aureus,* respectively; O&P, ova and parasite; PCR, polymerase chain reaction; SMAC, sorbitol-Mac Conkey.
Adapted from Centers for Disease Control and Prevention. Diagnosis and management of foodborne illnesses: a primer for physicians and other health care professionals. MMWR Morb Mortal Wkly Res 2004;53:1–33.
Additional data from Refs. [3,4,51]

SUMMARY

STEC (VTEC, EHEC) are important enteric pathogens worldwide, causing diarrhea with or without blood visibly present, and HUS. Children under the age of 10 years are at greatest risk. In children with STEC diarrhea, 15% develop HUS, which has 5% mortality rate. The STEC are unique among diarrheogenic *E coli* in producing Shiga toxin type 1 and type 2, the virulence factors responsible for bloody diarrhea and HUS. Cattle and other ruminants are the natural reservoir of STEC as their normal intestinal flora. Humans become infected by consumption of foods contaminated with cattle feces, notably undercooked ground (minced) beef, nonpasteurized products, and leafy vegetables that are consumed without cooking. The O157:H7 serotype of STEC predominates in human infections, and has been associated with outbreaks of diarrhea and HUS, but non-O157 STEC currently cause at least one third of STEC diarrhea and HUS. Diagnosis of STEC infection and of HUS is based on clinical signs; patient history; monitoring of renal function (especially in children); rapid testing of stool specimens for Shiga toxins; and isolation of STEC from stool cultures. Early diagnosis of STEC infection is important because of the contraindication for treating STEC using antimicrobial agents, and the intense supportive care needed if renal failure occurs.

REFERENCES

1. Hussein HS, Bollinger LM. Prevalence of Shiga toxin-producing *Escherichia coli* in beef cattle. J Food Prot 2005;68(10):2224–41.
2. Oporto B, Esteban JI, Aduriz G. *Escherichia coli* O157:H7 and non-O157 Shiga toxin-producing *E. coli* in healthy cattle, sheep and swine herds in Northern Spain. Zoonoses Public Health 2008;55(2):73–81.
3. Nataro JP, Bopp CS, Fields PI, et al. *Escherichia, Shigella,* and *Salmonella.* In: Murray PR, Baron EJ, Jorgensen JH, et al, editors. Manual of clinical microbiology. 9th edition. Washington, DC: American Society for Microbiology; 2007. p. 670–87.
4. Fontaine O, Griffin P, Henao O, et al. Diarrhea, acute. In: Heymann DL, editor. Control of communicable diseases manual. 19th edition. Washington, DC: American Public Health Association; 2008. p. 179–95.
5. CDC. Outbreak of Shiga toxin-producing *Escherichia coli* O157 infection associated with a day camp petting zoo—Pinellas County, Florida, May-June 2007. MMWR Morb Mortal Wkly Rep 2009;58(16):426–8.
6. Konowalchuk J, Speirs JI, Stavrik S. Vero response to a cytotoxin of *Escherichia coli.* Infect Immun 1977;18(3):775–9.
7. CDC. Diagnosis and management of foodborne illnesses: a primer for physicians and other health care professionals. MMWR Recomm Rep 2004;53(RR04):1–33.
8. Riley LW, Remis RS, Helgerson SD, et al. Hemorrhagic colitis associated with a rare *Escherichia coli* serotype. N Engl J Med 1983;308(12):681–5.
9. Tarr PI, Gordon CA, Chandler WL. Shiga-toxin-producing *Escherichia coli* and haemolytic uraemic syndrome. Lancet 2005;365(9464):1073–86.
10. Bielaszewska M, Stoewe F, Fruth A, et al. Shiga toxin, cytolethal distending toxin, and hemolysin repertoires in clinical *Escherichia coli* O91 isolates. J Clin Microbiol 2009;47(7):2061–6.
11. Hayashi T, Makino K, Ohnishi M, et al. Complete genome sequence of enterohemorrhagic *Escherichia coli* O157:H7 and genomic comparison with a laboratory strain K-12. DNA Res 2001;8(1):11–22.

12. Sandvig K. The Shiga toxins: properties and action on cells. In: Alouf JE, Popoff MR, editors. The comprehensive sourcebook of bacterial protein toxins. 3rd edition. Philadelphia: Elsevier Academic Press; 2006. p. 310–22.

13. Tarr PI. Shiga toxin-associated hemolytic uremic syndrome and thrombotic thrombocytopenic purpura: distinct mechanisms of pathogenesis. Kidney Int Suppl 2009;(112):S29–32.

14. Enter_Net. European Centre for Disease Prevention and Control (ECDC). Available at: http://ecdpc.europa.eu/Activities/surveillance/ENTER_NET/reports.html. Accessed July 30, 2009.

15. Gerner-Smidt P, Hise K, Kincaid J, et al. PulseNet USA: a five-year update. Foodborne Pathog Dis 2006;3(1):9–19.

16. CDC. Importance of culture confirmation of Shiga toxin-producing *Escherichia coli* infection as illustrated by outbreaks of gastroenteritis—New York and North Carolina, 2005. MMWR Morb Mortal Wkly Rep 2006;55(38):1042–5.

17. Karmali M. The way forward: what should we be doing? VTEC 2009, Buenos Aires, May 10th–13th, 2009. Meeting presentation. Available at: http://www.vtec2009.com.ar/index.cfm?fuseaction=main.home&seccion=1. Accessed August 18, 2009.

18. Leotta GA, Miliwebsky ES, Chinen I, et al. Characterization of Shiga toxin-producing *Escherichia coli* O157 strains isolated from humans in Argentina, Australia and New Zealand. BMC Microbiol 2008;9:46. Available at: http://www.biomedcentral.com/1471-2180/8/46. Accessed July 28, 2009.

19. McLaine PH, Rowe PC, Orrbine E. Experiences with HUS in Canada: what have we learned about childhood HUS in Canada? Kidney Int Suppl 2009;75(Suppl 112):S25–8.

20. Orth D, Grif K, Zimmerhackl LB, et al. Sorbitol-fermenting Shiga toxin-producing *Escherichia coli* O157 in Austria. Wien Klin Wochenschr 2009; 121(3-4):108–12.

21. Grys TE, Sloan LM, Rosenblatt JE, et al. Rapid and sensitive detection of Shiga toxin-producing *Escherichia coli* from non-enriched stool specimens by real-time PCR in comparison to enzyme immunoassay and culture. J Clin Microbiol 2009; 47(7):2008–12.

22. Karch H, Bielaszewska M. Sorbitol-fermenting Shiga toxin-producing *Escherichia coli* O157:H- strains: epidemiology, phenotypic and molecular characteristics, and microbiological diagnosis. J Clin Microbiol 2001;39(6):2043–9.

23. Bielaszewska M, Middendorf B, Koeck R, et al. Shiga toxin-negative attaching and effacing *Escherichia coli*: distinct clinical associations with bacterial phylogeny and virulence traits and inferred in-host evolution. Clin Infect Dis 2008;47(2):208–17.

24. Welch RA. The genus *Escherichia*. In: Dworkin M, Falkow S, Rosenberg E, editors. The prokaryotes, vol. 6. 3rd edition. New York: Springer Science, Business Media LLC; 2006. p. 60–71. Chapter 3.3.3.

25. Ogura Y, Ooka T, Asadulghani TJ, et al. Extensive genomic diversity and selective conservation of virulence-determinants in enterohemorrhagic *Escherichia coli* strains O157 and non-O157 serotypes. Genome Biol 2007; 8(7):R138. Available at: http://genomebiology.com/2007/8/7/R138. Accessed July 22, 2009.

26. Karama M, Gyles CL. Characterization of verotoxin-encoding phages from *Escherichia coli* O103:H2 strains of bovine and human origins. Appl Environ Microbiol 2008;74(16):5153–8.

27. Gavin PJ, Peterson LR, Pasquariello AC, et al. Evaluation of performance and potential clinical impact of Prospect Shiga toxin *Escherichia coli* microplate assay for detection of Shiga toxin-producing *E. coli* in stool samples. J Clin Microbiol 2004;42(4):1652–6.

28. Teel LD, Daly JA, Jerris RC, et al. Rapid detection of Shiga toxin-producing *Escherichia coli* by optical immunoassay. J Clin Microbiol 2007;45(10):3377–80.

29. CDC. Recommendations for diagnosis of Shiga toxin-producing *Escherichia coli* infections by clinical laboratories. MMWR Morb Mortal Wkly Rep 2009;58(RR12): 1–18.

30. Beutin L, Zimmermann S, Gleier K. Rapid detection and isolation of Shiga-like toxin (verocytotoxin)-producing *Escherichia coli* by direct testing of individual enterohemolytic colonies from washed sheep blood agar plates in the VTEC-RPLA assay. J Clin Microbiol 1996;34(11):2812–4.

31. Bitzan M. Treatment options for HUS secondary to *Escherichia coli* O157:H7. Kidney Int Suppl 2009;75(Suppl 112):S62–6.

32. Rivero MA, Padola NL, Etcheverría AI, et al. Enterohemorrhagic *Escherichia coli* and hemolytic-uremic syndrome in Argentina. Medicina (B Aires) 2004;64(4): 352–6 [in Spanish].

33. Hart J, Smith G. Verocytotoxin-producing *Escherichia coli* O157 outbreak in Wrexham, North Wales, July 2009. Euro Surveill 2009;14(32). Article 5. Available at: http://www.eurosurveillance.org/ViewArticle.aspx?ArticleId=19300. Accessed August 18, 2009.

34. ProMED. PRO/AH/EDR>E. COLI O157-UK: Wales dance camp, alert 17-Aug-2009. Archive Number 20090817.2915. Available at: http://www.promedmail. org. Accessed August 18, 2009.

35. CDC. Multistate outbreak of *E. coli* O157:H7 infections linked to eating raw refrigerated, prepackaged cookie dough. Updated June 30, 2009. Available at: http://www.cdc.gov/ecoli/2009/0630.html. Accessed August 18, 2009.

36. Greenland K, de Jager C, Heuvelink A, et al. Nationwide outbreak of STEC O157 infection in the Netherlands, December 2008-January 2009: continuous risk of consuming raw beef products. Euro Surveill 2009;14(8):19129.

37. CDC. Investigation of multistate outbreak of *E. coli* O157:H7 infections. Updated July 18, 2008. Available at: http://www.cdc.gov/ecoli/june2008outbreak/. Accessed August 19, 2009.

38. ProMED. PRO/AH/EDR>E. coli O157, restaurant - Canada, 2008: (ON), onions. Post June 23, 2009. Available at: http://www.promedmail.org. Accessed August 20, 2009.

39. Friesma I, Sigmundsdottir G, van der Zwaluw K, et al. An international outbreak of Shiga toxin-producing *Escherichia coli* O157 infection due to lettuce, September - October 2007. Euro Surveill 2008;13(50). Article 6. Available at: http://www. eurosurveillance.org/ViewArticle.aspx?Articleid=19065. Accessed August 19, 2009.

40. Webster D, Cowden J, Locking M. An outbreak of *Escherichia coli* O157 in Aberdeen Scotland, September, 2007. Euro Surveill 2007;12(39). Article 1. Available at: http://www.eurosurveillance.org/ViewArticle.aspx?Articleid=3273. Accessed August 19, 2009.

41. CDC. Update on multi-state outbreak of *E. coli* O157:H7 infections from fresh spinach, October 6, 2006. Available at: http://www.cdc.gov/ecoli/2006/ september/updates/100606.htm. Accessed August 18, 2009.

42. Schimmer B, Nygard K, Eriksen H-M, et al. Outbreak of haemolytic uraemic syndrome in Norway caused by stx2-positive *Escherichia coli* O103:H25 traced to cured mutton sausages. BMC Infect Dis 2008;8:41. Available at: http://ncbi.

nlm.nih.gov/pubmed/18387178?ordinalpos=1&itool=En..._Discovery_PMC&link
pos=1&logpos$=citedinpmarticles&logdbfrom=pubmed. Accessed August 19,
2009.

43. Sonoda C, Tagami A, Nagatomo D, et al. An enterohemorrhagic *Escherichia coli*
    O26 outbreak at a nursery school in Miyazaki, Japan. Jpn J Infect Dis 2008;61(1):
    92–3.

44. Muraoka R, Okazaki O, Fugimoto Y, et al. An enterohemorrhagic *Escherichia coli*
    O103 outbreak at a nursery school in Miyazaki Prefecture, Japan. Jpn J Infect Dis
    2007;60(6):410–1.

45. CDC. Summary of notifiable diseases—United States, 2007. MMWR Morb Mortal
    Wkly Rep 2009;56(53):1–94.

46. Bardiau M, Labrozzo S, Mainil JG. Putative adhesins of enteropathogenic and en-
    terohemorrhagic *Escherichia coli* of serogroup O26 isolated from humans and
    cattle. J Clin Microbiol 2009;47(7):2090–6.

47. Alpers CE. The kidney. In: Kumar V, Abbas AK, Fausto N, editors. Robbins and
    Cotran pathologic basis of disease. 7th edition. Philadelphia: Elsevier Saunders;
    2005. p. 955–1021.

48. Karmali MA. Host and pathogen determinants of verocytotoxin-producing
    Escherichia coli-associated hemolytic uremic syndrome. Kidney Int Suppl
    2009;75(Suppl 112):S4–7.

49. Fraser ME, Chernaia MM, Kozlov YV, et al. Shiga toxin. In: Parker MW, editor.
    Protein toxin structure. New York: Chapman and Hall; 1996. p. 173–90.

50. Fraser ME, Fujinaga M, Cherney MM, et al. Structure of Shiga toxin type 2 (Stx2)
    from *Escherichia coli* O157:H7. J Biol Chem 2004;279(26):27511–7.

51. Chen L, Crawford JM. The gastrointestinal tract. In: Kumar V, Abbas AK,
    Fausto N, editors. Robbins and Cotran pathologic basis of disease. 7th edition.
    Philadelphia: Elsevier Saunders; 2005. p. 797–875.

52. Garg AX, Suri S, Barrowman N, et al. Long-term renal prognosis of diarrhea-asso-
    ciated hemolytic uremic syndrome: a systematic review, meta-analysis, and
    meta-regression. JAMA 2003;290(10):1360–70.

West Nile Virus

Shannan L. Rossi, PhD, Ted M. Ross, PhD, Jared D. Evans, PhD*

KEYWORDS

- West Nile virus • Flavivirus • Infection
- Pathogenesis • Diagnosis

OVERVIEW

Since its isolation in Uganda in 1937, West Nile virus (WNV) has been responsible for thousands of cases of morbidity and mortality in birds, horses, and humans. Historically, epidemics were localized to Europe, Africa, the Middle East, and parts of Asia and primarily caused a mild febrile illness in humans. However, in the late 1990s, the virus became more virulent and spread to North America. In humans, the clinical presentation ranges from asymptomatic (approximately 80% of infections) to encephalitis/paralysis and death (<1% of infections). There is no FDA (Food and Drug Administration)-licensed vaccine for human use, and the only recommended treatment is supportive care. Individuals that survive infection often have a long recovery period. This article reviews the current literature summarizing the molecular virology, epidemiology, clinical manifestations, pathogenesis, diagnosis, treatment, immunology, and protective measures against WNV and WNV infections in humans.

VIROLOGY AND MOLECULAR BIOLOGY OF WNV

West Nile virus is a positive-stranded RNA virus in the family Flaviviridae (genus *Flavivirus*), that includes other human pathogens, such as dengue, yellow fever, and Japanese encephalitis viruses.[1,2] The virion consists of an envelope surrounding an icosahedral capsid approximately 50 nm in size. The 11-kilobase genome encodes a single open reading frame, which is flanked by 5′ and 3′ untranslated regions. The polyprotein of approximately 3000 amino acids is cleaved into 10 proteins by cellular and viral proteases (**Fig. 1**). Three of these proteins are the structural components required for virion formation (capsid protein [C]) and assembly into viral particles (pre-membrane [prM] and envelope [E] proteins). The other 7 viral proteins are nonstructural (NS) proteins (NS1, NS2A, NS2B, NS3, NS4A, NS4B, and NS5) and are all necessary for genome replication. NS3 contains an ATP-dependent helicase and in

This work was supported by T32 Grant #AI060525-04 from the National Institute of Heath (SR), W81XWH-BAA-06-1 and W81XWH-BAA-06-2 (TMR), and CVR Funds and Fine Foundation (JE). Department of Microbiology and Molecular Genetics, Center for Vaccine Research, University of Pittsburgh, 3501 Fifth Avenue, Pittsburgh, PA 15261, USA
* Corresponding author.
E-mail address: Evansj2@cvr.pitt.edu

Clin Lab Med 30 (2010) 47–65
doi:10.1016/j.cll.2009.10.006
0272-2712/10/$ – see front matter © 2010 Elsevier Inc. All rights reserved.

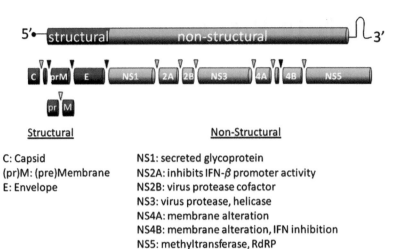

Fig. 1. WNV genome. A representation of the WNV genome including the 3 structural proteins that make up virion particle and the 7 nonstructural proteins necessary for virus replication and immune evasion.

conjunction with the NS2B protein, a serine protease, which is required for virus poly-protein processing. NS5 is a methyltransferase and RNA-dependent RNA polymerase. The other NS proteins are small, generally hydrophobic proteins of disparate functions. NS1 is a secreted glycoprotein implicated in immune evasion.[3] NS2A plays a role in virus assembly and inhibiting interferon (IFN)-β promoter activation.[4,5] NS4A is responsible for a rapid expansion and modification of the endoplasmic reticulum (ER) that helps establish replication domains.[5-8] NS4B blocks the IFN response.[9-12] All the NS proteins seem to be necessary for efficient replication.[13]

The flavivirus life cycle consists of 4 principal stages: attachment/entry, translation, replication, and assembly/egress (reviewed in Refs.[2,14]). WNV enters cells via receptor-mediated endocytosis, and is transported into endosomes. The WNV receptor is unknown. Several cell-surface proteins are potential WNV receptors (dendritic cell-specific intercellular adhesion molecule-3-grabbing non-integrin [DC-SIGN], integrin $\alpha_v\beta_3$),[15-17] and the receptor required for WNV binding and entry may vary by cell type. Acidification of the endosomal compartment causes a conformational change in the E protein, resulting in fusion of the viral and endosomal membranes and release of the virus nucleocapsid into the cytoplasm.[18,19] The viral RNA is translated and the polyprotein is processed. Genome replication is carried out in specific domains established by the viral proteins.[20,21] As stated earlier, viral proteins cause massive expansion and modification of the ER. Two domains are important in replication and virus protein processing: vesicle packets and convoluted membranes, respectively (Fig. 2).[21-26] Following replication and translation, genomes are packaged into virions, which mature through the ER-Golgi secretion pathway.[20,21,27,28] Progeny viruses are released by exocytosis.

PHYLOGENY

The most current phylogenetic studies based on complete or partial genome sequences indicate 5 lineages of WNV.[29] The virus that entered North America belongs to lineage I (clade Ia). This lineage also contains viruses found in Europe,

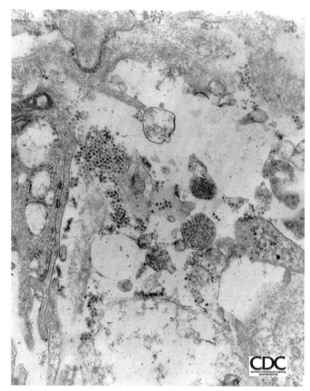

Fig. 2. WNV isolated from brain tissue from an infected crow. The tissue was cultured in a Vero cell for a 3-day incubation period. The Vero cells were fixed in glutaraldehyde, dehydrated, placed in an resin, thin sectioned, placed on a copper grid, and stained with uranyl acetate and lead citrate. The grids were then placed in the electron microscope and viewed. Total magnification, image 65,625x. (*Courtesy of* Dr Bruce Cropp, Microbiologist, Division of Vector-Borne Infectious Diseases, Centers for Disease Control and Prevention [CDC].)

the Middle East, and Africa. The genome of Kunjin virus, the Australian strain of WNV, is also in the lineage I group (clade Ib). Lineage II contains WNV mainly of African origin. Although there are exceptions, in general, lineage I (clade Ia) viruses can cause severe human neurologic disease, whereas lineage I (clade Ib) and lineage II viruses generally cause a mild, self-limiting disease. Not much is known about the viruses that comprise lineage III, IV, and V.

EPIDEMIOLOGY

WNV is maintained in nature in a cycle between birds and mosquitoes (**Fig. 3**). Although many different species of mosquito are capable of maintaining this cycle, the *Culex* species play the largest role in natural transmission (**Fig. 4**). Not all infected mosquitoes feed preferentially on birds, which can lead to other animals, including humans, becoming infected. Humans (and horses) are incidental or "dead-end" hosts in this cycle, because the concentration of virus within the blood (viremia) is insufficient to infect a feeding naïve mosquito. Other natural modes of WNV transmission have been documented but occur rarely. WNV transmission can occur between infected

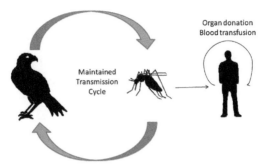

Fig. 3. The WNV transmission cycle. The maintenance of WNV in nature depends on many avian and mosquito species. Humans and other incidental hosts (like horses) become infected when WNV-infected mosquito takes a bloodmeal from them.

mother and newborn via the intrauterine route[30–32]or possibly by breast-feeding.[33] A recent study of pregnant women who became infected with WNV during the 2003 to 4 transmission in the United States suggested that adverse side effects in the newborn infant due to WNV infection of the mother are rare, and those cases with infant illness/infection/mortality may be associated with WNV infection that occurred while the mother was infected within 1 month prepartem.[34]

Within the human population, the virus can spread between individuals by more artificial means. In the early 2000s, patients that received tainted blood or organs from viremic donors became infected.[35–38] These events highlighted the need to safeguard blood and organ donations from potentially viremic, yet healthy, donors, and relatively few infections via this route of transmission have been reported since 2004.

The epidemiology of WNV is continuously changing. The virus was initially isolated from a febrile woman in Uganda in 1937.[39] Since then, few outbreaks of WNV in human or horse populations have been recorded until the beginning of the 1990s. When disease was observed in humans, symptoms were typically mild and neurologic complications were rare.[40,41] The exceptions were outbreaks in Israel in the early 1950s and France in the 1960s, which were characterized by encephalitis in humans and horses. A series of outbreaks in the 1990s brought WNV into the spotlight; epidemics in Algeria, Morocco, Tunisia, Italy, France, Romania, Israel, and Russia were associated with uncharacteristically severe human disease, including neurologic

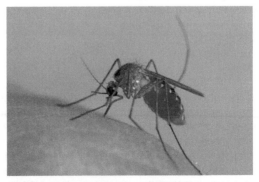

Fig. 4. *Culex* mosquito. The *Culex* species of mosquito, the most common vector of WNV, feeding. (*Courtesy of* US Geological Survey.)

complications and death.[40,42–44] In the summer of 1999, a cluster of patients with encephalitis in New York City signaled the entry of WNV into North America. The sequence of the 1999 New York strain of WNV is closest in identity to a viral isolate from Israel,[45] but how the virus traversed the Atlantic Ocean is still a mystery. In the past decade, there have been thousands of reported human cases of WNV disease (WN fever and WN encephalitis) accompanied by more than 1000 deaths (**Table 1**). The geographic range of the virus currently extends north into Canada, west across all 48 contiguous states, and south into Mexico, the Caribbean, and Central and South America (**Figs. 5** and **6**).[46] Since 2007, in addition to ongoing circulation of WNV in the Western Hemisphere, there have been outbreaks or isolations of WNV in Volograd (Russia),[47] South Africa,[48] Hungary,[49] Romania,[50] and Italy,[51] (see **Fig. 5**). In 2008 alone, there were 1338 cases of WNV disease reported to the Centers for Disease Control and Prevention (CDC) and resulted in 43 deaths within the United States (http://www.cdc.gov/ncidod/dvbid/westnile/surv&controlCaseCount08_detailed.htm).

CLINICAL PRESENTATION

It is difficult to accurately predict the incubation period of WNV in humans (time from mosquito bite/infection to the presentation of symptoms), but it is approximately 2 to 15 days.[35,52] The majority (>80%) of WNV infections are asymptomatic. Symptomatic infections manifest primarily as a mild, self-limiting febrile illness. However, approximately 1% of infected people develop neurologic infections and disease. Most symptomatic patients exhibit mild illness with fever, sometimes associated with headache, myalgias, nausea and vomiting, and chills.[35,53–56] Further, some patients briefly present with papular rash on the arms, legs, or trunk. These symptoms follow a fairly predictable pattern, with illness generally lasting less than 7 days. However, several patients experience severe fatigue and malaise during convalescence.

Approximately 5% of patients with symptomatic WNV infection develop neurologic disease. WNV neurologic symptoms include meningitis, encephalitis, and poliomyelitislike disease, presented as acute flaccid paralysis.[57] WNV encephalitis and meningitis are characterized by rapid onset of headache, photophobia, back pain, confusion, and continuous fever. The WNV poliomyelitis-like syndrome is characterized by acute onset of asymmetric weakness and absent reflexes without pain. Patients presenting with flaccid paralysis require further testing to determine nature and degree of disease. Diagnostic tests, including cerebrospinal fluid (CSF) examination, should be performed to differentiate WNV infection from stroke, myopathy, and Guillan-Barré syndrome. Other clinical symptoms may include tremor, myoclonus, postural instability, bradykinesia, and signs of parkinsonism.

PATHOGENESIS

Understanding the full range of WNV pathogenesis in humans has been difficult, mainly because of the difference in virulence between WNV strains, the high prevalence of asymptomatic or subclinical infections, and the relative infrequency of laboratory-confirmed human infections. Little has been published about human infections with WNV of limited virulence. Most of our current knowledge regarding WNV pathogenesis resulted from animal models (mostly rodent) infected under controlled conditions with a known amount of needle-inoculated virus, which may not accurately reflect the course of a natural infection in humans. Nevertheless, many documented accounts follow the course of infection in humans suffering from WN fever and WN encephalitis resulting from a virulent lineage I WNV infection.

Table 1
Summary of confirmed human cases of WN disease in the United States, 1999–2008[a]

Year	No. States Reporting[b]	Total Cases	Deaths	CFR[c]	Neurologic Involvement[d]	WN Fever[e]	Other Symptoms
1999	1	62	7	11.29%	59	3	0
2000	3	21	2	9.52%	19	2	0
2001	10	66	10	15.15%	64	2	0
2002	39 + DC	4156	284	6.83%	2946	1160	50
2003	45 + DC	9862	264	2.68%	2866	6830	166
2004	40 + DC	2539	100	3.94%	1142	1269	128
2005	43 + DC	3000	119	3.97%	1294	1607	99
2006	43 + DC	4269	177	4.15%	1459	2616	194
2007	43	3630	124	3.42%	1217	2350	63
2008	45 + DC	1356	44	3.24%	687	624	45

Abbreviations: CDC, Centers for Disease Control and Prevention; CFR, case fatality rate; DC, District of Columbia.
[a] Data obtained from the CDC, accessed May 13, 2009.
[b] The number of states reporting CDC-confirmed cases of WNV infections in humans.
[c] CFR determined as percentage of deaths from total CDC-confirmed reported cases.
[d] Neurologic involvement is comprised of encephalitis, meningitis.
[e] WN fever; febrile illness with no neurologic involvement.

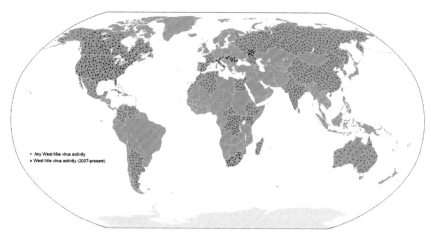

Fig. 5. Distribution of WNV. Countries with historic or recent (2007 to present) WNV activity (isolations from mosquitoes, birds, horses, or humans) are highlighted in red and blue, respectively.

WNV-infected mosquitoes transmit the virus to humans following a bloodmeal from the host. During this process, mosquito saliva contaminated with WNV is deposited in the blood and skin tissue. Virus contained within the skin is presumed to infect resident dendritic cells, such as Langerhans cells (MHCII+/NLDC145+/E-cadherin+ cells), which then traffic to the draining lymph node.[58,59] Shortly thereafter, virus amplifies in the tissues and results in a transient, low-level viremia lasting a few days, and it typically wanes with the production of anti-WNV IgM antibodies.[60] Following viremia, the virus infects multiple organs in the body of the host, including the spleen, liver, and kidneys. Eight days after onset of symptoms, WNV was detected in the urine (viruria) of a patient with encephalitis,[61] which is consistent with animal (hamster) experiments demonstrating viruria[61] and the presence of viral infection in the kidneys.[62,63]

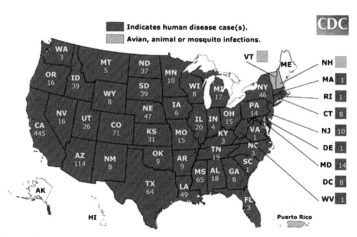

Fig. 6. The number of confirmed human cases of WNV disease in the United States in 2008. (*Courtesy of* CDC.)

On entering the central nervous system (CNS), WNV causes severe neurological disease. WNV may enter the brain through a combination of mechanisms that facilitates viral neuroinvasion, such as direct infection with or without a breakdown of the blood-brain barrier (BBB) or virus transport along peripheral neurons. High viremia may easily lead to an infection of the brain if the BBB is disrupted, and it is correlated with severity of infection in experimentally infected mice.[64] Viremia and high viral titers in the periphery alone do not predict neuroinvasion. Host proteins, such as death-associated protein kinase-related 2 (Drak2), intercellular adhesion molecule 1 (ICAM-1), macrophage migration inhibitory factor (MIF), and matrix metalloproteinase 9 (MMP-9), have all been implicated in altering BBB permeability during WNV infection.[65–68] The virus may pass into the CNS without disrupting the BBB.[69] The host's response to infection may also contribute to WNV pathogenesis. Studies from experimentally infected mice suggest that the innate immune sensing molecule toll-like receptor 3 (TLR3) may play a role in WNV invasion of CNS,[70] possibly by mediating the upregulation of tumor necrosis factor (TNF)-α, thereby resulting in capillary leakage and increased BBB permeability.[71] The proinflammatory chemokines/cytokines, monocyte chemoattractant protein 5 (MCP-5), MIF, IFN-γ–inducible protein 10 (IP-10), monokine induced by IFN-γ (MIG), IFN-γ, and TNF-α, were all upregulated in the brains of experimentally infected mice, suggesting that the host immune response may be at least partially responsible for neurologic symptoms of the disease.[65,72] However, an increase in BBB leakage does not accurately predict WNV-induced mortality in hamsters, nor does lethal infection increase BBB permeability in all strains of mice.[73] WNV may enter the brain by direct infection and retrograde spreading along neurons in the periphery.[74] Entering the brain via infected peripheral neurons is a likely route, because the level of viremia is low and leakage into the CNS by a breakdown of the BBB is less likely compared with animals with a high titer of circulating WNV in the blood. The discrepancies observed regarding BBB compromise suggest that further research is required to determine the exact mechanism through which WNV enters the CNS.

DIAGNOSIS

Diagnosis of WNV infection depends on several factors, including environmental conditions, behaviors, and clinical symptoms. Patient history provides crucial clues to diagnosis. For example, if a patient presents with clinical symptoms, including fever and headache, one must consider the distribution of WNV and its mosquito vector. WNV infection must be considered in endemic areas, especially during the summer months. Furthermore, the patient history should suggest exposure to mosquitoes through outdoor activities. An initial physical examination should confirm clinical symptoms of fever, headache, myalgia, or the more severe meningitis and flaccid paralysis. The presence of mosquito bites on the skin also helps diagnosis.

To confirm the initial diagnosis, specific laboratory tests must be ordered (**Table 2**). To date, the most consistent way to verify WNV infection is serology.[54,56] WNV antigen-specific enzyme-linked immunosorbent assay (ELISA) confirms infection. Serological tests include acute or convalescent samples of serum or CSF to determine the WNV-specific antibody profile by ELISA. The best test involves IgM-specific ELISA (MAC-ELISA) in which serum is collected within 8 to 21 days after the appearance of clinical symptoms. This test is commercially available and relatively inexpensive.[35] Also, serology can be performed to analyze immune responses. The presence of reactive lymphocytes or monocytes in CSF samples indicates WNV neurologic infection. More dramatically, a massive influx of polymorphonuclear cells occurs. In patients

Table 2
Laboratory tests and diagnosis of WNV infection

Test	Positive Results
CBC	Anemia, lymphopenia, thrombocytopenia
IgM-specific ELISA	WNV-specific IgM antibodies detected
PRNT	Known virus stock growth inhibited in tissue culture by serum, indicating neutralizing antibodies
NAT	PCR amplification shows presence of WNV genome RNA
Virus isolation/plaque assay	Serum or CSF contain virus as seen in plaque assay
CSF analysis	Antibodies and/or virus present in ELISA or plaque assay, Elevated protein and increased polymorphonuclear cells, negative gram stain
EMG/NCS	Severe effects on anterior horn cells

Abbreviations: CBC, complete blood count; ELISA, enzyme-linked immunosorbent assay; EMG, electromyogram; NAT, nucleic acid testing; NCS, nerve conduction studies; PCR, polymerase chain reaction; PRNT, plaque reduction neutralization test.

with WNV neuroinvasion, more than 40% of cells in the CSF are neutrophils.[75] Plaque reduction and neutralization tests allow for identification of virus specificity. A virology test can directly confirm the presence of virus. Serum or CSF is collected, and virus is amplified within permissive cells and sequenced. This test is time-consuming and expensive. Finally, molecular biological tools can be used to confirm the presence of virus. The nucleic acid test is a powerful tool for detecting WNV genomes. Serum or CSF collected during the initial phases of virus infection can be directly amplified or used to detect viral RNA by quantitative reverse transcription polymerase chain reaction with virus-specific primers.

Magnetic resonance imaging suggests abnormalities in the brain and meninges of WNV-infected patients presenting with CNS disease (**Fig. 7**).[53,76,77] The regions of the CNS most commonly affected are basal ganglia, thalami, brain stem, ventral horns, and spinal cord. However, most of these studies were performed retrospectively. Thus, the results do not provide predictive capabilities to WNV infection.

DIFFERENTIAL DIAGNOSIS

Several diseases manifest as symptoms similar to WNV, including bacterial meningitis and those caused by the encephalitides viruses, such as the Japanese and Murray Valley encephalitis viruses. Therefore, differential diagnosis is crucial to determining WNV infection. A differential diagnosis is required when a patient presents with unexplained febrile illness, encephalitis or extreme headache, or meningitis. Thus far, the only manner to differentiate between causes of encephalitis/meningitis is diagnostic and serological laboratory tests to identify the specific pathogen causing the symptoms.

TREATMENT AND LONG-TERM OUTCOMES

Currently, patients infected with WNV have limited treatment options. The primary course of action is supportive care. There is no FDA-licensed vaccine to combat WN disease in humans, despite the research of many laboratories and institutions and the vaccines available for use in horses.

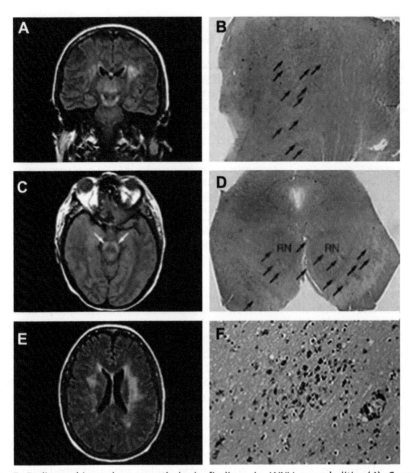

Fig. 7. Radiographic and neuropathologic findings in WNV encephalitis. (*A*) Coronal fluid-attenuated inversion recovery (FLAIR) magnetic resonance image shows an area of abnormally increased signal in the thalami, substantia nigra (extending superiorly toward the subthalamic nuclei), and white matter. (*B*) Corresponding tissue section from the same patient at autopsy 15 days later stained with Luxol fast blue-periodic acid Schiff for myelin shows numerous ovoid foci of necrosis and pallor throughout the thalamus and subthalamic nucleus (*arrows*). (*C*) Axial proton density image at the level of the midbrain shows a bilaterally increased signal in the substantia nigra (*arrows*). (*D*) Corresponding tissue section at autopsy stained with Luxol fast blue-periodic acid Schiff illustrates multifocal involvement of the substantia nigra (*arrows*), with nearly 50% of the area destroyed; the red nuclei are clearly affected. (*E*) Axial FLAIR image at the level of the lateral ventricle bodies shows a bilaterally increased signal within the white matter. A scan performed approximately 5 months earlier demonstrated an abnormal signal in the left periventricular white matter. This signal increased once WNV encephalitis developed, and the lesions in the right cerebral white matter (left side of photograph) were new. (*F*) Photomicrograph taken from the right periventricular white matter immunostained with the HAM56 antibody shows numerous macrophages in perivascular areas (*lower right*) and diffusely throughout the white matter (*center*). (*From* Kleinschmidt-DeMaster BK, Marder BA, Levi ME, et al. Naturally acquired West Nile virus encephalomyelitis in transplant recipients: clinical, laboratory, diagnostic, and neuropathological features. Arch Neurol 2004;61:1216; with permission. Copyright © 2004 American Medical Association. All rights reserved.)

Furthermore, there is no effective antiviral to combat WNV infection. Two classical antiviral compounds, IFN and ribavirin, showed promising results in vitro,[78,79] but it is unclear if these compounds are effective in patients.[80–84] Passively transferring anti-WNV immunoglobulin has been shown to be effective in mouse and hamster models[85] and may be helpful in patients.[86,87]

Long-term complications (1 year or more postinfection) are common in patients recovering from WNV infection. The most common self-reported symptom is fatigue and weakness, although myalgia, arthralgia, headaches, and neurologic complications, such as altered mental depression, tremors, and loss of memory and concentration, are not uncommon.[88] There is also evidence from animal models[62,89,90] and human autopsies[91,92] that the virus may persist in some individuals, as measured by isolation of virus or viral genomes or antigen months after infection or symptom presentation. Experimentally infected hamsters show long-term neurological sequelae, which seems to coincide with the presence of viral antigen and genome within areas of the brain showing neuropathology.[90] Although the direct evidence of persistence in humans is limited at this time, many patients have long-lasting WNV-specific IgM titers in the serum and CNS, suggesting that persistent infections may be more common than previously indicated.[93–95]

Table 3
WNV vaccines. A partial list of licensed and preclinical vaccines against WNV

Type	Antigen	Sponsor	Stage of Development
Chimeric (vector)			
Recombitek (canarypox)	WNV-prM-E	Merial	Licensed for horses
ChimeriVax (yellow fever virus)	WNV-prM-E	Acambis	Phase II
WNV-DENV4 (dengue virus 4)	WNV-prM-E	NIAID/NIH	Phase II
DNA			
WNV-DIII	WNV-DIII	Multiple laboratories	Preclinical
WNV-E	WNV-E	Multiple laboratories	Preclinical
WNV-prM-E	WNV-prM-E	Multiple laboratories	Preclinical
Inactivated/killed			
Innovator	Whole virus	Fort Dodge Animal Health	Licensed for horses
Subvirion particles/viruslike particles			
WNV-prM-E	WNV-prM-E	Multiple laboratories	Preclinical

Abbreviations: NIAID, National Institute of Allergy and Infectious Diseases; NIH, National Institutes of Health.

Data from http://www.fortdodgelivestock.com, http://www.merial.com, http://www.intervetusa.com, http://www.clinicaltrials.gov.

IMMUNITY

The innate and adaptive immune responses mounted against WNV are critically important for controlling infection. Type I IFNs (-α and -β) are important for limiting virus levels, reducing neuronal death, and increasing survival.[64] The amount of IFN made by the host in response to infection seems to be at least partly dependent on the strain or virulence of the virus; mice infected with lineage I WNV with attenuating mutations produce less type I IFN than mice infected with virulent lineage I WNV.[96] Furthermore, WNV strains that are more resistant to the affects of IFN (like some virulent lineage I viruses) are more virulent than IFN-sensitive strains (like lineage II strains).[97]

The adaptive immune response also plays a role in controlling infection. Studies using WNV-infected genetically engineered knockout mice indicate that T-[98–103]and B-[104] cells are critical for controlling infection. CD8+ T-cell recruitment to the brain by neurons expressing the chemokine CXCL10 and by CD40-CD40 ligand interactions help reduce the viral burden in the brain and increase survival in experimentally infected mice.[101,105] B cells are activated within the lymph nodes of WNV-infected mice 48 to 72 hours after infection in an IFN-α/-β–signaling dependent manner, and B cells secreting WNV-specific IgM were detected on day 7 postinfection.[106] IgM is critically important for the control of early WNV infection, and passive transfer of WNV-specific IgM could protect IgM-deficient mice from lethal WNV infection.[107] Approximately 3 to 4 days after WNV-specific IgM is detectable, anti-WNV IgG titers are measurable in patients.[60] IgG is the predominant antibody, most probably conferring long-term immunity against WNV re-infection. Although not enough data exist, immunity against WNV in convalescent patients is presumed to be lifelong.

VACCINATION

Although no FDA-approved vaccine exists for human use, there are effective, licensed vaccines for the treatment of horses. This success has encouraged others to develop these and other strategies for human vaccines. Currently, there are several ongoing clinical trials.

There are several strategies being pursued for WNV vaccine development (**Table 3**). The first strategy is inoculation of multiple doses of inactivated virus.[108,109] Fort Dodge Animal Health developed this strategy by formalin-inactivating whole virus. This formulation has been approved for horses. The second strategy involves the production of WNV antigens from a heterologous virus backbone. The vectors being used are canarypox (Recombitek), yellow fever virus (ChimeriVax), and dengue 4 (WNV-DEN4).[110–113] The Recombitek vaccine has been licensed for use in horses. The third approach is DNA vaccination. WNV structural antigens (prM-E) are expressed from DNA plasmids.[114] The final strategy is inoculation with purified viral proteins.[115–118] These proteins can be produced in mammalian cell culture, bacteria, or yeast. A recent study by Seino and colleagues[119] compared the efficacy of 3 available vaccines. Their study showed that horses vaccinated with the live, chimeric virus in the yellow fever or canarypox vectors had fewer clinical signs of WNV disease than animals receiving inactivated virus.

SUMMARY

In summary, WNV infection is a serious threat to public health, especially to the immunocompromised and the elderly. The virus is maintained in an enzootic cycle between mosquitoes and birds, with humans and other mammals as incidental hosts. Since its introduction to the Western hemisphere in 1999, WNV has spread across North and South America in fewer than 10 years. Most human infections are asymptomatic. However, clinical manifestations range from fairly mild febrile illness to very severe neurological sequelae, including acute flaccid paralysis and encephalitis. Currently, the virus is the most significant cause of viral encephalitis in the United States. Efficient diagnosis of WNV infection requires a detailed history, including potential exposure to contaminated mosquitoes, and sensitive serological and virology assays. Recent studies have explained virus-host interactions, including pathogenesis and immune evasion. Lastly, there are no prophylactic or therapeutic measures that exist to combat the diseases caused by WNV infection, which warrants future research.

REFERENCES

1. Gould EA, Solomon T. Pathogenic flaviviruses. Lancet 2008;371(9611):500–9.
2. Lindenbach BD, Rice CM. Flaviviridae: the viruses and their replication. In: HP, Knipe DM, editors. Fields virology. Philadelphia: Lippincott Williams, Wilkins; 2001. p. 991–1041.
3. Schlesinger JJ. Flavivirus nonstructural protein NS1: complementary surprises. Proc Natl Acad Sci U S A 2006;103(50):18879–80.
4. Leung JY, Pijlman GP, Kondratieva N, et al. Role of nonstructural protein NS2A in flavivirus assembly. J Virol 2008;82(10):4731–41.
5. Mackenzie JM, Khromykh AA, Jones MK, et al. Subcellular localization and some biochemical properties of the flavivirus Kunjin nonstructural proteins NS2A and NS4A. Virology 1998;245(2):203–15.
6. Egloff MP, Benarroch D, Selisko B, et al. An RNA cap (nucleoside-2'-O-)-methyltransferase in the flavivirus RNA polymerase NS5: crystal structure and functional characterization. EMBO J 2002;21(11):2757–68.
7. Khromykh AA, Kenney MT, Westaway EG. Trans-Complementation of flavivirus RNA polymerase gene NS5 by using Kunjin virus replicon-expressing BHK cells. J Virol 1998;72(9):7270–9.
8. Speight G, Coia G, Parker MD, et al. Gene mapping and positive identification of the non-structural proteins NS2A, NS2B, NS3, NS4B and NS5 of the flavivirus Kunjin and their cleavage sites. J Gen Virol 1988;69(Pt 1):23–34.
9. Evans JD, Seeger C. Differential effects of mutations in NS4B on West Nile virus replication and inhibition of interferon signaling. J Virol 2007;81(21):11809–16.
10. Liu WJ, Wang XJ, Mokhonov VV, et al. Inhibition of interferon signaling by the New York 99 strain and Kunjin subtype of West Nile virus involves blockage of STAT1 and STAT2 activation by nonstructural proteins. J Virol 2005;79(3):1934–42.
11. Munoz-Jordan JL, Laurent-Rolle M, Ashour J, et al. Inhibition of alpha/beta interferon signaling by the NS4B protein of flaviviruses. J Virol 2005;79(13):8004–13.
12. Munoz-Jordan JL, Sánchez-Burgos GG, Laurent-Rolle M, et al. Inhibition of interferon signaling by dengue virus. Proc Natl Acad Sci U S A 2003;100(24):14333–8.
13. Khromykh AA, Sedlak PL, Westaway EG. cis- and trans-acting elements in flavivirus RNA replication. J Virol 2000;74(7):3253–63.
14. Clyde K, Kyle JL, Harris E. Recent advances in deciphering viral and host determinants of dengue virus replication and pathogenesis. J Virol 2006;80(23):11418–31.
15. Chu JJ, Ng ML. Interaction of West Nile virus with alpha v beta 3 integrin mediates virus entry into cells. J Biol Chem 2004;279(52):54533–41.

16. Chu JJ, Ng ML. Infectious entry of West Nile virus occurs through a clathrin-mediated endocytic pathway. J Virol 2004;78(19):10543–55.
17. Medigeshi GR, Hirsch AJ, Streblow DN, et al. West Nile virus entry requires cholesterol-rich membrane microdomains and is independent of alphavbeta3 integrin. J Virol 2008;82(11):5212–9.
18. Modis Y, Ogata S, Clements D, et al. Structure of the dengue virus envelope protein after membrane fusion. Nature 2004;427(6972):313–9.
19. Mukhopadhyay S, Kuhn RJ, Rossmann MG. A structural perspective of the flavivirus life cycle. Nat Rev Microbiol 2005;3(1):13–22.
20. Mackenzie JM, Westaway EG. Assembly and maturation of the flavivirus Kunjin virus appear to occur in the rough endoplasmic reticulum and along the secretory pathway, respectively. J Virol 2001;75(22):10787–99.
21. Westaway EG, Ng ML. Replication of flaviviruses: separation of membrane translation sites of Kunjin virus proteins and of cell proteins. Virology 1980;106(1):107–22.
22. Westaway EG, Mackenzie JM, Khromykh AA. Replication and gene function in Kunjin virus. Curr Top Microbiol Immunol 2002;267:323–51.
23. Westaway EG, Mackenzie JM, Kenney MT, et al. Ultrastructure of Kunjin virus-infected cells: colocalization of NS1 and NS3 with double-stranded RNA, and of NS2B with NS3, in virus-induced membrane structures. J Virol 1997;71(9):6650–61.
24. Ng ML, Pedersen JS, Toh BH, et al. Immunofluorescent sites in Vero cells infected with the flavivirus Kunjin. Arch Virol 1983;78(3–4):177–90.
25. Bartenschlager R, Miller S. Molecular aspects of Dengue virus replication. Future Microbiol 2008;3:155–65.
26. Welsch S, Miller S, Romero-Brey I, et al. Composition and three-dimensional architecture of the dengue virus replication and assembly sites. Cell Host Microbe 2009;5(4):365–75.
27. Miyanari Y, Atsuzawa K, Usuda N, et al. The lipid droplet is an important organelle for hepatitis C virus production. Nat Cell Biol 2007;9(9):1089–97.
28. Miyanari Y, Hijikata M, Yamaji M, et al. Hepatitis C virus non-structural proteins in the probable membranous compartment function in viral genome replication. J Biol Chem 2003;278(50):50301–8.
29. Bondre VP, Jadi RS, Mishra AC, et al. West Nile virus isolates from India: evidence for a distinct genetic lineage. J Gen Virol 2007;88(Pt 3):875–84.
30. Centers for Disease Control and Prevention (CDC). Intrauterine West Nile virus infection–New York, 2002. MMWR Morb Mortal Wkly Rep 2002;51(50):1135–6.
31. From the Centers for Disease Control and Prevention. Intrauterine West Nile virus infection–New York, 2002. JAMA 2003;289(3):295–6.
32. Alpert SG, Fergerson J, Noel LP. Intrauterine West Nile virus: ocular and systemic findings. Am J Ophthalmol 2003;136(4):733–5.
33. Hinckley AF, O'Leary DR, Hayes EB. Transmission of West Nile virus through human breast milk seems to be rare. Pediatrics 2007;119(3):e666–71.
34. O'Leary DR, Kuhn S, Kniss KL, et al. Birth outcomes following West Nile Virus infection of pregnant women in the United States: 2003–2004. Pediatrics 2006;117(3):e537–45.
35. Petersen LR, Marfin AA. West Nile virus: a primer for the clinician. Ann Intern Med 2002;137(3):173–9.
36. Iwamoto M, Jernigan DB, Guasch A, et al. Transmission of West Nile virus from an organ donor to four transplant recipients. N Engl J Med 2003;348(22):2196–203.

37. Biggerstaff BJ, Petersen LR. Estimated risk of transmission of the West Nile virus through blood transfusion in the US, 2002. Transfusion 2003;43(8):1007–17.
38. Centers for Disease Control and Prevention (CDC). Detection of West Nile virus in blood donations–United States, 2003. MMWR Morb Mortal Wkly Rep 2003; 52(32):769–72.
39. Smithburn KC, Hughes TP, Burke AW, et al. A neurotropic virus isolated from the blood of a native of Uganda. Am J Trop Med Hyg 1940;20:471–92.
40. Murgue B, Murri S, Triki H, et al. West Nile in the Mediterranean basin: 1950–2000. Ann N Y Acad Sci 2001;951:117–26.
41. Hayes CG. West Nile virus: Uganda, 1937, to New York City, 1999. Ann N Y Acad Sci 2001;951:25–37.
42. Bin H, Grossman Z, Pokamunski S, et al. West Nile fever in Israel 1999–2000: from geese to humans. Ann N Y Acad Sci 2001;951:127–42.
43. Platonov AE, Shipulin GA, Shipulina OY, et al. Outbreak of West Nile virus infection, Volgograd Region, Russia, 1999. Emerg Infect Dis 2001;7(1):128–32.
44. Tsai TF, Popovici F, Cernescu C, et al. West Nile encephalitis epidemic in southeastern Romania. Lancet 1998;352(9130):767–71.
45. Lanciotti RS, Roehrig JT, Deubel V, et al. Origin of the West Nile virus responsible for an outbreak of encephalitis in the northeastern United States. Science 1999; 286(5448):2333–7.
46. Blitvich BJ. Transmission dynamics and changing epidemiology of West Nile virus. Anim Health Res Rev 2008;9(1):71–86.
47. Plantonov AE, Fedorova MV, Karan LS, et al. Epidemiology of West Nile infection in Volgograd, Russia, in relation to climate change and mosquito (Diptera: Culicidae) bionomics. Parasitol Res 2008;103(Suppl 1):S45–53.
48. Venter M, Human S, Zaayman D, et al. Lineage 2 West Nile virus as cause of fatal neurologic disease in horses, South Africa. Emerg Infect Dist 2009;15(6):877–84.
49. Krisztalovics K, Ferenczi E, Molnar Z, et al. West Nile virus infections in Hungary, August–September 2008. Euro Surveill 2008;13(45):pii, 19030.
50. Popovici F, Sarbu A, Nicolae O, et al. West Nile fever in a patient in Romania, August 2008: case report. Euro Surveill 2008;13(39):pii, 18989.
51. Rossini G, Cavrini F, Pierro A, et al. First human case of West Nile virus neuroinvasive infection in Italy, September 2008-case report. Euro Surveill 2008; 13(41):pii, 19002.
52. Mostashari F, Bunning ML, Kitsutani PT, et al. Epidemic West Nile encephalitis, New York, 1999: results of a household-based seroepidemiological survey. Lancet 2001;358(9278):261–4.
53. Brilla R, Block M, Geremia G, et al. Clinical and neuroradiologic features of 39 consecutive cases of West Nile Virus meningoencephalitis. J Neurol Sci 2004; 220(1–2):37–40.
54. Hayes EB, Sejvar JJ, Zaki SR, et al. Virology, pathology, and clinical manifestations of West Nile virus disease. Emerg Infect Dis 2005;11(8):1174–9.
55. Petersen LR, Roehrig JT, Hughes JM. West Nile virus encephalitis. N Engl J Med 2002;347(16):1225–6.
56. Tyler KL. West Nile virus infection in the United States. Arch Neurol 2004;61(8): 1190–5.
57. Campbell GL, Marfin AA, Lanciotti RS, et al. West Nile virus. Lancet Infect Dis 2002;2(9):519–29.
58. Byrne S, Halliday GM, Johnston LJ, et al. Interleukin-1 beta but not tumor necrosis factor is involved in West Nile virus-induced Langerhans cell migration from the skin in C57BL/6 mice. J Invest Dermatol 2001;117(3):702–9.

59. Johnston L, Halliday GM, King NJ. Langerhans cells migrate to local lymph nodes following cutaneous infection with an arbovirus. J Invest Dermatol 2000; 114(3):560–8.
60. Busch MP, Kleinman SH, Tobler LH, et al. Virus and antibody dynamics in acute West Nile virus infection. J Infect Dis 2008;198(7):984–93.
61. Tonry JH, Xiao SY, Siirin M, et al. Persistent shedding of West Nile virus in urine of experimentally infected hamsters. Am J Trop Med Hyg 2005;72(3):320–4.
62. Tesh RB, Siirin M, Guzman H, et al. Persistent West Nile virus infection in the golden hamster: studies on its mechanism and possible implications for other flavivirus infections. J Infect Dis 2005;192(2):287–95.
63. Ding X, Wu X, Duan T, et al. Nucleotide and amino acid changes in West Nile virus strains exhibiting renal tropism in hamsters. Am J Trop Med Hyg 2005; 73(4):803–7.
64. Samuel MA, Diamond MS. Alpha/beta interferon protects against lethal West Nile virus infection by restricting cellular tropism and enhancing neuronal survival. J Virol 2005;79(21):13350–61.
65. Arjona A, Foellmer HG, Town T, et al. Abrogation of macrophage migration inhibitory factor decreases West Nile virus lethality by limiting viral neuroinvasion. J Clin Invest 2007;117(10):3059–66.
66. Dai J, Wang P, Bai F, et al. Icam-1 participates in the entry of West Nile virus into the central nervous system. J Virol 2008;82(8):4164–8.
67. Wang P, Dai J, Bai F, et al. Matrix metalloproteinase 9 facilitates West Nile virus entry into the brain. J Virol 2008;82(18):8978–85.
68. Wang S, Welte T, McGargill M, et al. Drak2 contributes to West Nile virus entry into the brain and lethal encephalitis. J Immunol 2008;181(3):2084–91.
69. Verma S, Lo Y, Chapagain M, et al. West Nile virus infection modulates human brain microvascular endothelial cells tight junction proteins and cell adhesion molecules: transmigration across the in vitro blood-brain barrier. Virology 2009;385(2):425–33.
70. Wang T, Town T, Alexopoulou L, et al. Toll-like receptor 3 mediates West Nile virus entry into the brain causing lethal encephalitis. Nat Med 2004;10(12): 1366–73.
71. Diamond MS, Klein RS. West Nile virus: crossing the blood-brain barrier. Nat Med 2004;10(12):1294–5.
72. Garcia-Tapia D, Hassett DE, Mitchell WJ Jr, et al. West Nile virus encephalitis: sequential histopathological and immunological events in a murine model of infection. J Neurovirol 2007;13(2):130–8.
73. Morrey JD, Olsen AL, Siddharthan V, et al. Increased blood-brain barrier permeability is not a primary determinant for lethality of West Nile virus infection in rodents. J Gen Virol 2008;89(Pt 2):467–73.
74. Samuel MA, Wang H, Siddharthan V, et al. Axonal transport mediates West Nile virus entry into the central nervous system and induces acute flaccid paralysis. Proc Natl Acad Sci U S A 2007;104(43):17140–5.
75. Tyler KL, Pape J, Goody RJ, et al. CSF findings in 250 patients with serologically confirmed West Nile virus meningitis and encephalitis. Neurology 2006;66(3): 361–5.
76. Petropoulou KA, Gordon SM, Prayson RA, et al. West Nile virus meningoencephalitis: MR imaging findings. AJNR Am J Neuroradiol 2005;26(8): 1986–95.
77. Ali M, Safriel Y, Sohi J, et al. West Nile virus infection: MR imaging findings in the nervous system. AJNR Am J Neuroradiol 2005;26(2):289–97.

78. Rossi SL, Zhao Q, O'Donnell VK, et al. Adaptation of West Nile virus replicons to cells in culture and use of replicon-bearing cells to probe antiviral action. Virology 2005;331(2):457–70.

79. Anderson J, Rahal JJ. Efficacy of interferon alpha-2b and ribavirin against West Nile virus in vitro. Emerg Infect Dis 2002;8(1):107–8.

80. Chan-Tack KM, Forrest G. Failure of interferon alpha-2b in a patient with West Nile virus meningoencephalitis and acute flaccid paralysis. Scand J Infect Dis 2005;37(11–12):944–6.

81. Chowers MY, Lang R, Nassar F, et al. Clinical characteristics of the West Nile fever outbreak, Israel, 2000. Emerg Infect Dis 2001;7(4):675–8.

82. Kalil AC, Devetten MP, Singh S, et al. Use of interferon-alpha in patients with West Nile encephalitis: report of 2 cases. Clin Infect Dis 2005;40(5):764–6.

83. Sayao AL, Suchowersky O, Al-Khathaami A, et al. Calgary experience with West Nile virus neurological syndrome during the late summer of 2003. Can J Neurol Sci 2004;31(2):194–203.

84. Weiss D, Carr D, Kellachan J, et al. Clinical findings of West Nile virus infection in hospitalized patients, New York and New Jersey, 2000. Emerg Infect Dis 2001;7(4):654–8.

85. Morrey JD, Taro BS, Siddharthan V, et al. Efficacy of orally administered T-705 pyrazine analog on lethal West Nile virus infection in rodents. Antiviral Res 2008;80(3):377–9.

86. Ben-Nathan D, Gershoni-Yahalom O, Samina I, et al. Using high titer West Nile intravenous immunoglobulin from selected Israeli donors for treatment of West Nile virus infection. BMC Infect Dis 2009;9:18.

87. Saquib R, Randall H, Chandrakantan A, et al. West Nile virus encephalitis in a renal transplant recipient: the role of intravenous immunoglobulin. Am J Kidney Dis 2008;52(5):e19–21.

88. Sejvar JJ. The long-term outcomes of human West Nile virus infection. Clin Infect Dis 2007;44(12):1617–24.

89. Pogodina VV, Frolova MP, Malenko GV, et al. Study on West Nile virus persistence in monkeys. Arch Virol 1983;75(1–2):71–86.

90. Siddharthan V, Wang H, Motter NE, et al. Persistent West Nile virus associated with a neurological sequela in hamsters identified by motor unit number estimation. J Virol 2009;83(9):4251–61.

91. Penn RG, Guarner J, Sejvar JJ, et al. Persistent neuroinvasive West Nile virus infection in an immunocompromised patient. Clin Infect Dis 2006;42(5):680–3.

92. Brenner W, Storch G, Buller R, et al. West Nile Virus encephalopathy in an allogeneic stem cell transplant recipient: use of quantitative PCR for diagnosis and assessment of viral clearance. Bone Marrow Transplant 2005;36(4):369–70.

93. Kapoor H, Signs K, Somsel P, et al. Persistence of West Nile Virus (WNV) IgM antibodies in cerebrospinal fluid from patients with CNS disease. J Clin Virol 2004;31(4):289–91.

94. Prince HE, Tobler LH, Yeh C, et al. Persistence of West Nile virus-specific antibodies in viremic blood donors. Clin Vaccine Immunol 2007;14(9):1228–30.

95. Roehrig JT, Nash D, Maldin B, et al. Persistence of virus-reactive serum immunoglobulin m antibody in confirmed west nile virus encephalitis cases. Emerg Infect Dis 2003;9(3):376–9.

96. Rossi SL, Fayzulin R, Dewsbury N, et al. Mutations in West Nile virus nonstructural proteins that facilitate replicon persistence in vitro attenuate virus replication in vitro and in vivo. Virology 2007;364(1):184–95.

97. Keller BC, Fredericksen BL, Samuel MA, et al. Resistance to alpha/beta interferon is a determinant of West Nile virus replication fitness and virulence. J Virol 2006;80(19):9424–34.
98. Shrestha B, Diamond MS. Role of CD8+ T cells in control of West Nile virus infection. J Virol 2004;78(15):8312–21.
99. Shrestha B, Samuel MA, Diamond MS. CD8+ T cells require perforin to clear West Nile virus from infected neurons. J Virol 2006;80(1):119–29.
100. Shrestha B, Wang T, Samuel MA, et al. Gamma interferon plays a crucial early antiviral role in protection against West Nile virus infection. J Virol 2006; 80(11):5338–48.
101. Sitati EM, Diamond MS. CD4+ T-cell responses are required for clearance of West Nile virus from the central nervous system. J Virol 2006;80(24): 12060–9.
102. Wang T, Scully E, Yin Z, et al. IFN-gamma-producing gamma delta T cells help control murine West Nile virus infection. J Immunol 2003;171(5):2524–31.
103. Wang Y, Lobigs M, Lee E, et al. CD8+ T cells mediate recovery and immunopathology in West Nile virus encephalitis. J Virol 2003;77(24):13323–34.
104. Diamond MS, Shrestha B, Marri A, et al. B cells and antibody play critical roles in the immediate defense of disseminated infection by West Nile encephalitis virus. J Virol 2003;77(4):2578–86.
105. Klein RS, Lin E, Zhang B, et al. Neuronal CXCL10 directs CD8+ T-cell recruitment and control of West Nile virus encephalitis. J Virol 2005;79(17): 11457–66.
106. Purtha WE, Chachu KA, Virgin HW 4th, et al. Early B-cell activation after West Nile virus infection requires alpha/beta interferon but not antigen receptor signaling. J Virol 2008;82(22):10964–74.
107. Diamond MS, Sitati EM, Friend LD, et al. A critical role for induced IgM in the protection against West Nile virus infection. J Exp Med 2003;198(12):1853–62.
108. Ng T, Hathaway D, Jennings N, et al. Equine vaccine for West Nile virus. Dev Biol (Basel) 2003;114:221–7.
109. Samina I, Khinich Y, Simanov M, et al. An inactivated West Nile virus vaccine for domestic geese-efficacy study and a summary of 4 years of field application. Vaccine 2005;23(41):4955–8.
110. Arroyo J, Miller C, Catalan J, et al. ChimeriVax-West Nile virus live-attenuated vaccine: preclinical evaluation of safety, immunogenicity, and efficacy. J Virol 2004;78(22):12497–507.
111. Minke JM, Siger L, Karaca K, et al. Recombinant canarypoxvirus vaccine carrying the prM/E genes of West Nile virus protects horses against a West Nile virus-mosquito challenge. Arch Virol Suppl 2004;18:221–30.
112. Monath TP, Liu J, Kanesa-Thasan N, et al. A live, attenuated recombinant West Nile virus vaccine. Proc Natl Acad Sci U S A 2006;103(17):6694–9.
113. Pletnev AG, Claire MS, Elkins R, et al. Molecularly engineered live-attenuated chimeric West Nile/dengue virus vaccines protect rhesus monkeys from West Nile virus. Virology 2003;314(1):190–5.
114. Davis BS, Chang GJ, Cropp B, et al. West Nile virus recombinant DNA vaccine protects mouse and horse from virus challenge and expresses in vitro a noninfectious recombinant antigen that can be used in enzyme-linked immunosorbent assays. J Virol 2001;75(9):4040–7.
115. Chu JH, Chiang CC, Ng ML. Immunization of flavivirus West Nile recombinant envelope domain III protein induced specific immune response and protection against West Nile virus infection. J Immunol 2007;178(5):2699–705.

116. Ledizet M, Kar K, Foellmer HG, et al. A recombinant envelope protein vaccine against West Nile virus. Vaccine 2005;23(30):3915–24.
117. Lieberman MM, Clements DE, Ogata S, et al. Preparation and immunogenic properties of a recombinant West Nile subunit vaccine. Vaccine 2007;25(3): 414–23.
118. Qiao M, Ashok M, Bernard KA, et al. Induction of sterilizing immunity against West Nile Virus (WNV), by immunization with WNV-like particles produced in insect cells. J Infect Dis 2004;190(12):2104–8.
119. Seino KK, Long MT, Gibbs EP, et al. Comparative efficacies of three commercially available vaccines against West Nile Virus (WNV) in a short-duration challenge trial involving an equine WNV encephalitis model. Clin Vaccine Immunol 2007;14(11):1465–71.

Hantaviruses

Mohammed A. Mir, PhD

KEYWORDS

• Hantaviruses • Rodents • Reinfection • RNA

In 1978, the etiologic agent of Korean hemerologic fever was isolated from small infected field rodent *Apodemus agrarius* near the Hantan river in South Korea. The virus was named as Hantaan virus, after the name of the river Hantan. This initial discovery dates back to scientific approaches that were initiated after the Korean War (1950–1953), during which more than 3000 cases of Korean hemorrhagic fever were reported among United Nations (UN) troops. In 1981, Hantaan virus strain 76-118, isolated from *Apodemus agrarius,* was grown in A549 cell line, and its electron microscopic images revealed that the virus was a new member of the Bunyaviridae family. It was observed that hantaviruses, unlike other members of this family, do not have an arthropod vector, and exclusively establish a persistent infection in the population of their specific rodent hosts. In 1981, a new genus termed as hantavirus was introduced in the Bunyaviridae family, which included the viruses that cause hemorrhagic fever with renal syndrome (HFRS) (**Fig. 1**). It was initially thought that pathogenic hantaviruses are restricted to the Old World. Until 1993, the only native hantavirus found in the New World was nonpathogenic Prospect Hill virus (PHV). This myth ended after the hantavirus outbreak in the Four-Corners region of the southwestern United States that caused serious respiratory distress in infected patients and led to the discovery of a new hantavirus disease called hantavirus cardiopulmonary syndrome (HPS). An examination of frozen stored samples of lung tissue from people who had died of unexplained lung disease in the past revealed that HPS is an old disease with confirmed cases dating to at least 1959. Within a very short period, the virus causing HPS was isolated from a common dear mouse (*Peromyscus maniculatus,* see **Fig. 1**) and was later named Sin Nombre virus (SNV). Later on, it became clear that other hantaviruses similar to SNV, such as Andes virus (ANDV), are present throughout the United States. Currently, the hantavirus genus includes more than 21 species and more than 30 genotypes (**Table 1**).

Hantaviruses have coevolved for millions of years with their rodent and insectivore reservoirs. Rodent reservoirs include both Cricetidae rodents (subfamilies Arvicolinae, Neotominae, and Sigmodontinae) and Muridae rodents (subfamily Murinae). Cricetidae rodents include voles, lemmings of the northern hemisphere, and new world mice and rats. Muridae rodents include Old World mice and rats (**Fig. 2**). Hantavirus

Department of Microbiology, Molecular Genetics and Immunology, Kansas University Medical Center, 3901 Rainbow Boulevard, Kansas City, KS 66103, USA
E-mail address: mmir@kumc.edu

Clin Lab Med 30 (2010) 67–91
doi:10.1016/j.cll.2010.01.004
0272-2712/10/$ – see front matter. Published by Elsevier Inc.

labmed.theclinics.com

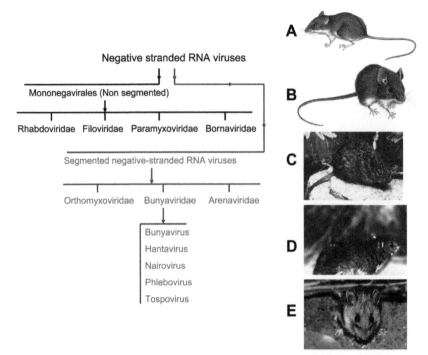

Fig. 1. Classification of negative stranded RNA viruses and the rodent reservoirs for the hantavirus genus. Left panel shows the classification of negative stranded RNA viruses in two groups, Mononegavirales and segmented negative stranded RNA viruses. Mononega-virales have a single copy of negative-sense RNA genome, and segmented RNA viruses have multiple copies of negative sense RNA genome. Segmented RNA viruses have been classified further into three families, Orthomyxoviridae, Bunyaviridae, and Arenaviridae. Viruses in the Bunyaviridae family have been classified into five genera, Bunyavirus, Hanta-virus, Nairovirus, Phlebovirus and Tospovirus. Right panel show the rodent reservoirs for hantaviruses. (*A*) Apodemus agrarius (reservoir for hantaan virus that cause HFRS); (*B*) deer mouse (*Peromyscus maniculatus*); (*C*) the cotton rat (*Sigmodon hispidus*); (*D*) the rice rat (*Oryzomys palustris*); (*E*) the white-footed mouse (*Peromyscus leucopus*). Rodents in *B, C, D,* and *E* cause HPS. All pictures in the right panel were obtained from the Centers for Disease Control and Prevention (CDC) Web site, http://www.cdc.gov/NCIDOD/DISEASES/HANTA/HPS/noframes/rodents.htm.

phylogeny follows closely that of their rodent hosts, suggesting long-term coevolution, although there is evidence of occasional host switches in the past. The phylogenetic tree suggests that cospeciation of hantaviruses with their host animals of four different rodent subfamilies appears to influence their ability to cause a specific clinical mani-festation in people. For example, most viruses in Neotominae and Sigmodontinae subfamilies are known to cause severe HPS with high mortality rates (40% to 50%). These viruses are distributed throughout North and South America in different rodent species of New World Neotominae and Sigmodontinae rodents. Old World hantavi-ruses that have coevolved with Murinae rodents cause severe HFRS that primarily affects kidney function, with a mortality of 0% to 15%. Although the disease caused by Murinae viruses has a lower mortality rate, it still poses a significant threat to human health because of severity of the disease and the ability of the viruses to cause large-scale epidemics. Among Arvicolinae-borne hantaviruses, only puumala virus (PUUV) causes a mild form of human disease often referred as nephropathia epidemica, with a mortality rate of less than 1%. Interestingly, most other members of this subfamily are nonpathogenic to people. Until recently, the only exception that did not have a confirmed rodent connection is Thottapalayam virus (TPMV), which was isolated from an Asian house shrew or musk shrew (*Suncus murinus*) captured in 1964 during a survey for Japanese encephalitis virus in southern India.[1]

MICROBIOLOGY

Electron microscopy revealed that hantaviruses are spherical or oval particles with a diameter of 80 to 210 nm (**Fig. 3**). They have tripartite negative sense RNA genome.[2,3] The large (L) segment genomic RNA encodes viral RNA-dependent RNA polymerase (RdRp); the medium-sized (M) segment encodes viral glycoprotein precursor (GPC), which is later cleaved into two glycoproteins, G1 and G2, and the small (S) segment encodes the viral nucleocapsid protein (N). The nucleotide sequence at 5' and 3' termini of each genome segment is complementary and undergoes base pairing to form panhandle structures (see **Fig. 3**). Inside the virus particle, the three genomic RNAs are complexed with N protein and form three individual nucleocapsids, which along with RdRp are packaged within a lipid envelope. Two glycoproteins, G1 and G2, remain embedded within the lipid envelope.

Like many other viruses, hantaviruses enter the host cells by the interaction between viral glycoproteins and cell surface integrin receptors (see **Fig. 3**). Interestingly, pathogenic and nonpathogenic hantaviruses use different integrin receptors to enter their host cells. Human integrin $\alpha IIa\beta3$ expressed by platelets, and $\alpha v\beta3$ expressed by endothelial cells, mediate the cellular entry for HFRS and HCP, causing hantaviruses.[4] In contrast, nonpathogenic hantaviruses, such as, PHV and TULV, use $\alpha5\beta1$ receptors for cellular entry. Once engaged on the host cell surface, hantaviruses enter the cells by clathrin-dependent endocytosis. Upon internalization, the three nucleocapsids are released into the cell cytoplasm along with viral RdRp. Subsequently, RdRp initiates transcription, and viral mRNAs encoding three viral proteins are synthesized. Viral mRNAs are around 100 nucleotides shorter than parent genomic viral RNAs and lack poly A tails. Viral RdRp uses a novel cap-snatching mechanism for transcription initiation. During cap snatching, 10- to14-nucleotide long 5' capped oligonucleotides are cleaved from host cell transcripts and used as primers by viral RdRp to initiate the viral mRNA synthesis, following a prime-and-realign mechanism.[5,6] Viral mRNAs are translated in the cell cytoplasm by the host cell translation machinery. Viral RdRp also replicates the genome via complementary cRNA synthesis. Complementary cRNAs are exact complements of genomic viral RNA (vRNA), and serve as templates for the synthesis of negative-sense viral genomes. Viral assembly and maturation take place either on the cell surface or on the Golgi apparatus. Virions that mature on the Golgi are transported to the cell surface via vesicular secretory pathways. Ultimately, new virions bud off the host cells from the plasma membrane.

NUCLEOCAPSID PROTEIN

N protein is the most abundant hantavirus protein found in the cytoplasm of infected cells. Its transcript is detected in infected cells 6 hours after infection. N protein is responsible for encapsidation and packaging of the viral genome. Recent studies, however, have shown that N is a multifunctional protein involved in diverse viral functions, including its role in the transcription and translation initiation of viral mRNA.[6,7] Trimeric N also recognizes the vRNA panhandle with specificity and likely facilitates the selective incorporation of viral genomic RNA into virions. N also has been found to interact with multiple host cell proteins, and the nature of such interaction remains unclear.

Table 1
Members of the genus _Hantavirus_, family _Bunyaviridae_

Species	Disease	Principal Reservoir	Distribution of Virus	Distribution of Reservoir
Hantaan (HTN)	HFRS	_Apodemus agrarius_ (striped field mouse)	China, Russia, Korea	Central Europe south to Thrace, Caucasus, and Tien Shan Mountains; Amur River through Korea to eastern Xizang and eastern Yunnan, western Sichuan, Fujiau, and Taiwan(China)
Dobrava-Belgrade (DOB)	HFRS	_Apodemus flavicollis_ (yellow-neck mouse)	Balkans	England and Wales, from northwest Spain, France, southern Scandinavia through European Russia to Urals, southern Italy, the Balkans, Syria, Lebanon, and Israel
Seoul (SEO)	HFRS	_Rattus norvegicus_ (Norway rat)	Worldwide	Worldwide
Puumala (PUU)	HFRS	_Clethrionomys glareolus_ (bank vole)	Europe, Russia, Scandinavia	Western Palearctic from France and Scandinavia to Lake Baikai, south to northern Spain, northern Italy, Balkans, western Turkey, northern Kazakhstan, Altai and Sayan Mountains, Britain and southwest Ireland
Thailand (THAI)	nd	_Bandicota indica_ (bandicoot rat)	Thailand	Sri Lanka, peninsular India to Nepal, Burma, northeast India, southern China, Laos, Taiwan, Thailand, Vietnam
Prospect Hill (PH)	nd	_Microtus pennsylvanicus_ (meadow vole)	United States, Canada	Central Alaska to Labrador, including Newfoundland and Prince Edward Island, Canada; Rocky Mountains to northern New Mexico, in Great Plains to northern Kansas, and in Appalachians to northern Georgia
Khabarovsk (KHB)	nd	_Microtus fortis_ (reed vole)	Russia	Transbaikalia Amur region, eastern China
Thottapalayam (TPM)	nd	_Suncus murinus_ (musk shrew)	India	Afghanistan, Pakistan, India, Sri Lanka, Nepal, Bhutan, Burma, China, Taiwan, Japan, Indomalayan region
Tula (TUL)	nd	_Microtus arvalis_ (European common vole)	Europe	Throughout Europe to Black Sea & NE to Kirov region, Russia
Sin Nombre (SN)	HPS	_Peromyscus maniculatus_ (deer mouse)	United States, Canada,	Alaska panhandle across northern Mexico, Canada, south through most of continental United States, excluding southeast and eastern seaboard, to southernmost Baja California Sur and to northcentral Oaxaca, Mexico

Virus	Disease	Reservoir host	Country	Distribution
New York (NY)	HPS	*Peromyscus leucopus* (white-footed mouse)	United States	Central and eastern United States to southern Alberta and southern Ontario, Quebec and Nova Scotia, Canada; to northern Durango and along Caribbean coast to Isthmus of Tehuantepec and Yucatan Peninsula, Mexico
Black Creek Canal (BCC)	HPS	*Sigmodon hispidus* (cotton rat)	United States	Southeastern United States, from southern Nebraska to central Virginia south to southeastern Arizona and peninsular Florida; interior and eastern Mexico through Middle America to central Panama; in South America to northern Colombia and northern Venezuela
El Moro Canyon (ELMC)[a]	nd	*Reithrodontomys megalotis* (western harvest mouse)	United States, Mexico	British Columbia and southeast Alberta, Canada; western and northcentral United States, southern to northern Baja California and interior Mexico to central Oaxaca
Bayou (BAY)[a]	HPS	*Oryzomys palustris* (rice rat)	United States	southeast Kansas to eastern Texas, eastward to southern New Jersey and peninsular Florida
Topografov (TOP)	nd	*Lemmus sibiricus* (Siberian lemming)	Siberia	Palearctic, from White Sea, western Russia, to Chukotski Peninsula, northeast Siberia, and Kamchatka; Nearctic, from western Alaska east to Baffin Island and Hudson Bay, southern Rocky Mountains to southern British Columbia, Canada
Andes (AND)	HPS	*Oligoryzomys longicaudatus*[c] (long-tailed pygmyrice rat)	Argentina	Northcentral to southern Andes, approximately to 50° south latitude, in Chile and Argentina
Isla Vista (ISLA)[a]	nd	*Microtus californicus* (California vole)	United States	Pacific coast, from southwestern Oregon through California, to northern Baja California; Mexico
Bloodland Lake (BLL)[a]	nd	*Microtus ochrogaster* (prairie vole)	United States	Northern and central Great Plains, eastcentral Alberta to southern Manitoba, Canada; southern to northern Oklahoma and Arkansas, eastern to central Tennessee and western West Virginia; relic populations elsewhere in the United States and Mexico
Muleshoe (MUL)[a]	nd	*Sigmodon hipidus* (cotton rat)	United States	See Black Creek Canal

(continued on next page)

Table 1
(continued)

Species	Disease	Principal Reservoir	Distribution of Virus	Distribution of Reservoir
Rio Segundo (RIOS)[a]	nd	*Reithrodontomys mexicanus* (Mexican harvest mouse)	Costa Rica	Southern Tamaulipas and westcentral Michoacan, Mexico; South through Middle American highlands to western Panama; Andes of western Colombia and northern Ecuador
Rio Mamore (RIOM)[a]	nd	*Oligoryzomys microtis* (small-eared pygmy rice rat)	Bolivia	Central Brazil south of Rios Solimoes–Amazon and contiguous lowlands of Peru, Bolivia, Paraguay, and Argentina
Oran virus[b]	HPS	*"Oligoryzomys longicaudatus"* (Northern Argentina)	South America	South America
Hu39694	HPS	*Oligoryzomys.[c] flavescens*	South America (Argentina)	South America (Argentina)
Laguna Negra virus	HPS	*Calomys laucha*	South America	South America
Choclo virus	HPS	*Oligoryzomys fulvescens*	South America	South America
Juquitiba virus	HPS	*Oligoryzomys nigripes*	South America (Brazil)	South America (Brazil)
Araraquara virus	HPS	*Bolomys lasiurus*	South America (Brazil)	South America (Brazil)
Castelo Dos Sonhos virus	HPS	*Oligoryzomyys ssp[c]*	South America (Brazil)	South America (Brazil)
Araucaria virus	HPS	*Bolomys lasiurus* or *Akodon ssp[c]*	South America (Brazil)	South America (Brazil)

Abbreviations: HFRS, hemorrhagic fever with renal syndrome; HPS, hantavirus pulmonary syndrome; nd, none documented.
[a] Not yet isolated in cell culture.
[b] Viruses for which incomplete characterization is available, but for which there is clear evidence indicating that they are unique.
[c] Suspected host, but not confirmed.

Data from Khaiboullina SF, Morzunov SP, St Jeor SC. Hantaviruses: molecular biology, evolution and pathogenesis. Curr Mol Med 2005;5:773–90; Schmaljohn C, Hjelle B. Hantaviruses: a global disease problem. Emerg Infect Dis 1997;3:95–104.

Cricetidae

Muridae

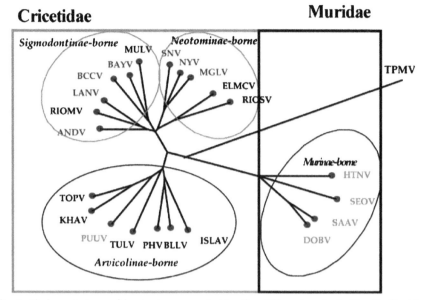

Fig. 2. Phylogenic tree of hantaviruses carried by the different rodents (Family Muridae, subfamily Murinae and Family Cricetidae, subfamilies Arvicolinae, Sigmodontinae and Neotominae) and insectivores. The tree is based on the complete coding region of the S segment. *Abbreviations:* ANDV, Andes virus; BAYO, Bayou virus; BCCV, Black Creek Canal virus; BLLV, Blood Land Lake virus; DOBV, Dobrava virus; ELMCV, El Moro Canyon virus; HTNV, Hantaan virus; ISLAV, Isla Vista virus; KHAV, Khabarovsk virus; LANV, Laguna Negra virus; MGLV, Monongahela virus; MULV, Muleshoe virus; NYV, New York virus; PHV, Prospect Hill virus; PUUV, Puumala virus; RIOMV, Rio Mamore virus; RIOSV, Rio Segundo virus; SAAV, Saaremaa virus; SEOV, Seoul virus; SNV, Sin Nombre virus; TOPV, Topografov virus; TPMV, Thottapalayam virus; TULV, Tula virus. In the figure, viruses causing HFRS are in red type, and those causing HCPS are in blue type. Viruses not associated with disease are in black type. (*From* Vaheri A, Vapalahti O, Plyusnin A. How to diagnose hantavirus infections and detect them in rodents and insectivores. Rev Med Virol 2008;18:279; with permission.)

GLYCOPROTEINS

Glycoprotein precursor (GPC) is synthesized on ribosomes associated with endoplasmic reticulum (ER) and is translocated to ER lumen by an endogenous signal peptide. In ER, GPC is post-translationally cleaved at a conserved WAASA site, and two glycoproteins, G1 and G2, are generated, which are later glycosylated and translocated to the Golgi. Glycoproteins facilitate the attachment of virions with the integrin receptors located on the host cell surface.

RDRP

Hantavirus RdRp is a huge protein with a molecular weight of 250 to 280 KDa. Because of its high molecular weight, RdRp is difficult to express in bacteria, and thus it remains the most uncharacterized protein in hantaviruses. RdRp mediates both transcription and replication of viral genome. During transcription, RdRp synthesizes viral mRNA from negative-sense vRNA template. During replication, RdRp replicates vRNA genome via a cRNA intermediate. Thus it is likely that hantavirus RdRp has multiple activities, including endonuclease, replicase, transcriptase, and RNA helix unwinding activities. Recent studies, however, have shown that viral RdRp

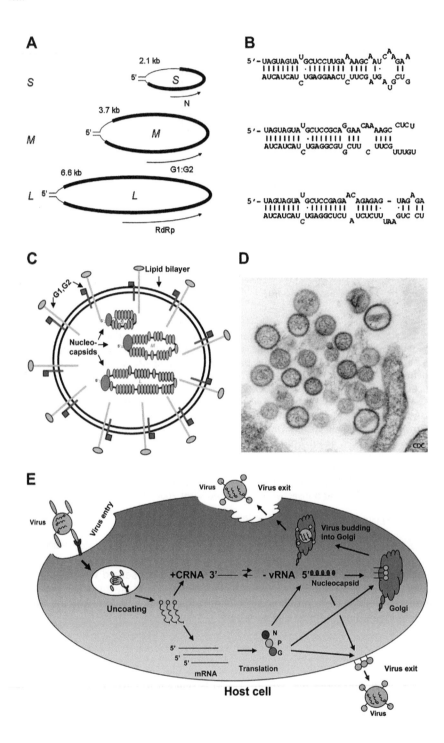

requires N protein for function. For example, short-capped primers generated from host cell mRNAs by the process of cap snatching are used by RdRp to initiate the transcription. Hantavirus N protein has been found to be involved in the generation of such capped primers.[6]

EPIDEMIOLOGY

The geographic distribution of hantavirus hosts mirrors the hantavirus epidemiology and geographic distribution (see **Table 1**). Hantavirus infection to people is considered a spill over infection that causes two types of serious illnesses, HFRS and HPS. The primary root of infection for both these illnesses is the inhalation of live virus through the lungs. In general people get hantavirus infection by direct contact with infected rodents or their aerosolized excreta; although there are reports documenting the spread of ANDV from person to person.[8,9] HFRS is caused by Old World hantaviruses and most of its cases are found in eastern Asia (China, Korea, and Eastern part of Russia and Europe, including the European part of Russia). Annually, more than 100,000 HFRS cases are reported in China alone,[10] and over 900 cases are reported in Korea and eastern Russia.[11] In Europe, most HFRS cases are registered in Russia, Finland, and Sweden (**Fig. 4**; see **Table 1**). Most HFRS patients are males between the ages of 20 and 50 years. The HFRS mortality rate depends upon the type of virus, and in general it varies from 0.1% to 10%. HRFS patients mostly live in rural areas where the hantaviral rodent hosts are thickly inhabited. The only hantavirus that causes diseases in urban areas is the Seoul virus (SEOV), because its host is a domestic rat (*Rattus norvegicus* and *Rattus rattus*). HPS has a mortality of 40% to 50% and is caused by New World hantaviruses, including SNV, ANDV, Monongahela virus, New York virus, Black Creek Canal virus, Bayou virus, Oran virus, and numerous other newly identified strains. Although HPS is found throughout the United States, most cases are registered in the western region and are caused by SNV. In fact, SNV is the predominantly found viral species that causes HPS in patients. HPS outbreaks in North America are associated with increased population of the host deer mouse (*Peromyscus maniculatus*). HPS also has been reported in other countries in South and Central America, including Argentina, Brazil, Chile, Bolivia, Paraguay, Uruguay, and Panama.

PATHOGENESIS

It is not yet exactly clear how hantaviruses spread in the human body after their inhalation through lungs. Immature dendritic cells (DCs), however, likely play a significant role in their dissemination. Immature DCs express β3 integrins, the receptors that hantaviruses use for attachment and entry. In the airways and alveoli of lungs, the DCs located in the vicinity of epithelial cells serve as primary targets for pathogen

---

Fig. 3. Hantaviral genome. (*A*) Hantaviral genome comprises of three negative sense RNAs, S segment encodes nucleocapsid protein (N), M segment encodes glycoproteins G1 and G2, and L segment encodes viral RdRp. (*B*) Panhandle structures of three hantaviral genomic RNAs are formed by the base pairing of complementary bases at 5′ and 3′ terminus of each genome segment. (*C*) Pictorial representation of hantavirus particle, showing three nucleocapsids enveloped in a lipid bilayer. (*D*) Thin-section electron micrograph of Sin Nombre virus isolate, a causative agent of hantavirus pulmonary syndrome (HPS) http://www.cdc.gov/ncidod/diseases/hanta/hps/noframes/hpsem.htm. (*E*) Pictorial representation of hanta virus life cycle.

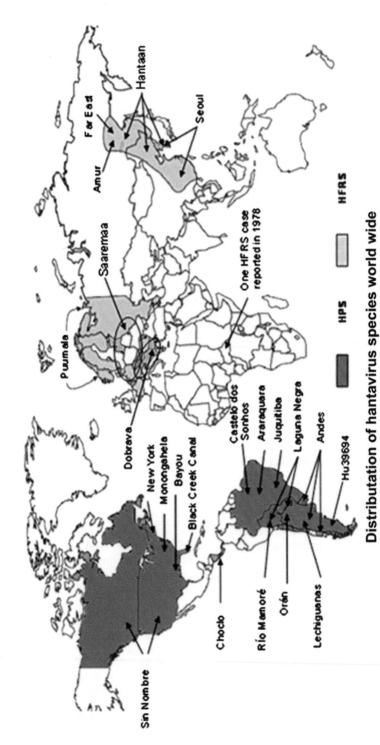

Fig. 4. Worldwide distribution of hantavirus species.

pick-up. Hantaviruses infect both immature and mature DCs, which likely serve as vehicles for the transport of virions through the lymphatic vessels to the regional lymph nodes, where they get opportunity to infect other immune cells, such as macrophages and monocytes. After further replication, the free or cell bound virions can infect the endothelial cells, the ultimate targets for viruses, causing hemorrhagic fever.[12]

Increased vascular permeability and decreased platelet count are the hallmarks of hantavirus-associated disease, and the mechanics of such pathogenesis are poorly understood. Unlike other hemorologic fever viruses such as the Ebola virus, the hantaviruses do not increase the permeability of endothelial cell monolayers in vitro, nor do they cause any cytopathic effects in the host endothelial cells. This points toward the role of the host immune system in hantavirus pathogenesis.

Invading viruses are detected early during infection by nonimmune cells and DCs located at host pathogen interface.[13] Pathogen recognition receptors (PRRs) for virus detection in host cells include TLRs and RIG-I like helicases (RIG-I and MDA5). RIG-I detects viruses from multiple families, including Orthomyxoviridae, Paramyxoviridae, Rhabdoviridae and Flaviviridae. However, the PRR that senses hantaviruses in host cells remains to be identified. Type 1 interferon (IFN) and other proinflammatory responses triggered by PRR signaling induce host resistance for viral infection and activation of innate immune cells, such as natural killer (NK) cells or NKT cells for host defense. These early responses are aimed to reduce the viral dissemination during the lag phase before adaptive immune response is ready to strike. It is established that treatment of cells with type 1 INF induces the expression of several hundred INF-stimulating genes (ISGs), including the well characterized MxA protein that has antiviral activity against the viruses of the Bunyaviridae family.[14,15] Interestingly, most pathogenic hantaviruses have evolved the strategies to sabotage the INF-induced host defense mechanisms. For example, pathogenic hantaviruses (HTNV, NYV) delay the type 1 INF response, including MxA expression in endothelial cells. This virus-programmed delay in the establishment of the antiviral state in host cells generates a window of opportunity for rapid replication and spread of pathogenic hantaviruses through the endothelial cell layer.

Inflammatory cytokines/chemokines produced by antiviral innate immune response represent a double-edged sword. On one hand, they play a role in virus elimination, but on the other hand, if not properly regulated, they can facilitate a virus-associated disease. For example, tumor necrosis factor (TNF)α can purge viruses from infected cells without causing cell lysis. At the same time, however, TNFα can modulate the endothelial barrier functions by promoting vascular leakage by increasing leukocyte adhesion and transendothelial migration.[16] TNFα and other cytokines are suspected to play a role in Ebola virus (EBOV)-mediated septic shock during EBOV hemorologic fever. Although hantavirus infection to DCs in vitro produces substantial amount of TNFα, which is consistent with increased plasma levels of this cytokine in hantavirus-infected patients during the acute phase of HFRS. However, there is no evidence of such a harmful innate immune response, producing a cytokine storm similar to the 1918 strain of influenza virus, that could contribute to the hantavirus immunopathogenesis.

In general, DCs are the prime targets for viruses to evade immune system. For example, human cytomegalovirus and herpes simplex viruses (DNA viruses) impair the function of DCs and induce their apoptosis by different mechanisms.[17] Filoviruses, such as EBOV and Marburg virus infect immature human DCs and inhibit their transition to antigen-presenting cells and also impair their ability to produce T cell stimulatory cytokines.[18] On the other hand, hantaviruses infect immature DCs and activate their maturation and transition into antigen-presenting cells without causing any cytopathic effects. Mature DCs after hantavirus infection had increased T cell stimulatory capacity, explaining the elicitation of vigorous T cell response with long-lasting memory in patients during the acute phase of hantavirus infection.[19] Although epitopes are defined for all three hantavirus proteins, N protein is the major viral target antigen recognized by T cells, likely because of its higher comparative abundance in infected cells. In recent years, the concept that cytotoxic lymphocytes (CTL) response directed against hantavirus-infected endothelial cells mediates increased capillary permeability has gained more and more support from multiple indirect evidences. For example, T cell-attracting chemokines CCL5 and CXCL10 are secreted by human lung microvascular endothelial cells after infection by either HTNV or SNV in vitro.[20] Hantavirus-specific CTLs efficiently lyse human endothelial cells leading to the increased vascular permeability.[21] In addition, PUUV-infected patients show a peak CTL response at the onset of disease with increased serum levels of perforin, gran- zyme B, and the epithelial cell apoptosis marker caspase-cleaved cytokeratin- 18.[22,23] The number of CD8 + T cells in PUUV-infected patients strongly increase during the acute phase of HFRS, and leave a strong long-lived CTL memory against the PUUV N protein.[19] It is likely that a strong unusual primary response accounts for such a long-lived hantavirus-specific CTL memory. These observations suggest that the strength of antiviral CTL response and the number of available CTL targets in endothelial cell layer could determine the severity of damage to the vascular bed in hantavirus-infected patients. An interesting question of how the reservoir host rodents escape the vascular damage during persistent hantavirus infection remains to be answered. Recent studies, however, have suggested that regulatory T cells may play an important role in limiting immunopathology in the natural reservoir host, but this response may interfere with viral clearance. It is hypothesized that in people the immune mechanisms that down-regulate the hantavirus-specific CTL response and facilitate the viral clearance by noncytolytic means are missing, leading to a CTL storm for rapid elimination of virus at the expense of costly damage to the endo- thelial barrier that causes fatal capillary leakage. In contrast, rodent hosts have elevated regulatory T cell response that controls the CTL activity, leading to viral persistence without immunopathology (**Fig. 5**). The quality of T cell response triggered against hantaviruses is determined by DCs, which are programmed through PRRs during early stages of infection. Thus, further investigation is required to identify the PRRs that detect hantaviruses in rodent hosts and people. It is probable that PRRS for hantaviruses in people and rodents are different and program DCs differently, leading to a fatal disease in people and viral persistence in rodent hosts. Similar to cellular immunity, hantaviruses induce a stable and long-lasting humoral immune response involving antibodies of all immunoglobulin (Ig) subclasses (IgA, IgM, IgG). Antibodies against N protein appear soon after the onset of the disease, and anti- bodies against G1 and G2 appear later during the progress of the disease. High titers of antibodies have been found in individuals who experienced HCPS years ago. People infected with PUUV show the presence of neutralizing antibodies in blood decades after infection, suggesting that previously infected individuals are protected for life from the infection. **Tables 2** and **3** summarize the immune response in people and rodents by hantavirus infection.

CLINICAL PRESENTATION

As described by the Centers for Disease Control and Prevention (CDC), patients with HCPS typically present a short febrile prodrome of 3 to 5 days.[20] In addition to fever and myalgias, early symptoms include headache, chills, dizziness, nonproductive cough, nausea, vomiting, and other gastrointestinal symptoms. Malaise, diarrhea,

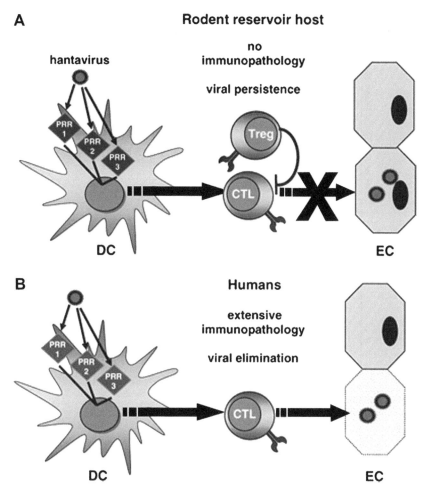

Fig. 5. Working hypothesis of differential regulation of hantavirus-specific immune responses in rodent reservoir hosts and people. During their encounter with viruses, DCs integrate different signals received through several PRRs (eg, PRR 1, PRR 2, PRR3), which determine the quality of the ensuing T cell response. (*A*) In their rodent reservoir host, hantavirus-associated PRR signaling could program DCs to stimulate Treg cells that can suppress virus-specific CTLs, leading to viral persistence and at the same time preventing virus-induced immunopathology. (*B*) In people, who are not adapted to hantaviruses, PRR signaling in DCs results in a dominant antiviral CTL response. As a consequence, hanta-virus-infected endothelial cells (EC) are immediately eliminated leading to immunopa-thology. (*From* Schonrich G, Rang A, Lutteke N, et al. Hantavirus-induced immunity in rodent reservoirs and humans. Immunol Rev 2008;225:180; with permission.)

and lightheadedness are reported by approximately half of all patients, with less frequent reports of arthralgias, back pain, and abdominal pain. Patients may report shortness of breath, (respiratory rate usually 26 to30 times per minute). Typical find-ings on initial presentation include fever, tachypnea, and tachycardia, with usually a normal physical examination.

The analysis of clinical, laboratory, and autopsy data of 17 patients with confirmed hantavirus infection during a 1993 hantavirus outbreak reveled the mean duration of

Table 2
Summary of immune response in humans during hantavirus infection

Categorical Response	Immune Marker	Effect on Infection	Virus Species	In Vitro/in Vivo	Tissue or Cell Typev Phase of Infection[a]
Innate	RIG-I	Elevated	SNV	In vitro	HUVEC, ≤24 h p.i
		Reduced	NY-I	In vitro	HUVEC, ≤24 h p.i
	TLR3	Elevated	SNV	In vitro	HUVEC, ≤24 h p.i
	INF-β	Elevated	PUUV, PHV, ANDV	In vitro	HSVEC, HMVEX, ≤24 h p.i
		Reduced	TULV, PUUV NSs	In vitro	COS-7 and MRC5 cells, ≤24 h p.i
	INF-α	Elevated	PUUV, HTNV	In vitro	Mφ, DCs, 4 days p.i
		No change	HTNV	In vitro	Blood, acute
	IRF-3, IRF-7	Elevated	SNV, HTNV, PHV	In vitro	HMVEC-L, ≤24 h p.i.
	MxA	Elevated	HTNV, NY-IV, PHV, PUUV, ANDV, SNV	In vitro	Mφ, HUVEC, HMVEC-L, 6 h 4 days p.i
	MCH I & II	Elevated	HTNV	In vitro	DCs, 4 days p.i
	CD 11b	Elevated	PUUV	In vitro	Blood, acute
	CD-40, CD80, CD86	Elevated	HTNV	In vitro	DCs, 4 days p.i
	Nk cells	Elevated	PUUV	In vitro	Bal, acute
Proinflammatory/ adhesion	IL-1β	Elevated	SNV, HTNS	In vitro	Blood, lungs, acute
	IL-6	Elevated	SNV, PUUV	In vitro	Blood, lungs, acute
	NF-α	Elevated	PUUV, SNV, HTNV	In vitro	Blood, lungs, acute, kidney
	CCL5	Elevated	SNV, HTNV	In vitro	HMVEC-L, HUVEC, 3–4 days p.i
	CXCL8	Elevated	PUUV	In vitro	Blood, acute
		Elevated	PUUV	In vitro	Men, blood, acute
		Elevated	TULV, PHV, HTNV	In vitro	HUVEC, Mφ, 4–2 days p.i
	CXCL10	Elevated	SNV, HTNV, PHV	In vitro	HUVEC-L, HUVEC, 3–4 days p.i
		Elevated	PUUV	In vitro	Men, blood, acute
	IL-2	Elevated	SNV, HTNV, PUUV	In vitro	Blood, lungs, acute
	Nitric oxide	Elevated	PUUV	In vitro	Blood, acute
	GM-CSF	Elevated	PUUV	In vitro	Women, blood, acute
	ICAM, VCAM	Elevated	HTNV, PHV	In vitro	Kidney acute
		Elevated	HTNV	In vitro	HUVEC, 3–4 days p.i
	E- selectin	Elevated	PUUV	In vitro	Blood, acute

CD8+ and CD4 + T cells	INF-γ	Elevated	HTNV, SNV	In vitro	Blood, CD4+, CD8+, lungs, acute
	CD8+	Elevated	DOBV, PUUV, HTNV	In vitro	Blood, BAL, acute
	Virus specific INF-γ+CD8+	Elevated	PUUV, SNV	In vitro	PBMC, acute
	Perforin, granzyme B	Elevated	PUUV	In vitro	Blood acute
	CD4+CD25+ activated	Elevated	DOB, PUUV	In vitro	PBMC, acute
	IL-4	Elevated	SNV	In vitro	Lungs, acute
Regulatory	Suppressor T cells[b]	Reduced	HTNV	In vitro	Blood, acute
	IL-10	Elevated	PUUV	In vitro	Blood, acute
	TGF-β	Elevated	PUUV	In vitro	Kidney, acute
Humoral	IgM, IgA, IgG, IgE	Elevated	All hantaviruses	In vitro	Blood

Abbreviations: ANDV, Andes virus; Bal, bronchoalveolar lavage; COS-7, African green monkey kidney fibroblast transformed with Siman virus 40; DCs, dendritic cells; DOBV, Dobrava virus; HMVEC-L, human lung microvascular endothelial cells; HSVEC, human saphenous vein endothelial cells; HTNV, Hantaan virus; HUVEC, human umbilical vascular endothelial cells; MRC5, human fetal lung fibroblasts; Mφ, macrophages; NY-IV, New York -1; PHV, Prospect Hill virus; p.i., post infection; PMBC, human peripheral blood mononuclear cells; PUUV, Puumala virus; SNV, Sin Nombre virus; TULV, Tula virus.

[a] Acute infection is during symptomatic disease in patients.

[b] Suppressor T cells likely represent cells currently referred to as regulatory T cells.

Data from Easterbrook JD, Klein SL. Immunologic mechanisms mediating hantavirus persistence in rodent reservoirs. PLoS Pathog 2008;4:e1000172.

Table 3
Summary of immune response in rodents during hantavirus infection

Categorical Response	Immune Marker	Effect on Infection	Virus Species	Host, Tissue, or Cell Type	Phase of Infection[a]
Innate	TLR7	Reduced	SEOV	Male Norway rats, lungs	Acute persistent
		Elevated	SEOV	Female Norway rats, lungs	Acute persistent
	RIG-I	Elevated	SEOV	Female Norway rats, lungs	Acute persistent
		Elevated	SEOV	Norway rats, Thalamus	Acute
	TLR3	Elevated	SEOV	Male Norway rats, lungs	Acute persistent
	INF-β	Reduced	SEOV	Male Norway rats, lungs	Acute persistent
		Elevated	SEOV	Female Norway rats, lungs	Acute
	MX2	Reduced	SEOV	Male Norway rats, lungs	Acute persistent
		Elevated	SEOV	Female Norway rats, lungs	Acute persistent
		Elevated	HTN, SEOV	Mice,[b] fibroblast transfected with MX2	3–4 days p.i
	JAK2	Elevated	SEOV	Female Norway rats, lungs	Acute
	MHC II	Elevated	PUUV,	Bank voles	Genetic susceptibility
Proinflammatory/adhesion	IL-1β	Reduced	SEOV,	Male Norway rats, lungs	Persistent
	IL-6	Reduced	SEOV	Male and female Norway rats, lungs	Acute persistent
		Elevated	SEOV	Male rats spleen	Acute
	TNF-α	Reduced	HTNV	Newborn mice,[b] CD8+, Spleen	Acute
		Reduced	SEOV	Male Norway rats, lungs	Acute persistent
		Elevated	SEOV	Female Norway rats, lungs	Acute
	CXCL1/	Reduced	SEOV	Male Norway rats, lungs	Acute persistent
	CXCL10	Elevated	SEOV	Male Norway rats, Spleen	Acute
	CCL2/CCL5	Elevated	SEOV	Male Norway rats, Spleen	Acute
	NOS2	Reduced	SEOV	Male Norway rats, lungs	Acute persistent
		Elevated	SEOV	Male Norway rats, spleen	Acute
		Elevated	HTNV	Mouse Mφ,[b] in vitro	6 h p.i
	VCAM/VGF	Elevated	SEOV	Male Norway rats, spleen	Acute

Category	Marker	Change	Virus	Host	Infection
CD8+ and CD4 + T cells	CD8+	Reduced	HTNV,	Newborn mice,[b] spleen	Persistent
		Elevated	HTNV,	SCID mice,[b] CD8+ transferred	Persistent
	INF-γ	Elevated	SEOV	Female Norway rats, lungs	Persistent
		Elevated	SEOV	Female Norway rats, lungs	Acute
		Elevated	SEOV	Male Norway rats, lungs	Acute
		Elevated	SNV	Female & male Norway rats Deer mice, CD4 + T cells	Acute
		Elevated	HTNV	Newborn mice[b] CD4 + T cells	Acute
		Reduced	HTNV	Newborn mice[b] CD4 + T cells	Persistent
	INF-γR	Elevated	SEOV	Female Norway rats, lungs	Acute persistent
		Reduced	SEOV	Male Norway rats, lungs	Persistent
	T cells	Elevated	SEOV	Nude rat	Persistent
		Elevated	HTNV	Nude mice[b]	Persistent
	IL-4	Reduced	SEOV	Male Norway rats, lungs	Acute persistent
		Elevated	SNV	Deer mice, CD4 + T cells	Acute
		Elevated	SEOV	Female & male Norway rats	Acute
Regulatory	Regulatory T cells	Elevated	SEOV	Male Norway rats, lungs	Persistent
	FoxP3	Elevated	SEOV	Male Norway rats, lungs	Persistent
		Elevated	SEOV	Male Norway rats, lungs	Persistent
	TGF-β	Reduced	SNV	Deer mice, CD4 + T cells	Persistent
	IL-10	Elevated	SEOV	Male Norway rats, lungs, spleen	Persistent
			SNV	Deer mice, CD4 + T cells	Persistent
Humoral	IgG	Elevated	SNV	Deer mice	Persistent
		Elevated	SEOV	Norway rats	Persistent
		Elevated	HTNV	Field mice	Persistent
		Elevated	PUUV	Banl Voles	Persistent
		Elevated	BCCV	Cotton rats	Persistent

Abbreviations: BCCV, Black Creek Canal virus; HTNV, Hantaan virus; Mφ, macrophages; p.i., post infection; PUUV, Puumala virus; SEOV, Seoul virus; SNV, Sin Nombre virus.

[a] Acute infection is <30 days p.i and persistent infection is ≥30 days p.i.

[b] *Mus musculus*, non-natural reservoir host for hantaviruses.

Data from Easterbrook JD, Klein SL. Immunologic mechanisms mediating hantavirus persistence in rodent reservoirs. PLoS Pathog 2008;4:e1000172.

symptoms before hospitalization was 5.4 days. The most common symptoms at the time of hospitalization were fever, myalgia, headache, cough, and nausea or vomiting (**Tables 4** and **5**), with myalgia being the most frequently reported initial symptom. The most common physical findings were tachypnea and tachycardia. Fifty percent of the patients had a respiratory rate of 28 or more breaths per minute, and 50% had a heart rate of 120 or more beats per minute. No patient had conjunctival hemorrhage, petechial rash, clinical signs of internal hemorrhage (including a guaiac-positive stool specimen), or peripheral or periorbital edema. Notable hematologic findings included an elevated white cell count with increased neutrophils, myeloid precursors, and atypical lymphocytes

The partial-thromboplastin time was 40 seconds or longer in 67% of the patients at the time of admission (**Tables 6** and **7**). Although minimal abnormalities of renal function were common, the serum creatinine levels did not rise above 2.5 mg/dL (220 μmol/L) in any patient (see **Tables 6** and **7**). The mean specific gravity of urine at the time of admission was 1.024 plus or minus 0.010. Forty percent of patients had proteinuria on admission. Urine dipstick tests for blood were positive in 57% of tested patients at the time of admission.

The initial chest radiograph showed interstitial or interstitial and alveolar infiltrates (**Fig. 6**) in 65% of patients, fluffy alveolar infiltrates in 12% of patients, and no abnormalities in 24% of patients. Subsequently, 94% of patients had rapidly evolving, bilateral, diffuse infiltrates, and 6% of patients had interstitial infiltrates confined to the lower lobes. Pleural effusions were noted during the course of the illness in four patients. Eleven of 12 patients (92%) who underwent chest radiography and arterial

Table 4
Symptoms in 17 patients with hantavirus infection

Symptom	Number of Patients (%)
Fever	17 (100)
Myalgia	17 (100)
Headache	12 (71)
Cough	12 (71)
Nausea or vomiting	12 (71)
Chills	11 (65)
Malaise	10 (59)
Diarrhea	10 (59)
Shortness of breath	9 (53)
Dizziness or lightheadedness	7 (41)
Arthralgia	5 (29)
Back pain	5 (29)
Abdominal pain	4 (24)
Chest pain	3 (18)
Sweats	3 (18)
Distrait or frequent urination	3 (18)
Rhinorrhea or nasal congestion	2 (12)
Sore throat	2 (12)

Data from Duchin JS, Koster FT, Peters CJ, et al. Hantavirus pulmonary syndrome: a clinical description of 17 patients with a newly recognized disease. The Hantavirus Study Group. N Engl J Med 1994;330:949–55.

Table 5
Symptoms in 10 pediatric patients (age ≤16 years) with SNV infection

Symptom	Number of Patients (%)
Fever	10 (100)
Myalgia	8 (80)
Headache	10 (100)
Cough	9 (90)
Nausea or vomiting	9 (90)
Chills	3 (30)
Diarrhea	4 (40)
Shortness of breath	8 (80)
Dizziness or lightheadedness	3 (30)
Back pain	5 (50)
Abdominal pain	5 (50)
Chest pain	3 (30)
Sore throat	4 (40)

Data from Ramos MM, Overturf GD, Crowley MR, et al. Infection with Sin Nombre hantavirus: clinical presentation and outcome in children and adolescents. Pediatrics 2001;108:E27.

Table 6
Results of laboratory studies during hospitalization in patients with hantavirus infection

Test[a,b]	Admission Value	Maximal [Minimal] Value
White cells-X10^3/mm^3	10.4 (3.1–65.3)	26.0 (5.6–65.3)
Band forms - %	22 (8–62)	27 (4–67)
Hematocrit -%		
Men	51.3 (49.9–60.0)	56.3 (49.9–67.7)
Women	46.4 (35.0–55.8)	48.5 (36.5–60.3)
Platelets – ×10^3/mm^3	84 (26–320)	[64] (12–148)
Prothrombin time – sec	13.0 (11.2–21.1)	14 (12.6–21.1)
Partial-thromboplastin time – seconds	42.5 (30.0–150.0)	54.4 (31.0–150.0)
Bicarbonate – mmol/L	18 (12–25)	[14] (8–20)
Lactate dehydrogenase IU/L	362 (209–1525)	568 (324–1525)
Aspartate aminotransferase IU/liter	112 (28–432)	148 (62–432)
Alanine aminotransferase IU/L	55 (25–148)	63 (27–149)
Albumin – g/dL	3.0 (1.5–4.6)	[2.5] (1.5–3.5)
Blood urea nitrogen – g/dL	11 (3–23)	17 (8–32)
Creatinine – mg/dL	1.1 (0.6–2.5)	1.4 (0.6–2.5)
Lactate – mmol/L	4.4 (2.2–11.0)	—
Creatine kinase – 1U/L	46 (19–1026)	—

[a] Maximal normal values: Lactate dehydrogenase, 180 to 232 IU/L; aspartate aminotransferase, 35 to 40 IU/L; alanine aminotransferase, 35 to 60 IU/L; Lactate, 2.2 mmol/L; creatine kinase, 180 to 269 IU/L. To convert values fro creatinine to μmol/L, multiply by 88.4
[b] Two of 10 patients tested had elevated creatine kinase concentrations: 1026 IU/L with an MB fraction of 16 (2%) in 1 patient, and 814 IU/Lwith an MB fraction of 87 (11%) in another patient, who was undergoing cardiopulmonary resuscitation when the sample was obtained.
Data from Duchin JS, Koster FT, Peters CJ, et al. Hantavirus pulmonary syndrome: a clinical description of 17 patients with a newly recognized disease. The Hantavirus Study Group. N Engl J Med 1994;330:949–55.

Table 7
Results of laboratory studies at the time of admission in pediatric patients with Sin Nombre hantavirus infection.

Test	Admission Value (Median [Range])
White cells × 10³/mm³	9.0 (3.4–59.2)
Mematocrit %	
Patients 10–12 y (n = 5)	42.0 (34.9–45.2)
Males 13–16 y (n = 2)	54.3 (47.6–61)
Females 13–16 y (n = 4)	41.9 (40–48.4)
Platelets × 10³/mm³	67 (43–98)
Creatinine (mg/dL)	0.7 (0.4–3.9)
Prothrombin time (seconds)	13.1 (11.0–29.8)
Partial thromboplastin time (seconds)	38 (27–212)
Carbon dioxide (mmol/L)	20 (15–27)
Blood urea nitrogen (mg/dL)	10 (8–26)
Aspartate aminotransferase (IU/L)	98 (39–129)
Albumin (g/dL)	2.8 (1.2–3.5)
Alanine aminotransferase (IU/L)	55 (21–80)
Lactate dehydrogenase (IU/L)	1243 (382–1724)
Lactate (mmol/L)	2.5 (1.5–18.4)

Data from Ramos MM, Overturf GD, Crowley MR, et al. Infection with Sin Nombre hantavirus: clinical presentation and outcome in children and adolescents. Pediatrics 2001;108:E27.

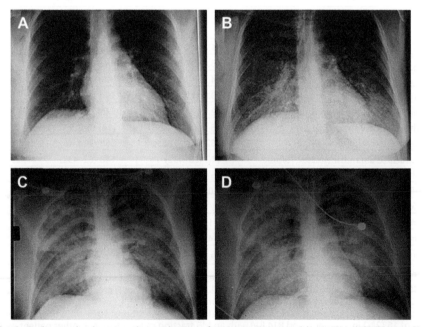

Fig. 6. Radiographs showing the evolution of HPS in a 30-year-old woman. (*A*) Chest radiograph before onset of illness. (*B*) Admission radiograph. (*C*) Radiograph after intubation. (*D*) Radiograph just before death. (*From* Graziano KL, Tempest B. Hantavirus pulmonary syndrome: a zebra worth knowing. Am Fam Physician 2002;66:1015–20.)

measurement of oxygen saturation at the time of admission had either pulmonary infiltrates or arterial oxygen saturation under 90 mm Hg. Similar observations were made in other hantavirus-infected cases [24,25]

Since the emergence of HCPS in United States in 1993, only 5.5% of the cases reported to CDC were children younger than 16 years. Due to minimum causalities in younger children and adolescents, it is hypothesized that hantavirus infection in children is less likely to develop into serious illness as compared with adults. The analysis of clinical data of 10 SNV pediatric cases is presented in **Tables 4** to **9**.

DIAGNOSTICS

Hantavirus infection is diagnosed on the basis of a positive serologic test and the confirmation of viral antigen in the tissue of infected patient or the presence of viral RNA sequences in patient's blood or tissue, along with a compatible history of the disease.

SEROLOGIC ASSAYS

During the 1993 hantavirus outbreak, cross-reactive antibodies to the previously known hantaviruses such as, Hantaan, Seoul, Puumala, and Prospect Hill virus were found in the acute- and convalescent-phase sera of some HPS patients. Since then, tests based on specific viral antigens from SNV have been developed and are used widely for the routine diagnosis of HPS. Enzyme-linked immunosorbent assay (ELISA) is the popular test for the detection of IgM antibodies in patient's blood that are raised against hantaviruses during infection.

An IgG test in conjunction with the IgM-capture test is also used for the diagnosis of hantavirus disease. Acute- and convalescent-phase sera should reflect a fourfold rise in IgG antibody titer or the presence of IgM in acute-phase sera for a positive hantavirus infection. It may be noted that acute-phase serum used as an initial diagnostic specimen may not yet have IgG. IgG is a long-lasting antibody, retained for many years after infection. Thus, SNV IgG ELISA has been used in serologic investigations of the epidemiology of the disease and appears to be appropriate for this purpose. Rapid immunoblot strip assay (RIBA) is an investigational prototype assay for the identification of serum antibodies to recombinant proteins and peptides specific for SNV and other hantaviruses. Also, neutralizing plaque assays recently have been performed

Table 8
Clinical findings at the time of admission in 17 patients with hantavirus infection

Sign	Percentage of Patients	Median (Range)
Respiratory rate ≥20/min	100	28 (20–70)
Heart rate ≥ 100 beats per minute	94	120 (90–150)
Temperature ≥38.1°C	75	38.8 (35.4–40.4)
Systolic or rales on lung examination	31	
Abdominal tenderness	24	
Cool, clammy, or mottled skin	18	
Injection or suffusion of conjunctiva	18	

Data from Duchin JS, Koster FT, Peters CJ, et al. Hantavirus pulmonary syndrome: a clinical description of 17 patients with a newly recognized disease. The Hantavirus Study Group. N Engl J Med 1994;330:949–55.

Table 9
Clinical findings at the time of admission in nine pediatric patients with SNV infection.

Sign	Percentage of Patients
Tachypnea	67
Fever (temperature $\geq 38.0°C$)	56
Crackles or rales on lung examination	44
Abdominal tenderness	44
Hypotension[a]	33
Tachycardia (heart rate >20 beats per minute)	22
Cool, clammy, or mottled skin	11

Respiratory rate >25 beats/min (10–13 years old). Respiratory rate >20 breaths/min (≥ 14 years old). Includes two patients mechanically ventilated before admission.

[a] Systolic blood zpressure <95 mm Hg (10–13 years old). Systolic blood pressure <100 mm Hg (≥ 14 years old).

Data from Ramos MM, Overturf GD, Crowley MR, et al. Infection with Sin Nombre hantavirus: clinical presentation and outcome in children and adolescents. Pediatrics 2001;108:E27.

for the serologic confirmation of SNV infections. However, these specific assays are not commercially available. Isolation of hantaviruses from human sources is difficult, and no isolates of SNV-like viruses have been recovered from people. Thus, isolation of hantavirus is not considered for diagnostic purposes.

IMMUNOHISTOCHEMISTRY

Immunohistochemistry (IHC) testing of formalin-fixed tissues with specific monoclonal and polyclonal antibodies can be used to detect hantavirus antigens and has proven to be a sensitive method for laboratory confirmation of hantaviral infections. IHC has an important role in the diagnosis of HPS in patients from whom serum samples and frozen tissues are unavailable for diagnostic testing and in the retrospective assessment of disease prevalence in a defined geographic region.

POLYMERASE CHAIN REACTION

Reverse transcriptase polymerase chain reaction (RT-PCR) is a very sensitive assay that can be used for the detection of hantaviral RNA in infected samples such as lung tissues and blood clots from infected patients. RT-PCR, however, is very prone to cross-contamination and should be considered an experimental technique with a limited use for diagnostic purposes of hantavirus infections.

DIFFERENTIAL DIAGNOSIS

Various infectious etiologies, such as, pneumonia, sepsis with acute respiratory distress syndrome (ARDS), and acute bacterial endocarditis often can be confused with HPS. Other conditions commonly found in the southwest United States have presentations similar to HPS such as septicemic plague, tularemia, histoplasmosis, and coccidioidomycosis. In addition, noninfectious conditions, including myocardial infarction with pulmonary edema and Goodpasture syndrome also should be considered.

TREATMENT

Apart from supportive care, there is no treatment for hantavirus infection at present. Patients receive broad-spectrum antibiotics while awaiting the results of laboratory diagnostic tests for the confirmation of hantavirus-associated disease. Initial supportive care includes the use of antipyretics and analgesics. Patients are transferred immediately to intensive care unit (ICU) if preliminary symptoms indicate a higher probability of HPS. ICU management should include careful assessment, monitoring, and adjustment of volume status and cardiac function, including inotropic and vasopressor support if needed. Fluids should be administrated carefully because of higher chances of capillary leakage. Supplemental oxygen is necessary for hypoxic patients. Because of high risks of respiratory failure, ICU management should keep equipment and materials for intubation and mechanical ventilation readily available. Patients with severe HPS quickly progress to respiratory failure, and in absence of ECMO (extracorporeal membrane oxygenation), almost all patients die within 24 to 48 hours of the onset of this severe phase.

Antiviral therapy including the use of ribavirin, a guanosine analog, has not been shown to be effective for the treatment of HPS. Efficacy trials in HFRS patients in China, however, have shown significant beneficial effects of ribavirin if started early in the disease course. Although ribavarin perturbs SNV replication in vitro, neither an open-label trial conducted during the 1993 outbreak nor an attempted placebo-controlled trial demonstrated clinical benefit for HPS. It has been suggested, however, that ribavirin efficacy may depend on phase of infection and the severity of the disease at the time of administration. Ribavirin is not recommended for treating HPS, and it is not available for this use.

Examination of neutralizing antibody titers in patients at the time of admission has revealed low antibody titers for the patients with severe disease and higher antibody titers for patients with mild disease. These observations provide clues toward the use of human neutralizing antibodies during the acute phase of HPS that might prove effective for the treatment or prophylaxis of hantaviral infections.

There is no US Food and Drug Administration-approved vaccine for hantavirus infection in the United States. A killed-virus vaccine against hantavirus infection has been developed in Korea and China. Such approaches, however, are not pursued in the United States for many reasons. Efforts are underway to develop a DNA vaccine, based on the gene gun approach for the transport of an expression plasmid-containing M segment gene to the individual, which upon expression will generate neutralizing antibodies against glycoproteins G1 and G2.

IMMUNITY AND REINFECTION

High titers of neutralizing antibodies have been found in individuals who experienced HPS years ago.[26,27] Neutralizing antibodies against PUUV have been detected in individuals decades after infection.[28] These observations suggest that previously infected individuals are protected for life from reinfection. There are no known reinfections with the homologous hantavirus. Closely related hantaviruses, such as Seoul and Hantaan viruses, seem to cross-protect against reinfection in experimental animals, and one might expect cross-protection among the hantaviruses derived from sigmodontine rodents.

REFERENCES

1. Carey DE, Reuben R, Panicker KN, et al. Thottapalayam virus: a presumptive arbovirus isolated from a shrew in India. Indian J Med Res 1971;59:1758–60.

2. Johnson KM. Hantaviruses: history and overview. Curr Top Microbiol Immunol 2001;256:1–14.
3. Schmaljohn CS. Bunyaviridae: the viruses and their replication. In: Fields BN, Knipe DM, Howley PN, editors. Fields virology. Philadelphia: Lippencott-Raven; 1996. p. 1581–602.
4. Gavrilovskaya IN, Gorbunova EE, Mackow NA, et al. Hantaviruses direct endo-thelial cell permeability by sensitizing cells to the vascular permeability factor VEGF, while angiopoietin 1 and sphingosine 1-phosphate inhibit hantavirus-directed permeability. J Virol 2008;82:5797–806.
5. Elliott RM, Schmaljohn CS, Collett MS. Bunyaviridae genome structure and gene expression. Curr Top Microbiol Immunol 1991;169:91–141.
6. Mir MA, Duran WA, Hjelle BL, et al. Storage of cellular 5' mRNA caps in P bodies for viral cap-snatching. Proc Natl Acad Sci U S A 2008;105:19294–9.
7. Mir MA, Panganiban AT. A protein that replaces the entire cellular eIF4F complex. EMBO J 2008;27:3129–39.
8. Enria D, Padula P, Segura EL, et al. Hantavirus pulmonary syndrome in Argentina. Possibility of person-to-person transmission. Medicina (B Aires) 1996;56:709–11.
9. Padula PJ, Edelstein A, Miguel SD, et al. Epidemic outbreak of hantavirus pulmo-nary syndrome in Argentina. Molecular evidence of person to person transmis-sion of Andes virus. Medicina (B Aires) 1998;58(Suppl 1):27–36.
10. Khan A, Khan AS. Hantaviruses: a tale of two hemispheres. Panminerva Med 2003;45:43–51.
11. Lee HW. Hemorrhagic fever with renal syndrome in Korea. Rev Infect Dis 1989; 11(Suppl 4):S864–76.
12. Marty AM, Jahrling PB, Geisbert TW. Viral hemorrhagic fevers. Clin Lab Med 2006;26:345–86.
13. Banchereau J, Steinman RM. Dendritic cells and the control of immunity. Nature 1998;392:245–52.
14. Frese M, Kochs G, Feldmann H, et al. Inhibition of bunyaviruses, phleboviruses, and hantaviruses by human MxA protein. J Virol 1996;70:915–23.
15. Kochs G, Janzen C, Hohenberg H, et al. Antivirally active MxA protein sequesters La Crosse virus nucleocapsid protein into perinuclear complexes. Proc Natl Acad Sci U S A 2002;99:3153–8.
16. Bradley JR. TNF-mediated inflammatory disease. J Pathol 2008;214:149–60.
17. Larsson M, Beignon AS, Bhardwaj N. DC-virus interplay: a double edged sword. Semin Immunol 2004;16:147–61.
18. Pollara G, Kwan A, Newton PJ, et al. Dendritic cells in viral pathogenesis: protec-tive or defective? Int J Exp Pathol 2005;86:187–204.
19. Van Epps HL, Terajima M, Mustonen J, et al. Long-lived memory T lymphocyte responses after hantavirus infection. J Exp Med 2002;196:579–88.
20. Sundstrom JB, McMullan LK, Spiropoulou CF, et al. Hantavirus infection induces the expression of RANTES and IP-10 without causing increased permeability in human lung microvascular endothelial cells. J Virol 2001;75:6070–85.
21. Hayasaka D, Maeda K, Ennis FA, et al. Increased permeability of human endothe-lial cell line EA.hy926 induced by hantavirus-specific cytotoxic T lymphocytes. Virus Res 2007;123:120–7.
22. Klingstrom J, Hardestam J, Stoltz M, et al. Loss of cell membrane integrity in puu-mala hantavirus-infected patients correlates with levels of epithelial cell apoptosis and perforin. J Virol 2006;80:8279–82.
23. Tuuminen T, Kekalainen E, Makela S, et al. Human CD8 + T cell memory gener-ation in Puumala hantavirus infection occurs after the acute phase and is

associated with boosting of EBV-specific CD8+ memory T cells. J Immunol 2007; 179:1988–95.

24. Centers for Disease Control and Prevention. Case definitions for infectious conditions under public health surveillance. MMWR Morb Mortal Wkly Rep 1997;46: 1–55.

25. Bruno P, Hassell LH, Joel Brown J, et al. The protean manifestations of hemorrhagic fever with renal syndrome. Ann Intern Med 1990;113:385–91.

26. Valdivieso F, Vial P, Ferres M, et al. Neutralizing antibodies in survivors of Sin Nombre and Andes hantavirus infection. Emerg Infect Dis 2006;12:166–8.

27. Ye C, Prescott J, Nofchissey R, et al. Neutralizing antibodies and Sin Nombre virus RNA after recovery from hantavirus cardiopulmonary syndrome. Emerg Infect Dis 2004;10:478–82.

28. Settergren B, Ahlm C, Juto P, et al. Specific Puumala IgG virus half a century after haemorrhagic fever with renal syndrome. Lancet 1991;338:66.

Malaria

Lynne S. Garcia, MS, MT, CLS

KEYWORDS

• Malaria • *Plasmodium* spp • Parasitic infections
• Infectious diseases

Malaria represents an ancient human disease, and deadly periodic fevers and spleno-megaly have been mentioned as early as 2700 BC in both Egyptian and Chinese writings. Malaria arrived in the Rome by 200 BC, spread throughout Europe during the twelfth century, and arrived in England by the fourteenth century. It is assumed that European explorers, conquistadors, and colonists imported *Plasmodium malariae* and *Plasmodium vivax* to the Americas. The arrival of *Plasmodium falciparum* coincided with the importation of African slaves, and by the early 1800s malaria was found worldwide.

Malaria has had a greater impact on world history than any other infectious disease, impacting the outcome of wars, population movements, and the development and decline of various nations. Before the American Civil War, malaria was found as far north as southern Canada; however, by the early 1950s it was no longer an endemic disease within the United States.

More than 300 to 500 million individuals worldwide are infected with *Plasmodium* spp, and 1.5 to 2.7 million people a year, most of whom are children, die from the infection. Malaria is endemic in over 90 countries in which 2400 million people live; this represents 40% of the world's population.[1] Approximately 90% of the malaria deaths occur in Africa. Despite continuing efforts in vaccine development, malaria prevention is difficult, and no drug is universally effective.

Of the 4 most common species that infect humans, *P vivax* and *P falciparum* cause 95% of infections. Data suggest that *P vivax* may be responsible for 80% of the infections, because this species also has the widest distribution, throughout the tropics, subtropics, and temperate zones. *P falciparum* is generally confined to the tropics, *P malariae* is sporadically distributed, and *Plasmodium ovale* is confined mainly to central West Africa and some South Pacific islands. As recently as 2004, a fifth malaria was implicated in human disease; *Plasmodium knowlesi*, a malaria parasite of long-tailed macaque monkeys, has been confirmed in several human cases from Malaysian Borneo, Thailand, Myanmar, and the Philippines.[2,3] Although it has been known for more than 50 years that under laboratory conditions some monkey malarias could be transmitted to humans, it is now well established that *P knowlesi* is emerging as

LSG & Associates, 512 12th Street, Santa Monica, CA 90402-2908, USA
E-mail address: Lynnegarcia2@verizon.net

Clin Lab Med 30 (2010) 93–129
doi:10.1016/j.cll.2009.10.001
0272-2712/10/$ – see front matter © 2010 Elsevier Inc. All rights reserved.

an important zoonotic human pathogen. *P knowlesi*, as well as some other simian malarias, may present additional concerns in the future.[4]

Although malaria is often associated with travelers to endemic areas, other situations resulting in infection include blood transfusions, use of hypodermic needles contaminated by prior use, bone marrow transplantation, congenital infection, and transmission within the United States by indigenous mosquitoes that acquired the parasites from imported infections.[5–11]

In nonendemic areas, it is important for health care personnel to understand the difficulties related to malarial diagnosis, specifically the fact that symptoms are often nonspecific and may mimic other conditions. Travelers are susceptible to malarial infection when they return to an endemic area, and prophylaxis may be recommended. Also, due to an increase in the number of people traveling from the tropics to malaria-free areas, the number of imported malaria cases is also increasing.

It is possible that mosquitoes can transmit the infection among people who live or work near international airports; these mosquitoes can also reach areas far removed from the airports.[12] This situation has been termed "airport malaria," and diagnostic testing for malaria should be considered in patients who work or live near an international airport and who present with an acute febrile illness. In addition to asking a patient, "where have you been, and when were you there?" one should also ask, "where do you live?"

Contributing factors to malaria-related fatalities in United States travelers include: (1) failure to seek pretravel advice, (2) failure to prescribe correct chemoprophylaxis, (3) failure to obtain prescribed chemoprophylaxis, (4) failure to adhere to chemoprophylaxis regimen, (5) failure to seek medical care promptly for illness, (6) failure to take adequate patient history, (7) delay in diagnosis of malaria, and (8) delay in initiating treatment of malaria.[13] One or more of these potential problems can lead to the death of the patient.

MICROBIOLOGY

The female anopheline mosquito is the vector for *Plasmodium* spp When the mosquito takes a blood meal, sporozoites contained in the salivary glands are discharged into the puncture wound.[14] Within approximately 60 min, the sporozoites are carried via the blood to the liver hepatocytes, thus initiating the preerythrocytic or primary exoerythrocytic cycle. The round or oval sporozoites begin dividing repeatedly, resulting in large numbers of exoerythrocytic merozoites. Once these merozoites leave the liver, they invade the red blood cells (RBCs), thus initiating the erythrocytic cycle. A secondary or dormant schizogony occurs in *P vivax* and *P ovale*, which remain quiescent in the liver until a later time. These resting stages have been termed hypnozoites.[15] Delayed schizogony apparently does not occur in *P falciparum*, *P malariae*, or *P knowlesi*.

Recrudescence refers to a situation in which the RBC infection is not eliminated by the immune system or by therapy, and the parasite numbers in the RBCs begin to increase again with subsequent clinical symptoms. All species may cause a recrudescence. A recurrence or true relapse refers to a situation in which the erythrocytic infection is eliminated, and a relapse occurs later because of a new invasion of the RBCs from liver merozoites; theoretically this occurs only in *P vivax* and *P ovale* infection.

Once the RBCs have been invaded, the parasites continue to grow and feed on hemoglobin. The merozoite (or young trophozoite) is vacuolated, ring shaped, more or less ameboid, and uninucleate (an exception would be the "headphone" rings seen primarily in *P falciparum* infections). The excess protein, an iron porphyrin, and hematin left over from the metabolism of hemoglobin combine to form malarial pigment.

As the nucleus begins to divide, the trophozoite is now called a developing schizont. The mature schizont contains merozoites that are released into the bloodstream. Although many merozoites are destroyed by the immune system, others immediately invade RBCs, in which a new cycle of erythrocytic schizogony begins. After several erythrocytic generations, some of the merozoites begin to develop into the male and female gametocytes. These changes may be predetermined genetically, as a response to some specific stimulus or some other unknown factors.[16]

The asexual and sexual forms circulate in the blood during infections by 4 of the *Plasmodium* species. However, in *P falciparum* infections, as the parasite continues to grow, the RBC membrane becomes sticky and the cells tend to adhere to the endothelial lining of the capillaries of the internal organs. Thus, only the ring forms and the gametocytes (occasionally mature schizonts) normally appear in the peripheral blood.

When gametocytes are ingested with the vector's blood meal, they mature into gametes within the mosquito gut. The male microgametes undergo nuclear division by a process called exflagellation. The microgametes break out of the RBC, become motile, and penetrate the female macrogamete, with the fertilized stage being called the zygote. As the zygote elongates and becomes motile, it is now called the ookinete. This stage migrates to the mosquito midgut, secretes a thin wall, and grows into the oocyst, which extends into the insect's hemocele. Within days to weeks, the oocyst matures, with the development of hundreds of sporozoites. Within the mosquito the oocyst ruptures, then the sporozoites are released into the hemocele and dispersed throughout the body, including the salivary glands. When the mosquito next takes a blood meal, the sporozoites are injected with saliva into the host.

EPIDEMIOLOGY

Malaria is endemic in close to 100 countries in which 2400 million people reside, almost half of whom are located in Africa south of the Sahara (**Fig. 1**). More than 90% of malaria deaths occur in Africa, primarily among young children. The number of cases outside tropical Africa may be as high as 20 million, with about 80% being found in Asia where severe drug resistance has developed in the Indochinese peninsula. Although in most of Asia and the Americas the risk of malaria is relatively low, problems still remain in certain areas. Approximately two-thirds of malaria infections in the Americas occur in the Amazon basin. Also, malaria has reemerged in areas where control had been achieved in the past; these areas include Azerbaijan, Tajikistan, Iraq, and Turkey.

Disease prevention is difficult, and there are no drugs that are universally effective. Malaria is primarily a rural disease, and the parasite is transmitted by the female anopheline mosquito. Although appropriate vectors may be present in an area, an average number of bites per person per day must be sustained or the infection gradually dies out. This critical requirement for sustained infection can be influenced by several factors, including the vector preference for human blood and habitation, and the duration of infection in a specific area. Once an area is clear of the infection there may also be a drop in population immunity, a situation that may lead to a severe epidemic if the infection is reintroduced into the population.[17]

Global Warming

Climate change effects on African malaria vectors shift their distributional potential from west to east and south, which has implications for overall numbers of people

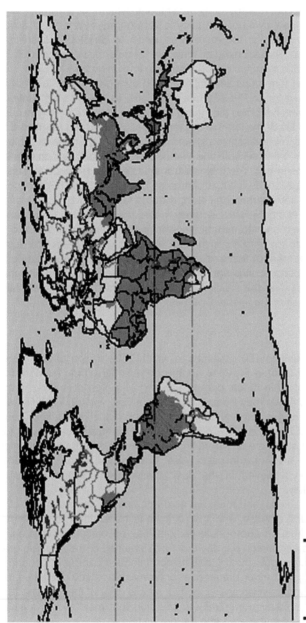

Legend

No Malaria Cases Reported in Region

Malaria Cases Reported in Region

Fig. 1. World map of *Plasmodium* spp endemic areas. (*Courtesy of the Centers for Disease Control and Prevention.*)

exposed to these vector species. Although the total population exposed may be reduced, malaria is likely to pose new public health problems in areas where it has not previously been common.[18] Development of malaria parasites in their mosquito hosts and the development of their vector mosquitoes are inhibited at temperatures higher than 23° to 24°C. If global warming progresses further, the present center of malarial endemicity in sub-Saharan Africa will move to an area with an optimum temperature for both the vector and the parasite, migrating to avoid the hot environment.[19] Based on projections made by the Inter-Governmental Panel on Climate Change (IPCC 2001), by 2050 and 2100 increases in temperature will be approximately 1.4° to 5.9°C with a 7% increase in rainfall. With these climate and rainfall changes in mind, the malaria situation in India is projected to see changes including a faster rate of development of mosquitoes, faster rate of digestion of blood meal, and an increased frequency of vector feeding. As a result, malaria will continue to spread into new areas.[20] Estimates of an increase of 3°C by the year 2100 could increase the world annual incidence of malaria by 50 to 80 million from the current 300 to 500 million. Temperature and humidity are among the most important factors for malaria transmission. Parasite multiplication inside the cold blooded mosquito reduces dramatically at temperatures between 20° and 27°C and parasite development ceases below 16°C, so that malaria is confined by a 16°C minimum temperature line. Therefore, within the next few decades tertiary spread of infection may occur in the United Kingdom.[21]

However, not everyone believes global warming is the key factor in malaria estimates of change. Future changes in climate may alter the prevalence and incidence of malaria, but the major emphasis on "global warming" as a dominant parameter may not reflect the total picture; the principal determinants are also linked to ecological and societal change, politics, and economics.[22] The histories of 3 diseases, malaria, yellow fever, and dengue, indicate that climate has rarely been the principal determinant of their prevalence or range; human activities and their impact on local ecology have generally been much more significant.

Populations at Risk

In areas of high transmission, children younger than 5 years and women pregnant with their first child are most vulnerable. In areas of low transmission, all ages are at risk, particularly due to low immunity. Also refugees are very vulnerable, primarily due to poor living conditions; specific areas include Afghanistan, Angola, Cambodia, Ethiopia, Rwanda, Somalia, and the Democratic Republic of the Congo. In certain areas of India, Pakistan, and Africa, some urban and periurban centers contribute from 10% to 20% of the overall incidence of malaria. Another vulnerable group is represented by nonimmune travelers visiting endemic areas, with visitors to tropical Africa representing the highest risk group in the northern hemisphere.

Controls

Several programs have gained attention and success during the last few years. Insecticide-impregnated bed nets have become more widely used, with the success of such an approach depending on insect susceptibility to the particular insecticide used (often pyrethroids), high coverage with impregnated bed nets, high malaria incidence, good community participation at an acceptable sustained level, high mosquito densities when people go to bed, and a high proportion of P falciparum.[23–25]

The use of permethrin-impregnated clothing has also been found to reduce the incidence of both malaria and leishmaniasis by a large percentage. In addition to use by the military,[26] permethrin-impregnated clothing for travelers is also beneficial. This insecticide kills mosquitoes, flies, and ticks on contact. Also, impregnated clothing fibers remain effective even after 3 months of repeated machine washing.

Another control issue involves the safety of the blood supply. Many factors impact the blood supply worldwide, including government policies and regulations, professional society standards, the donor pool (voluntary or paid), ability of health care personnel to order blood when necessary, infectious disease screening, post-transfusion adverse effects monitoring, and product-related side effects.[27]

Unfortunately, there are several reasons why overall control efforts are not as successful as hoped. In many areas, there is a shortage of people with sufficient knowledge to handle issues related to epidemiology and the overall planning and management of control. Often, health services are inadequate to deal with diagnosis and treatment needs. Increased drug resistance continues to be a major issue, with ongoing problems related to drug quality, availability, and cost. Collaboration across political and geographic boundaries is not only desirable, but necessary if surveillance programs are to be successfully sustained.

Vaccines

With the development of in vitro culture of *P falciparum*, genetic engineering techniques, serologic immunofluorescence, and other newer techniques, progress toward vaccine production may lead to effective protection against malarial infections.[28-33]

A perfect malaria vaccine will induce immune responses against every life cycle stage of *Plasmodium*. Different and distinct immune mechanisms operate against the different stages in the life cycle. Therefore, a multistage vaccine must be a multi-immune response vaccine. Development of these types of vaccines will be required to reduce significantly the increasing malaria infections and deaths seen each year.[29,31] Various vaccine targets include the preerythrocytic, erythrocytic, and sexual stages. For a malaria vaccine to induce optimal and sustainable protection, both cellular and humoral responses will have to be elicited against multiple targets from the different life cycle stages.

CLINICAL PRESENTATION

From the time of the original mosquito bite until approximately a week later, the patient remains asymptomatic. During the time the patient is asymptomatic, the parasites are undergoing multiplication in the preerythrocytic cycle in the liver. Although several broods will begin to develop when the liver merozoites invade the RBCs, one will eventually dominate and suppress the others, thus beginning the process of periodicity. Once the cycle is synchronized, the simultaneous rupture of a large number of RBCs and liberation of metabolic waste by-products into the bloodstream precipitate the typical paroxysms of malaria. Before the onset of synchrony, the patient's symptoms may be mild, somewhat vague, and may include a low fever that exhibits no periodicity.

Symptoms of malaria include anemia, splenomegaly, and the classic paroxysm, with its cold stage, fever, and sweats. Although the febrile paroxysms strongly suggest a malaria infection, many patients who are seen in medical facilities in the early stages of the infection do not exhibit a typical fever pattern. Patients may have a steady low-grade fever or several small, random peaks each day. Because the symptoms associated with malaria in the early stages are so nonspecific, the diagnosis should be considered in any symptomatic patient with a history of travel to an endemic area. During the primary infection in a nonimmune host, the early fever episodes can affect density-dependent regulation of the parasite population, maintaining cycles of parasitemia and promoting synchronous parasite growth. The typical paroxysm begins with the cold stage and rigors lasting 1 to 2 hours. During the next few hours, the patient spikes a high fever and feels very hot, and the skin is warm and dry. The last several hours are characterized by marked sweating and a subsequent drop in body temperature to normal or subnormal.

Anemia seen in malarial infections can be caused by several mechanisms, such as (1) direct RBC lysis as a function of the parasite life cycle, (2) splenic removal of both infected and uninfected RBCs (coated with immune complexes), (3) autoimmune lysis of coated infected and uninfected RBCs, (4) decreased incorporation of iron into heme, (5) increased fragility of RBCs, and (6) decreased RBC production from bone marrow suppression.

Malaria can mimic many other diseases, such as gastroenteritis, pneumonia, meningitis, encephalitis, or hepatitis. Other possible symptoms include lethargy, anorexia, nausea, vomiting, diarrhea, and headache. Leukopenia can also be seen in malaria, as can an occasional elevated white blood cell count with a left shift. Eosinophilia and thrombocytopenia may also be seen but are much less frequent. A clinical comparison of some of the features of the 5 different malarias is presented in **Table 1**. Parasite morphology can be seen in **Table 2** and **Box 1**.

Plasmodium vivax (Benign Tertian Malaria)

The primary clinical attack usually occurs 7 to 10 days after infection, although there are strain differences, with a much longer incubation period being possible (months to years). In some patients, particularly those who have never been exposed to malaria before, symptoms such as headache, photophobia, muscle aches, anorexia, nausea, and sometimes vomiting occur before organisms can be detected in the bloodstream. In other patients, usually those with prior exposure to the malaria, the parasites can be found in the bloodstream several days before symptoms appear.

After an irregular periodicity of a few days, a regular 48-hour cycle is established. An untreated primary attack may last from 3 weeks to 2 months or longer. Over time, the paroxysms become less severe and more irregular in frequency and then stop altogether. In approximately 50% of patients infected with P vivax, relapses occur after weeks, months, or up to 5 years (or more).

Severe complications are rare in P vivax infections, although coma and sudden death or other symptoms of cerebral involvement have been reported, particularly in patients with varying degrees of primaquine resistance. These patients can exhibit cerebral malaria, renal failure, circulatory collapse, severe anemia, hemoglobinuria, abnormal bleeding, acute respiratory distress syndrome, and jaundice.[34–36] Molecular studies confirmed that these were single species infections with P vivax and not mixed infections with P falciparum.

P vivax infects only the reticulocytes, so the parasitemia is usually limited to around 2% to 5% of the available RBCs (**Table 3**). During the first few weeks of infection, the spleen will progress from being soft and palpable to hard, with continued enlargement during a chronic infection. However, the spleen will return to its normal size if the infection is treated during the early phases.

Although leukopenia is normally seen, leukocytosis may be present during the febrile episodes. Concentrations of total plasma proteins usually remain unchanged, although the albumin level may be low and the globulin fraction may be elevated. The development of antibodies results in an increase in the gammaglobulins. The level of potassium in serum may also be increased as a result of RBC lysis.

Table 1
Plasmodium spp: clinical characteristics of the 5 human infections

Infection	P vivax	P ovale	P malariae	P falciparum	P knowlesi	Comments
Incubation period	8–17 d	10–17 d	18–40 d	8–11 d	9–12 d	All may be extended for months to years
Prodromal symptoms						
Severity	Mild to moderate	Mild	Mild to moderate	Mild	Mild to moderate	All may mimic influenza symptoms
Initial fever pattern	Irregular (48 h)	Irregular (48 h)	Regular (72)	Continuous remittent	Regular (24 h)	Early symptoms may reflect lack of regular periodicity
Symptom periodicity	48 h	48 h	72 h	36–48 h	24–27 h	
Initial paroxysm						
Severity	Moderate to severe	Mild	Moderate to severe	Severe	Moderate to severe	P knowlesi might increase/ lose virulence on passage in humans
Mean duration	10 h	10 h	11 h	16–36 h	Not available	
Duration of untreated primary attack	3–8+ wk	2–3 wk	3–24 wk	2–3 wk	Not available	
Duration of untreated infection	5–7 y	12 mo	20+ y	6–17 mo	Not available	
Parasitemia limitations	Young RBCs	Young RBCs	Old RBCs	All RBCs	All RBCs	
Anemia	Mild to moderate	Mild	Mild to moderate	Severe	Moderate to severe	P knowlesi can be as dangerous as P falciparum
CNS involvement	Rare	Possible	Rare	Very common	Possible	
Nephrotic syndrome	Possible	Rare	Very common	Rare	Probably common	

Plasmodium ovale (Ovale Malaria)

Although *P ovale* and *P vivax* infections are clinically similar, *P ovale* malaria is usually less severe, tends to relapse less frequently, and usually ends with spontaneous recovery after approximately 6 to 10 paroxysms. The incubation period is similar to that seen in *P vivax* malaria, but the frequency and severity of the symptoms are much less, with a lower fever and a lack of typical rigors. *P ovale* infects only the reticulocytes (as does *P vivax*), so that the parasitemia is generally limited to around 2% to 5% of the available RBCs[37] (see **Table 3**). The geographic range is usually described as being limited to tropical Africa, the Middle East, Papua New Guinea, and Irian Jaya in Indonesia. However, *P ovale* infections in Southeast Asia may cause benign and relapsing malaria in this area. In both Southeast Asia and Africa, 2 different types of *P ovale* circulate in humans. Human infections with variant-type *P ovale* are associated with higher parasitemias, thus having possible clinical relevance.[38]

Plasmodium malariae (Quartan Malaria)

P malariae invades primarily the older RBCs, so that the number of infected cells is somewhat limited. The incubation period prior to symptoms may be much longer than that seen with *P vivax* or *P ovale* malaria, ranging from about 27 to 40 days. Parasites can be found in the bloodstream several days before the initial attack, and the prodromal symptoms may resemble those of *P vivax* malaria. Regular periodicity is established early in the infection, with a more severe paroxysm, including a longer cold stage and more severe symptoms during the hot stage. Collapse during the sweating phase is not uncommon.

Proteinuria is common in *P malariae* infections and in children may be associated with clinical signs of the nephrotic syndrome. With a chronic infection, kidney problems result from deposition within the glomeruli of circulating antigen-antibody complexes in an antigen excess situation.[39] The nephrotic syndrome associated with *P malariae* infections is apparently unaffected by the administration of steroids. A membranoproliferative type of glomerulonephritis with relatively sparse proliferation of endothelial and mesangial cells is the most common type of lesion seen in quartan malaria. Because chronic glomerular disease associated with *P malariae* infections is usually not reversible with therapy, genetic and environmental factors may play a role in the nephrotic syndrome.

The patient may experience a spontaneous recovery, or there may be a recrudescence or series of recrudescences over many years (>50 years). In these cases, patients are left with a latent infection and persisting low-grade parasitemia.

Plasmodium falciparum (Malignant Tertian Malaria)

P falciparum invades all ages of RBCs, and the proportion of infected cells may exceed 50%. Schizogony occurs in the internal organs (spleen, liver, and bone marrow) rather than in the circulating blood. Ischemia caused by the plugging of vessels within these organs by parasitized RBCs will produce various symptoms, depending on the organ involved. A decrease in the ability of the RBCs to change shape when passing through capillaries or the splenic filter may apparently lead to plugging of the vessels.[40] Also, only *P falciparum* causes cytoadherence, a feature that is associated with severe malaria.

The onset of a *P falciparum* malaria attack occurs 8 to 12 days after infection and is characterized by 3 to 4 days of vague symptoms such as aches, pains, headache, fatigue, anorexia, or nausea. This stage is followed by fever, a more severe headache, and nausea and vomiting, with occasional severe epigastric pain. At the onset of fever,

Table 2
***Plasmodia* in Giemsa-stained thin blood smears[a]**

	P vivax	P malariae	P falciparum	P ovale	P knowlesi
Persistence of exoerythrocytic cycle	Yes	No	No	Yes	No
Relapses	Yes	No, but long-term recrudescences are recognized	No long-term relapses	Possible, but usually spontaneous recovery	No
Time of cycle	44–48 h	72 h	36–48 h	48 h	24 h
Appearance of parasitized red blood cells; size and shape	1.5–2 times larger than normal; oval to normal; may be normal size until ring fills one-half of cell	Normal shape; size may be normal or slightly smaller	Both normal	60% of cells larger than normal and oval; 20% have irregular, frayed edges	Normal shape, size
Schüffner dots (eosinophilic stippling)	Usually present in all cells except early ring forms	None	None; occasionally comma-like red dots are present (Maurer dots)	Present in all stages including early ring forms, dots may be larger and darker than in P vivax	No true stippling; occasional faint dots
Color of cytoplasm	Decolorized, pale	Normal	Normal, bluish tinge at times	Decolorized, pale	Normal
Multiple rings/cell	Occasional	Rare	Common	Occasional	Common
All developmental stages present in peripheral blood	All stages present	Ring forms few, as ring stage brief; mostly growing and mature trophozoites and schizonts	Young ring forms and no older stages; few gametocytes	All stages present	All stages present

Appearance of parasite; young trophozoite (early ring form)	Ring is one-third diameter of cell, cytoplasmic circle around vacuole; heavy chromatin dot	Ring often smaller than in P vivax, occupying one-eighth of cell; heavy chromatin dot; vacuole at times "filled in"; pigment forms early	Delicate, small ring with small chromatin dot (frequently 2); scanty cytoplasm around small vacuoles; sometimes at edge of red cell (appliqué form) or filamentous slender form; may have multiple rings per cell	Ring is larger and more ameboid than in P vivax, otherwise similar to P vivax	Rings one-third to one-half diameter of RBC; double chromatin dots; appliqué forms rare; multiple rings per RBC
Growing trophozoite	Multishaped irregular ameboid parasite; streamers of cytoplasm close to large chromatin dot; vacuole retained until close to maturity; increasing amounts of brown pigment	Nonameboid rounded or band-shaped solid forms; chromatin may be hidden by coarse dark brown pigment	Heavy ring forms; fine pigment grains	Ring shape maintained until late in development; nonameboid compared with P vivax	Slightly ameboid and irregular; band forms seen; very little pigment
Mature trophozoite	Irregular ameboid mass; 1 or more small vacuoles retained until schizont stage; fills almost entire cell; fine brown pigment	Vacuoles disappear early; cytoplasm compact, oval, band shaped, or nearly round almost filling cell; chromatin may be hidden by peripheral coarse dark brown pigment	Not seen in peripheral blood (except in severe infections); development of all phases following ring form occurs in capillaries of viscera	Compact; vacuoles disappear; pigment dark brown, less than in P malariae	Denser cytoplasm (slightly ameboid) band forms seen; little to no malaria pigment (scattered, fine brown grains)
Schizont (presegmenter)	Progressive chromatin division; cytoplasmic bands containing clumps of brown pigment	Similar to P vivax except smaller; darker; larger pigment granules peripheral or central	Not seen in peripheral blood (see above)	Smaller and more compact than P vivax	Between 2 and 5 divided nuclear chromatin masses; abundant pigment granules; occupy two-thirds of RBC

(continued on next page)

Table 2
(continued)

	P vivax	P malariae	P falciparum	P ovale	P knowlesi
Mature schizont	Merozoites, 16 (12–24) each with chromatin and cytoplasm, filling entire red cell, which can hardly be seen	8 (6–12) merozoites in rosettes or irregular clusters filling normal-sized cells, which can hardly be seen; central arrangement of brown-green pigment	Not seen in peripheral blood	Three-quarters of cells occupied by 8 (8–12) merozoites in rosettes or irregular clusters	RBCs normal size; distorted/fimbriated RBCs very rare; occupy whole RBC; maximum of 16 merozoites; no rosettes; grapelike clusters
Macroga-metocyte	Rounded or oval homogeneous cytoplasm; diffuse delicate light brown pigment throughout parasite; eccentric compact chromatin	Similar to P vivax, but fewer in number, pigment darker and more coarse	Sex differentiation difficult; "crescent" or "sausage" shapes characteristic; may appear in "showers," black pigment near chromatin dot, which is often central	Smaller than P vivax	Occupy most of RBC; bluish cytoplasm; dense pink chromatin at periphery of parasite

Microga-metocyte	Large pink to purple chromatin mass surrounded by pale or colorless halo; evenly distributed pigment	Similar to P vivax, but fewer in number, pigment darker and more coarse	Same as macrogametocyte (described above)	Smaller than P vivax	Occupy most of RBC; cytoplasm pinkish-purple; early forms similar to mature trophs
Main criteria	Large pale red cell; trophozoite irregular; pigment usually present; Schüffner dots not always present; several phases of growth seen in one smear; gametocytes appear as early as third day	Red cell normal in size and color; trophozoites compact, stain usually intense; band forms not always seen; coarse pigment; no stippling of red cells; gametocytes appear after a few weeks	Development following ring stage takes place in blood vessels of internal organs; delicate ring forms and crescent-shaped gametocytes are only forms normally seen in peripheral blood; gametocytes appear after 7–10 days	Red cell enlarged, oval, with fimbriated edges; Schüffner dots seen in all stages; gametocytes appear after 4 days or as late as 18 days	Ring forms compact; single/double chromatin dots, appliqué forms, multiple rings/RBC (mimic P falciparum); overall RBCs not enlarged; developing stages mimic P malariae (band forms, 16 merozoites in mature schizont, but no rosettes

[a] Other blood stains are perfectly acceptable; if the PMNs look acceptable/normal on the stained blood films, any parasites present will also exhibit typical morphology. Other acceptable stains include: Wright stain, Wright/Giemsa combination, Field stain, and rapid stains (Diff-Quik, American Scientific Products, McGraw Park, IL and Wright's Dip Stat Stain Set, Medical Chemical Corp, Torrance, CA, USA). Color variation is normal, even using Giemsa stain.

> **Box 1**
> **Malaria characteristics with fresh blood or blood collected using ethylenediamine tetra-acetic acid (EDTA) with no extended lag time (preparation of thick and thin blood films within <60 min of collection)**
>
> *Plasmodium vivax (benign tertian malaria)*
> 1. 48-hour cycle
> 2. Tends to infect young cells
> 3. Enlarged RBCs
> 4. Schüffner dots (true stippling) after 8–10 hours
> 5. Delicate ring
> 6. Very ameboid trophozoite
> 7. Mature schizont contains 12–24 merozoites
>
> *Plasmodium malariae (quartan malaria)*
> 1. 72-hour cycle (long incubation period)
> 2. Tends to infect old cells
> 3. Normal size RBCs
> 4. No stippling
> 5. Thick ring, large nucleus
> 6. Trophozoite tends to form "bands" across the cell
> 7. Mature schizont contains 6–12 merozoites
>
> *Plasmodium ovale*
> 1. 48-hour cycle
> 2. Tends to infect young cells
> 3. Enlarged RBCs with fimbriated edges (oval)
> 4. Schüffner dots appear in the beginning (in RBCs with very young ring forms in contrast to *P vivax*)
> 5. Smaller ring than *P vivax*
> 6. Trophozoite less ameboid than that of *P vivax*
> 7. Mature schizont contains average 8 merozoites
>
> *Plasmodium falciparum (malignant tertian malaria)*
> 1. 36–48-hour cycle
> 2. Tends to infect any cell regardless of age, thus very heavy infection may result
> 3. All sizes of RBCs
> 4. No Schüffner dots (Maurer dots: may be larger, single dots, bluish)
> 5. Multiple rings/cell (only young rings, gametocytes, and occasional mature schizonts are seen in peripheral blood)
> 6. Delicate rings, may have 2 dots of chromatin/ring, appliqué or accolé forms
> 7. Crescent-shaped gametocytes
>
> *Plasmodium knowlesi (simian malaria)[a]*
> 1. 24-hour cycle
> 2. Tends to infect any cell regardless of age, thus very heavy infection may result

3. All sizes of RBCs, but most tend to be normal size

4. No Schüffner dots (faint, clumpy dots later in cycle)

5. Multiple rings/cell (may have 2–3)

6. Delicate rings, may have 2 or 3 dots of chromatin/ring, appliqué forms

7. Band form trophozoites commonly seen

8. Mature schizont contains 16 merozoites, no rosettes

9. Gametocytes round, tend to fill the cell

[a] Early stages mimic P falciparum; later stages mimic P malariae

there may be a feeling of chilliness. As with the other Plasmodium spp, periodicity of the cycle will not be established during the early stages. At this point, any presumptive diagnosis is often totally unrelated to a possible malaria infection. In P falciparum malaria, if the fever does develop a synchronous cycle, it is usually a cycle of somewhat less than 48 hours. An untreated primary attack of P falciparum malaria usually ends within 2 to 3 weeks. True relapses from the liver do not occur, and after a year, recrudescences are rare.

Severe or fatal complications of P falciparum malaria can occur at any time and are related to the plugging of vessels in the internal organs. The severity of the complications may not correlate with the peripheral blood parasitemia, particularly in P falciparum infections. Acute lung injury is more likely to occur in patients with severe, multisystemic P falciparum malaria. Patients who present with acute lung injury and septic shock should be suspected of a bacterial coinfection and should be treated empirically.

Disseminated intravascular coagulation is a rare complication and is associated with a high parasitemia, pulmonary edema, anemia, and cerebral and renal complications. Vascular endothelial damage from endotoxins and bound parasitized blood cells may lead to clot formation in small vessels.

Cerebral malaria is more common in P falciparum malaria, but can occur in the other species as well. If the onset is gradual, the patient becomes disoriented or violent or may develop severe headaches and pass into coma. Some patients, including those with no prior symptoms, may suddenly become comatose. Physical signs of central nervous system involvement vary, and there is no correlation between the severity of the symptoms and the parasitemia. Patients with cerebral malaria are generally infected with RBC rosette-forming P falciparum, and the plasma from these patients generally has no antirosetting activity. A rosette usually consists of a parasitized RBC surrounded by 3 or more uninfected RBCs. Interaction with adjacent uninfected RBCs in rosettes appears to be mediated by knobs seen on the parasitized RBC.[41] However, P falciparum parasites from cases of mild malaria lack the rosetting phenotype or have a much lower rosetting rate. Also in these cases of mild malaria, antirosetting activity is present in the plasma. Thus, it seems that RBC rosetting contributes to the pathogenesis of cerebral malaria, while antirosetting antibodies in the plasma offer protection against this clinical complication.

Many factors, including free oxygen radicals and other mediators of inflammation, are also involved in the pathogenesis of cerebral malaria.[1,42] Tumor necrosis factor-α and other pyrogenic cytokines play a role in the regulation of parasite density in the host; cerebral malaria is also thought to be related to excessive tumor necrosis factor-α.

Table 3
Parasitemia determined from conventional light microscopy: clinical correlation

Parasitemia (%)	No. of Parasites/μL	Clinical Correlation
0.0001–0.0004	5–20	Number of organisms required for positive thick film (sensitivity) Examination of 100 thick-blood-film (TBF) fields (0.25 μL) may miss up to 20% of infections (sensitivity 80%–90%); at least 300 fields should be examined before reporting a negative result Examination of 100 thin-blood-film fields (THBF) (0.005 μL); at least 300 fields should be examined before reporting a negative result; both thick and thin blood films should be examined for every specimen submitted for a suspect malaria case (report final results using 100 × oil immersion objective) **One set (TBF + THBF) of negative blood films does not rule out a malaria infection**
0.002	100	**Patients may be symptomatic below this level, particularly if they are immunologically naïve** (no prior exposure to malaria)
0.02	1,000	Level seen in travelers (immunologically naïve)—results may also be lower than this
0.1	5,000	Minimum sensitivity of the BinaxNOW rapid lateral flow method (dipstick); (review package insert)
0.2	10,000	Level above which immune patients will exhibit symptoms
2	100,000	Maximum parasitemia of *P vivax* and *P ovale* (which infect young RBCs only)
2–5	100,000–250,000	Hyperparasitemia, severe malaria[a]; increased mortality
10	500,000	Exchange transfusion may be considered; high mortality

[a] World Health Organization criteria for severe malaria are parasitemia of >10,000/μL and severe anemia (hemoglobin, <5 g/L). Prognosis is poor if >20% of parasites are pigment-containing trophozoites and schizonts and/or if >5% of neutrophils contain visible pigment.

In patients with cerebral malaria, magnetic resonance imaging demonstrates an increased brain volume, which probably results from sequestration of parasitized RBCs and compensatory vasodilatation rather than from edema. Although brain stem herniation may occur, its relation to brain death in patients with cerebral malaria remains unclear. In fatal *P falciparum* infections, ultrastructural brain morphology confirms that parasitized RBC sequestration in cerebral microvessels is much higher in patients with cerebral malaria (cerebrum, cerebellum, and medulla oblongata) than with patients with noncerebral malaria.[1]

Extreme fevers, 41.7°C (107°F) or higher, may develop in a relatively uncomplicated malaria attack or may develop in cases of cerebral malaria. Without vigorous therapy, the patient usually dies. Cerebral malaria is considered to be the most serious complication and the major cause of death with *P falciparum*, and accounts for up to 10% of all *P falciparum* patients admitted to the hospital and for 80% of fatal cases.

Bilious remittent fever involves the liver; symptoms include abdominal pain, nausea, and severe and persistent vomiting, with the vomitus containing bile or fresh blood. Dehydration may result from severe diarrhea or dysentery. The liver is large and tender, the skin becomes icteric, and the urine contains bile.

Diarrhea or dysentery without liver involvement or jaundice also occurs; malabsorption is characterized by decreased absorption of D-xylose and vitamin B_{12}, and a low carotene level. Jejunal biopsy reveals edema, round cell infiltration of the lamina propria, and blunting of villi, which have also been found at autopsy.

Symptoms of algid malaria involving the adrenal glands include circulatory collapse, low blood pressure, hypothermia, rapid, thready pulse, and pale, cold, clammy skin. There may be severe abdominal pain, vomiting and diarrhea, and muscle cramps. At autopsy, the adrenal glands are congested, necrotic, and hemorrhagic. In the subacute stage of algid malaria and after recovery, some patients develop symptoms resembling Addison disease.

Although uncommon, blackwater fever is usually associated with *P falciparum* malaria, and often there is a history of previous malarial attacks. Sudden, intravascular hemolysis results in dark-colored urine (acidic urine with a high methemoglobin content). Because the hemoglobinuria does not necessarily cause symptoms, the onset may be missed. Quinine sensitivity has been suggested as one factor leading to blackwater fever, while another has been the presence of antibodies acting as hemolysins against RBC antigens. The parasitemia in these patients may be relatively low. With the increased use of quinine in patients with chloroquine-resistant malaria, more cases of blackwater fever may be seen in these areas.

Acute renal failure may also occur unrelated to blackwater fever and hemolytic anemia. Renal anoxia is believed to lead to tubular necrosis. The nephrotic syndrome caused by acute glomerulonephritis has also been reported in some patients with *P falciparum* malaria, although it is more commonly seen in cases of *P malariae* infection.

Independent risk factors contributing to anemia in falciparum malaria in patients presenting with anemia on admission include: age less than 5 years, a palpable spleen, a palpable liver, recrudescent infections, being female, a history of prolonged history of illness (>2 days) before admission, and pure *P falciparum* infections rather than mixed infections with *P falciparum* and *P vivax*. It seems that coinfection with *P vivax* can modify the severity of the disease.

In African children with malaria, impaired consciousness or respiratory distress can identify those at high risk of death. Evidence of hepatic and renal dysfunction also suggests a poor prognosis. However, unlike malaria in adults, children with severe malaria do not always have acute renal failure.

It is estimated that approximately 100,000 infant deaths in Africa could be attributed to malaria during pregnancy resulting in low-birth-weight babies.[43] Antimalarial preventive treatment during pregnancy has been estimated to prevent 22,000 deaths of children younger than 5 years, through reduced numbers of preterm deliveries. However, if one assumes an efficacy rate of 80% in preventing placental malaria, the number of deaths prevented may be closer to 80,000.

Plasmodium knowlesi (Simian Malaria)

A relatively large focus of human infections with the simian malaria, *P knowlesi*, has been reported in Malaysian Borneo; cases have also been reported from Thailand, Myanmar, China, Philippines, and Singapore. The early blood stages of *P knowlesi* resemble those of *P falciparum*, whereas the mature blood stages and gametocytes resemble those of *P malariae* (see **Box 1** and **Table 2**). Unfortunately, these infections are often misdiagnosed as the relatively benign *P malariae*; however, infections with *P knowlesi* can be fatal.

P knowlesi infection should be considered in patients with a travel history to forested areas of Southeast Asia, especially if *P malariae* is diagnosed, unusual forms are seen with microscopy, or if a mixed infection with *P falciparum/P malariae* is diagnosed.

Because the disease is potentially fatal, proper identification to the species level is critical.

Patients exhibit chills, minor headaches, and daily low-grade fever. Patients who present with *P malariae* hyperparasitemia diagnosis by microscopy should receive intensive management as appropriate for severe falciparum malaria, assuming the infection is actually caused by *P knowlesi*.

Mixed Infections

Coincident infection with more than one species of malaria is more common than previously suspected.[44] In Thailand, up to 30% of patients who present with severe *P falciparum* malaria also are infected with *P vivax*. In Africa, dual infections with *P falciparum* and *P malariae* have also been found. In Gambian children, the prevalence of mixed species varies from less than 1% to more than 60%, and these figures may be underestimates. A rare quadruple malaria infection has even been reported in a remote area in the western half of New Guinea Island (Irian Jaya Province, Indonesia), and this infection was confirmed using nested polymerase chain reaction (PCR) and species-specific primer pairs (*P vivax*, *P falciparum*, *P ovale*, *P malariae*).[45] In Africa, *P ovale* occurs commonly in areas with Duffy-negative populations who are refractory to *P vivax*, thus appearing to prevent the natural coexistence of the 2 species. However, the Duffy blood group negative trait that protects many African populations from *P vivax* is considered very rare or nonexistent in New Guinea. Because *P ovale* is considered a very unusual finding outside of Africa, the natural occurrence of *P ovale* and *P vivax* together in the same patient is considered a very rare finding.

It is generally accepted that *P falciparum* predominates over *P vivax* in mixed infections. *P ovale* has been found in mixed infections and has been established in persons carrying *P falciparum*, *P vivax*, and *P malariae* at the same time.[45] Simultaneous patent infections with 3 or 4 *Plasmodium* species are not entirely rare findings in the blood of healthy carriers in regions of hyperendemic infection.

Detection of mixed infections can be difficult due to different levels of parasitemia, low organism densities, and confusion among various morphologic criteria for identification to the species level; these problems have been well documented. Using PCR methods, it is likely that a higher detection rate of chronic and mixed malarial species will be possible.[45]

PATHOGENESIS

Although malaria parasites differ in ways that might be related to pathogenicity, it is difficult to prove that these characteristics are consistently linked with virulence. The severity of infections depends on several parasite and host factors.

Multiplication Capacity

It is well known that some patients can die with a relatively low parasitemia, whereas others will survive with a much higher parasitemia. However, there is a general correlation between the parasitemia and prognosis, particularly in *P falciparum* malaria (can infect any age RBC, leading to higher parasitemias). There also seems to be a positive correlation between the number of sequestered parasitized RBCs and the severity of *P falciparum* malaria.

Red Cell Selectivity

Because both *P vivax* and *P ovale* prefer younger RBCs, this automatically limits the level of parasitemia; the same limitations apply to *P malariae* that prefers to infect older

RBCs. In the case of *P falciparum* and *P knowlesi*, both of these species have no age preference in terms of RBC infectivity; thus, very heavy parasitemias may result.

Cytoadherence and Rosetting Ability

Malarial parasites with both these adhesive characteristics tend to be more pathogenic. Although all human malarial species can induce rosetting, only *P falciparum* causes fatal infections. Rosetting has been linked to cerebral malaria. Cytoadherence is caused only by *P falciparum*.

Cytokine Release

It has been demonstrated that parasite products, host cellular material, malarial pigment, and antibody complexes stimulate macrophages, monocytes, and endothelium to release inflammatory cytokines in malaria. Cytokines are thought to be involved in placental dysfunction, suppression of red cell production, hepatic dysfunction, inhibition of gluconeogenesis, and the cause of fever. Cytokines are also important mediators of parasite killing; they activate leukocytes and probably other cells to release toxic oxygen species, nitric oxide, generating parasitocidal lipid peroxides, and cause fever.[46]

Immunologic Processes

Acquired immunity apparently can act in 3 ways: reducing the probability of clinical disease, speeding the clearance of parasites, and increasing tolerance to subpatent infections. One form of clinical immunity reduces susceptibility to clinical disease and develops with age and exposure (with half-life of the order of 5 years or more), and another form of antiparasite immunity results in more rapid clearance of parasitemia, is acquired later in life, and is longer lasting (half-life of >20 years).

Potential regulatory mechanisms include regulatory T cells, which have been shown to significantly modify cellular immune responses to various protozoan infections, including leishmania and malaria; neutralizing antibodies to proinflammatory malarial toxins such as glycosylphosphatidylinositol and malarial pigment; and self-regulating networks of effector molecules. Innate and adaptive immune responses are moderated by the total immunologic environment, which is influenced by the genetic background of the host and by possible coinfection with other pathogens.

In hyperendemic or holoendemic malaria areas, residents have hypergammaglobulinemia; however, most of this antibody is not directed against malaria antigens. In nonimmune individuals, IgM and IgG2 isotypes represent the acute antibody response; but they fail to arm cytotoxic cells, thus being unable to kill the parasites.[10]

Drug Resistance

Drug resistance to *Plasmodium* spp can develop through several mechanisms, including changes in drug permeability or transport, drug conversion to an alternate form that becomes ineffective, increased expression of the drug target, or changes in the enzyme target that decrease the binding affinity of the inhibitor.[47–52] Compliance with prescribed drug regimens remains a problem when trying to document actual drug resistance; without confirmation that therapeutic drug levels are reached, actual resistance is impossible to validate. Current antimalarial drugs and associated problems are listed in **Table 4**.

Table 4
Antimalarial drugs, primary use, and associated problems

Antimalarial Drug	Primary Use	Associated Problems
Artemisinin	Asexual erythrocytic stages, particularly on young, ring forms; not effective against liver stages; short elimination half-life	Recrudescence, may be some neurotoxicity; reproductive safety concerns; high cost
Atovaquone-Proguanil (Malarone)	Atovaquone: blocks nucleic acid synthesis, inhibits replication (asexual erythrocytic stages) Proguanil: asexual erythrocytic stages, lowers concentration at which atovaquone causes collapse of mitochondrial membrane potential; treatment and prophylaxis of *P falciparum* (overall effective against sexual and asexual stages); primary prophylaxis in areas with chloroquine-resistant or mefloquine-resistant *P falciparum*	Atovaquone: associated with recrudescence when used alone Malarone: well tolerated; mild side effects (anorexia, nausea, vomiting, abdominal pain, diarrhea, pruritus, headache; not recommended during pregnancy or lactation); contraindicated in persons with severe renal impairment
Chloroquine	Treatment and prophylaxis all species; nonenzymatic inhibition of heme polymerization; primary prophylaxis in areas endemic for chloroquine-sensitive *P falciparum*; *pfcrt* major chloroquine resistance gene	Bitter taste; generally well tolerated; side effects include nausea, abdominal discomfort, dizziness, retinal pigmentation, blurred vision, electrocardiographic changes, muscular weakness; resistance worldwide, except Central America; safe to take during pregnancy; may exacerbate psoriasis; cumulative dose >100 g over time leads to irreversible retinopathy
Doxycycline	Used in combination with quinine sulfate; primary prophylaxis in areas with chloroquine-resistant or mefloquine-resistant *P falciparum*	Phototoxicity; not used in pregnancy or in children; gastrointestinal intolerance
Fansidar (pyrimethamine-sulfadoxine)	Asexual erythrocytic stages; inhibition of enzyme dihydrofolate reductase; main target blood schizonts; very limited gametocytocidal effects	Rapid resistance develops to *P falciparum*; limited use as single agent; no longer recommended for prophylaxis (adverse effects); not recommended for *P vivax*; allergic reactions to sulfa drugs well known

(continued on next page)

Table 4
(continued)

Antimalarial Drug	Primary Use	Associated Problems
Halofantrine	Asexual erythrocytic stages; exact mechanism unknown; P vivax and P falciparum; limited data for other species	Not recommended for prophylaxis (toxicity); cardiotoxicity, poor absorption, sporadic resistance; contraindicated in pregnancy
Mefloquine	Erythrocytic schizonts of all species; related to quinine; interacts with ferriprotoporphyrin IX and host cell phospholipids (exact mechanism not known); may interfere with digestion of hemoglobin; no effect on tissue schizonts or gametocytes	Psychoses; resistance in Indochina and Africa; can enhance dysrhythmias in patients on beta blockers; very expensive
Primaquine	Very active against preerythrocytic sporozoites and exoerythrocytic tissue schizonts, and gametocytes; main use is to prevent relapses of P vivax and P ovale	Narrow therapeutic index; not used in glucose-6-phosphate dehydrogenase–deficient patients; resistance or tolerance demonstrated; not used in pregnancy or lactation
Quinine sulfate	Blood schizonticides; all 4 species; chloroquine-resistant P falciparum	Usually given in combination with other agents; associated with tinnitus, dysphoria, reversible high-tone deafness; also associated with massive hemolysis in heavy P falciparum infections (blackwater fever); resistance in Brazil, Indochina
Quinidine gluconate	Blood schizonticides; all 4 species	Limited availability; requires cardiac monitoring in intensive care setting; same problems as seen with quinine

Data from Lou J, Lucas R, Grau GE. Pathogenesis of cerebral malaria: recent experimental data and possible applications for humans. Clin Microbiol Rev 2001;14:810–20. Tran VB, Tran VB, Lin KH. Malaria infection after allogeneic bone marrow transplantation in a child with thalassemia. Bone Marrow Transplant 1997;19:1259–60.

DIAGNOSIS

Infections with *Plasmodium* spp can be life-threatening, and laboratory requests, processing, examination, and reporting for blood smear examination and organism identification should be treated as "STAT" requests.[53–55] In terms of health care personnel training, it is important to recognize that parasite recovery and identification often tend to be more difficult than expected. Patient history details should be available to the laboratorian (**Table 5**).

Conventional Light Microscopy

Single-draw blood films or specimens are not sufficient to exclude the diagnosis of malaria, especially when the patient has received partial prophylaxis or therapy. Partial use of antimalarials reduces the parasitemia, which complicates making the correct diagnosis, even when serious disease is present. Patients with a relapse case or an early primary case may also have few organisms in the blood smear (see **Fig. 2** and **Table 3**).

Regardless of the presence or absence of any fever periodicity, both thick and thin blood films should be prepared immediately, and at least 200 to 300 oil immersion fields should be examined on both films before a negative report is issued.[53] One set of negative films will not rule out malaria; additional blood specimens should be examined over a 36-hour time frame. Although Giemsa stain is recommended for all parasitic blood work, the organisms can also be seen if other blood stains, such as Wright stain, are used (see **Box 1** and **Table 2**). Blood collected using EDTA anticoagulant is preferred over heparin; however, if the blood remains in the tube for any length of time, after staining Schüffner dots may not be visible (*P vivax*, as an example) and other morphologic

Table 5 Patient information required for the diagnostic laboratory	
Question	**Comment**
Where has the patient been, and what was the date of return to the United States?	May be helpful in suggesting particular species and/or resistance information
Where do you live? This is particularly relevant if the patient lives by an airport	Well documented that mosquitoes can be transmitted to nonendemic areas through airplanes and/or baggage
Has malaria ever been diagnosed in the patient before? If so, what species was identified?	If the response is "yes"—often a relapse case may exhibit a lower parasitemia; species will dictate therapy if *P vivax* or *P ovale* involved (potential relapse)
What medication (prophylaxis or otherwise) has the patient received, and how often? When was the last dose taken?	Prophylaxis tends to reduce the parasitemia; thus microscopic examination of blood films may need to be extended; dose information will influence microscopic examination, as well
Has the patient ever received a blood transfusion? Is there a possibility of other needle transmission (drug user)?	Both situations represent malaria parasite transmission possibilities—may have nothing to do with being in an endemic area
When was the blood specimen drawn, and was the patient symptomatic at the time? Is there any evidence of a fever periodicity?	If periodicity present, will influence interpretation of blood film findings; if no periodicity, may represent an early infection with very low parasitaemia

changes in the parasites will be seen. Also, the proper ratio between blood and antico-agulant is required for good organism morphology, so each collection tube should be filled to the top. Finger-stick blood is recommended, particularly when the volume of blood required is minimal (ie, when no other hematologic procedures have been ordered). The blood should be free-flowing when taken for smear preparation, and should not be contaminated with alcohol used to clean the finger prior to the stick. However, the use of finger-stick blood is much less common than in the past, and venipuncture blood is the normal specimen obtained. Identification to the species level determines which drug(s) is recommended. In early infections, patients with *P falciparum* infections may not have the crescent-shaped gametocytes in the blood. Low parasitemias with the delicate ring forms may be missed; consequently, oil immersion examination at 1000× is mandatory. Some microscopists may use the 50× or 60× oil immersion objectives to screen the blood films; however, oil immersion examination using the 100× objective is required before reporting the final results.

Peripheral parasitemia does not always reflect the number of sequestered para-sites, but usually correlates with disease severity (see **Table 3**). Malaria pigment may serve as an indicator for parasite density, because the pigment can be seen within monocytes and polymorphonuclear leukocytes (PMNs) during microscopic examination of the blood films. Malaria pigment also correlates with severe disease compared with uncomplicated malaria. Pigmented neutrophils (PMNs, monocytes) have been associated with cerebral malaria and with death in children with severe malaria.[56]

Routine microscopy occasionally reveals ookinetes of *Plasmodium* spp; this repre-sents a potential "artifact" that could lead to the incorrect diagnosis of *P falciparum* infection. The ookinetes tend to resemble the crescent-shaped gametocytes seen in infections with *P falciparum*. The appearance of these stages in the peripheral blood, rather than the mosquito gut, is due to the delay between blood collection using EDTA anticoagulant and smear preparation. It has been documented that some gameto-cytes (*P falciparum*) will exflagellate at room temperature (pH 7.4). In this case, the microgametes could resemble spirochetes.[53,57] It is important to understand the potential for artifacts when handling/storing these specimens for blood parasite diagnosis.[53,54]

Malaria is considered to be immediately life-threatening, and a patient with the diag-nosis of *P falciparum* or *P knowlesi* malaria should be considered a medical emer-gency because the disease can be rapidly fatal. This approach to the patient is also recommended in situations where *P falciparum* or *P knowlesi* cannot be "ruled out" as a possible diagnosis. Any laboratory providing the expertise to identify malarial parasites should do so on a 24-hour basis, 7 days a week.

Laboratory personnel must be aware of the "STAT" nature of diagnostic blood work for malaria requests, as well as the importance of obtaining patient history information (see **Table 5**). The typical textbook presentation of the blood smears from an endemic area patient may not be seen, particularly if the patient has been traveling and has never been exposed to malaria before (immunologically naïve with a very low parasi-temia). It becomes very important that the smears be examined at length and under oil immersion using the 100× objective. Although a low parasitemia may be present on the blood smears, the patient may still be faced with a serious, life-threatening disease.

Other Diagnostic Methods

Giemsa-stained thick and thin blood films have been used to diagnose malaria for many years, and have always been considered the "gold standard." Alternative methods have been developed, including different approaches to staining, microscopy, flow cytometry, biochemical methods, immunoassay, and molecular methods (**Table 6**). These procedures have been developed to reduce cost, reduce the need for expensive equipment, increase sensitivity, and provide simple, rapid methods that do not require conventional microscopy.[58,61–69]

Microhematocrit centrifugation, using the QBC tube (glass capillary tube and closely fitting plastic insert; QBC malaria blood tubes, Becton Dickinson, Sparks, MD, USA), has been used for the detection of blood parasites. After centrifugation of capillary or venous blood, parasites or RBCs containing parasites are concentrated into a small region near the top of the RBC column and are held close to the wall of the tube by the plastic float, thereby making them readily visible by microscopy. Tubes precoated with acridine orange provide a stain that induces fluorescence in the parasites. The tube is placed into a plastic holder, a drop of oil is applied to the top of the hematocrit tube, a coverslip is added, and the tube is examined with a 40× to 60× oil immersion objective (the objective must have a working distance of 0.3 mm or greater). Although *Plasmodium* spp parasites can be detected using this method (which is more sensitive than use of the thick

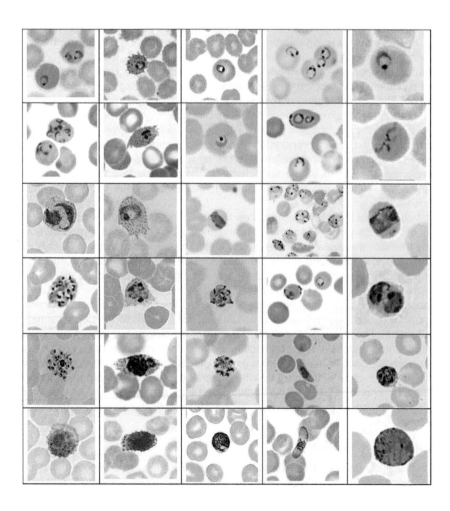

or thin blood smear), appropriate thick and thin blood films must be examined to accurately identify organisms at the species level.

With the development of newer, more expensive drugs, their effective use requires rapid, accurate, and inexpensive diagnostic procedures so that directed therapy can be provided. Several of these rapid malaria tests (RMTs) are now commercially available, some of which use monoclonal antibodies against the histidine-rich protein 2 (HRP2) whereas others detect species-specific parasite lactate dehydrogenase (pLDH). These procedures are based on an antigen capture approach in dipstick or cartridge formats (see **Table 6**). Note that only one of these RMTs is Food and Drug Administration approved for use within the United States.

Other methods include a dot blot assay or direct detection of *P falciparum* by using a specific DNA probe after PCR amplification of target DNA sequences. Recent studies recommend using PCR for detection of malaria; the high sensitivity, rapidity, and simplicity of some of the methods are relevant for epidemiology studies, therapy follow-up, and immunization trials. Detection is possible for as few as 5 or 10 parasites per microliter of blood, with confirmation that PCR detects many more cases of low-level parasitemia than do thick blood films.[70,71] This approach is also valuable when the determination of species is questionable, or in situations where mixed infections are suspected.

Laboratory personnel using automated differential instruments need to be aware of potential limitations related to the diagnosis of blood parasite infections.[72,73] *Plasmodium* spp and *Babesia* infections have been completely missed using these instruments. Even if the slide is "flagged," the number of fields scanned by

---

Fig. 2. Morphology of malaria parasites. Column 1 (*left to right*): *Plasmodium vivax* (note enlarged infected RBCs). (1) Early trophozoite (ring form) (note one RBC contains 2 rings—not that uncommon); (2) older ring, note ameboid nature of rings; (3) late trophozoite with Schüffner dots (note enlarged RBC); (4) developing schizont; (5) mature schizont with 18 merozoites and clumped pigment; (6) microgametocyte with dispersed chromatin. Column 2: *Plasmodium ovale* (note enlarged infected RBCs). (1) Early trophozoite (ring form) with Schüffner dots (RBC has fimbriated edges); (2) early trophozoite (note enlarged RBC, Schüffner dots, and RBC oval in shape); (3) late trophozoite in RBC with fimbriated edges; (4) developing schizont with irregular-shaped RBC; (5) mature schizont with 8 merozoites arranged irregularly; (6) microgametocyte with dispersed chromatin. Column 3: *Plasmodium malariae* (note normal or smaller than normal infected RBCs). (1) Early trophozoite (ring form); (2) early trophozoite with thick cytoplasm; (3) late trophozoite (band form); (4) developing schizont; (5) mature schizont with 9 merozoites arranged in a rosette; (6) macrogametocyte with compact chromatin. Column 4: *Plasmodium falciparum*. (1) Early trophozoites (the rings are in the headphone configuration with double chromatin dots); (2) early trophozoite (accolé or appliqué form); (3) early trophozoites (note the multiple rings/cell); (4) late trophozoite with larger ring (accolé or appliqué form); (5) crescent-shaped gametocyte; (6) crescent-shaped gametocyte. Column 5: *Plasmodium knowlesi*—with the exception of image 5, these were photographed at a higher magnification (note normal or smaller than normal infected RBCs). (*Courtesy of* the Centers for Disease Control and Prevention.) (1) Early trophozoite (ring form); (2) early trophozoite with slim band form; (3) late trophozoite (band form); (4) developing schizont; (5) mature schizont with merozoites arranged in a rosette; (6) microgametocyte with dispersed chromatin. *Note*: Without the appliqué form, Schüffner dots, multiple rings per cell, and other developing stages, differentiation among the species can be very difficult. It is obvious that the early rings of all 4 species can mimic one another very easily. *Remember*: One set of negative blood films cannot rule out a malaria infection.

Table 6
Alternative approaches to malaria diagnosis[a]

Principle of the Method	Method	Comments	Pros	Cons
Giemsa-stained blood films[b]; Light microscopy	Thick (TBF) and thin blood films (THBF);	Traditional method	TBF used to screen larger amount of blood THBF allow visualization of parasite within RBC; generally thought to be more sensitive than rapid antigen tests, particularly for identification to the species level	TBF unable to see parasite within RBC THBF provides less blood per examination
	Cytocentrifugation (100 µL lysed blood centrifuged onto slide, stained with Giemsa or other blood stain)	Commercially available (used in histopathology labs)	Amount of blood examined is increased	Blood lysed; unable to see parasite within RBC
Fluorescent DNA/RNA stains	TBF and THBF films (eg, acridine orange)		Sensitivity good	Requires expertise in reading
	After centrifugation (QBC)	Commercially available	Saves time, fairly sensitive	Expensive, species ID may be difficult
	Flow cytometry	Commercially available, low sensitivity	Automated counts	Low sensitivity due to "background noise"

Molecular methods	DNA/RNA hybridization	Poor sensitivity	"New approach"	Low sensitivity, cumbersome procedures
	PCR	Sensitive	Detect low numbers; species ID with mixed infections; used with blood spot collection	Lengthy procedure; automation may solve this problem
	Real-time PCR (QT-PCR)	Sensitive	Sensitivity of 20 parasites/mL blood	Requires 500 μL blood; takes 12 h longer than QT-NASBA
	Real-time nucleic acid sequence-based (QT-NASBA)	Sensitive	Sensitivity of 20 parasites/mL blood	Requires 50 μL blood; takes 12 h less than QT-PCR; lends itself to testing large numbers of samples
Malaria pigment detection	Dark-field microscopy	Inferior to TBF	Pigment in WBCs sensitive indicator of prognosis	Not as sensitive as TBF
	Automated blood cell analyzers	Commercially available; detection of cases not suspected as having malaria	Detects malaria pigment (WBCs, schizonts, gametocytes)	Nonspecific findings per species and parasitemia; not effective in low parasitemia cases
	Depolarizing monocytes containing malarial pigment	Related to duration of symptoms before testing	Malarial pigment in monocytes	More obvious if parasitemia ≥0.5%
	Pseudoreticulocytosis	Related to *P falciparum*	Nuclear material from intraerythrocytic parasites	More obvious if parasitemia ≥0.5%

(continued on next page)

Table 6
(continued)

Principle of the Method	Method	Comments	Pros	Cons
Antigen detection	HRP-2 Assays; *P falciparum* only Paracheck Pf (Orchid Biomedical Systems)	Commercially available	Simple, rapid dipstick format; good correlation with conventional microscopy; may detect *P falciparum* (chloroquine resistant) after patient treated for *P vivax* (mixed infections)	*P falciparum* only; drop in sensitivity at low levels of parasitemia (<100/µL); misses cases of only mature gametocytes (no HRP-2); false positives seen
	ParaHIT (Span Diagnostic f Ltd)	Commercially available	Simple, rapid dipstick format, good sensitivity and specificity	False positives seen; occasional failure to detect high parasitemias; persistent positive results in treated patients
	MAKROmed (Makro Medical Pty Ltd)	Commercially available	Antigen capture immunochromatographic strip format; may be more sensitive than conventional microscopy	Highly sensitive in detecting placental malaria, lower than expected specificity
	HRP-2 Assays; *P falciparum* and panmalaria tests BinaxNOW Malaria (Binax Inc, Inverness)	Commercially available (FDA Approved)	Simple, rapid dipstick format; lower false positive rate; good sensitivity (*P falciparum*, *P vivax*), especially when coupled with microscopy	Some reagents must be stored at 2–8°C; cost may be a factor; more sensitive for placental malaria than microscopy; insensitive for *P ovale* and *P malariae*;
	pLDH assay: OptiMAL-IT (DiaMed AG)	Commercially available; test only positive with viable organisms	Simple, rapid dipstick format; also picks up *P vivax*; few false positives; good test of cure (picks up viable parasites only)	Similar limitations at low parasitemias (<0.01%); mixed infection ID difficult; cannot replace microscopy
	CareStart Malaria (AccessBio Inc); several formats Pf (LDH and non-*P falciparum* LDH) Pf (HRP-2)	Commercially available	Excellent specificity and sensitivity; room temp storage; become negative more quickly than HRP2 formats	Decreased sensitivity with low parasitemia

Abbreviations: HRP-2, histidine-rich protein 2; ID, identification; pLDH, parasite lactate dehydrogenase; RBC, red blood cell; TBF, thick blood film; THBF, thin blood film; WBCs, white blood cells.

^a *Data from* Refs.[53–73]

^b Other blood stains can also be used; quality control is built into the system (if WBCs look good, then parasites will look good).

a technologist on instrument-read smears is small. Failure to detect a light parasite-mia is almost guaranteed. In these cases, after diagnosis had been made on routine thick and thin blood films submitted to the parasitology laboratory, all previous smears examined by the automated system were reviewed using routine micros-copy and found to be positive for parasites. Unfortunately, failure to make the diag-nosis resulted in delayed therapy. Although the majority of these instruments are not designed to detect intracellular blood parasites, the inability of the automated systems to discriminate between uninfected RBCs and those infected with parasites may pose serious diagnostic problems in situations where the parasitemia is 0.5% or less.

TREATMENT, PROGNOSIS, AND LONG-TERM OUTCOME

Antimalarial drugs are classified by the stage of malaria against which they are effec-tive. These drugs are often referred to as tissue schizonticides (which kill tissue schiz-onts), blood schizonticides (which kill blood schizonts), gametocytocides (which kill gametocytes), and sporonticides (which prevent formation of sporozoites within the mosquito) (see **Table 4**).[74] Malaria continues to be a serious health problem, both in residents of areas where the disease is endemic and in travelers returning to areas where it is not endemic.[60] Unfortunately, travelers may obtain medications from friends or purchase over-the-counter drugs in foreign countries, some of which have proven to be diluted or totally ineffectual.[75] Even when appropriate drugs are obtained, compliance with defined dosing regimens remains a problem, particularly when trying to confirm actual drug resistance. Side effects are often a problem with many drugs, including those for treating *Plasmodium* spp infections (see **Table 4**).

Therapy has become more complex because of the increase in resistance of *P falciparum* to a variety of drugs and because of advances in treatment of severe disease complications (see **Table 4**). To ensure proper therapy, the clinician should know what species of *Plasmodium* is involved, the estimated parasitemia, and the geographic and travel history of the patient, to determine the area where infection was probably acquired and the possibility of drug resistance. The use of oral or paren-teral therapy will be determined by the clinical status of the patient.

Development of resistance to the inexpensive antimalarials, such as chloroquine and Fansidar, has had a tremendous financial and public health impact on developing coun-tries. In the late 1980s, chloroquine-resistant *P falciparum* completely covered Africa. Resistance to pyrimethamine has also spread rapidly since the introduction of this drug. Fansidar is no longer effective in many areas of Indochina, Brazil, and Africa.

Although chloroquine-resistant *P falciparum* is well recognized, chloroquine has generally been effective for both chemoprophylaxis and treatment of *P vivax*, *P ovale*, and *P malariae* infections. Cases of chloroquine-resistant *P vivax* (CRPV) malaria have now been identified in Papua New Guinea, Indonesia, Malaysia, Vietnam, the Republic of Korea, Myanmar, and Ethiopia. CRPV is now endemic in Malaysia, Myanmar, and Vietnam. However, there is no evidence of CRPV from Thailand, Cambodia, Laos, China, or the Philippine archipelago.[76] Although CRPV has been documented in a few areas within South America (Guyana, Colombia, Brazil, Peru), it is at a very low frequency, with a risk of less than 5%. Population-based epidemiologic studies will be necessary to define the geographic range and prevalence of CRPV. At this time, it is not clear whether this development represents a newly emerging public health problem; however, clinicians need to be aware that possible therapeutic or prophylactic failures with chloroquine may result with *P vivax* infections in people who have been in Indonesia or Oceania.

Table 7
Host genetic factors in resistance to malaria

Factor	Comments
Hemoglobin disorders	
Sickling disorders	Includes sickle cell disease (SS), heterozygous states for sickle cell gene and those for hemoglobin C (SC) or β-thalassemia (S-thal); carrier state for sickle cell gene is AS; widely distributed throughout tropical Africa, parts of the Mediterranean, the Middle East, and central India; hemoglobin S confers protection against *P falciparum* malaria (parasite cannot complete life cycle due to cell sickling and destruction; reduced oxygen levels result in diminished parasite growth; reduced rosetting of red blood cells (RBCs) in sickle carriers; protection also be related to hemoglobin structure and parasite inability to metabolize)
Hemoglobins C, E	Data for selective advantage against malaria less convincing than hemoglobin S; reduced parasite invasion and impaired growth has been documented; data for hemoglobin E have shown inconsistent results
Hemoglobin F	Growth of *P falciparum* reduced in presence of hemoglobin F, thought to be due to hemoglobin itself rather than RBC properties; higher levels of hemoglobin F during first year of life might offer protection (newborn infants and adults with persistent fetal hemoglobin production)
Thalassemia (α and β)	Distribution of β-thalassemia coincides with that of malaria; 70% reduction in clinical malaria and 50% reduction in risk; although not seen in all geographic areas, in Papua, New Guinea, high protective effect of homozygous state for α-thalassemia against complications of *P falciparum* malaria; babies under 2 (homozygous for α^+-thalassemia) had higher frequency of both *P vivax* and *P falciparum*, but were resistant from age 2 on
Erythrocyte polymorphisms	
Glucose-6-phosphate dehydrogenase deficiency	Both female heterozygotes and male hemizygotes have reduced risk (around 50%) of developing severe malaria
Duffy-negative RBCs	Resistant to invasion by *P vivax*
Ovalocytosis	Patients subject to severe malarial infection with high parasitemias; however, strong protection against cerebral malaria; structural change in RBC membrane interferes with binding of infected RBCs to vascular endothelium
Immunogenetic variants	
Human leukocyte antigen (HLA) genes	Each protective HLA type associated with 40%–50% decrease in risk; these HLA types are common
HLA Class I	HLA-A, -B, -C determine specificities of $CD8^+$ T cells (cytotoxic, major role in defense against intracellular pathogens); HLA-B35 frequency reduced in children with cerebral malaria and those with severe malarial anemia
HLA Class II	HLA-DR, -DQ, DP determine specificities of $CD4^+$ T cells that secrete cytokines and provide T cell help for antibody production and action of other T cells; HLA-DRB1*1302-HLA-DQB1*1501frequency reduced in children with severe malarial anemia

(continued on next page)

Table 7 (continued)	
Factor	**Comments**
Cytokine, other immune response genes	
TNF	Tumor necrosis factor (TNF) major mediator of malaria fever; TNF increased in children with cerebral malaria and markedly so in children with fatal cerebral malaria
MBL	Mannose-binding lectin (MBL); deficiency may be associated with increased susceptibility to infectious diseases; effect on malaria may be small to none
CD35	Also called complement receptor 1 (CR1) plays a role in rosetting; African variant of CR1 may protect against severe malaria.

Adapted from Hill AVS, Weatheral DJ. Host genetic factors in resistance to malaria. In: Sherman IW, editor. Malaria: parasite biology, pathogenesis, and protection. Washington, DC: ASM Press; 1998. p. 445–55; with permission.

Primaquine is the only available drug against the hypnozoites within the liver (*P vivax, P ovale*). However, this drug has been in use for almost 60 years and may no longer be as effective as before.[36] Rather than use the term "resistant" for these documented problems with primaquine therapy, the terms "primaquine tolerant" or "primaquine refractory" are preferred.[76] Current recommended regimens require 2 weeks of daily dosing; unfortunately the drug may cause potentially fatal hemolytic anemia in some individuals with glucose-6-phosphate dehydrogenase deficiency.

Suppressive Therapy

Chemoprophylactic agents to prevent clinical symptoms are given to individuals who are going into areas where malaria is endemic.[13] These drugs are effective only against the erythrocytic forms and do not prevent the person from getting malaria; that is, they do not prevent sporozoites from entering the liver and beginning the pre-erythrocytic cycle of development. The most commonly used drugs for this purpose are quinine, chloroquine, hydroxychloroquine, and amodiaquine, all of which are effective when the organisms enter the RBCs from the liver and begin the erythrocytic cycle. Fansidar, which is a combination of pyrimethamine and sulfadoxine, is recommended for prophylaxis only for travelers who are staying for a long time in high-transmission areas where chloroquine-resistant malaria is endemic. This recommendation was based on revisions in response to increased numbers of adverse reactions to Fansidar prophylaxis, including severe mucocutaneous reactions, some of which were fatal (see **Table 4**). In general, chloroquine is still the choice for prophylaxis against *P falciparum*, but it is not totally effective against *P vivax*. Resistance to Fansidar was reported in Thailand as early as 1981. Quinine is normally used in these situations; however, quinine-resistant *P falciparum* has been reported in Africa, with little to no information on previous chloroquine intake. A combination of quinine and tetracycline is recommended for chloroquine- and Fansidar-resistant *P falciparum*.

With the introduction of chloroquine, with its high potency, long half-life, and low toxicity, continued research into the chemoprophylactic potential of other antimalarial agents such as primaquine was drastically reduced. Resistance to the newer chemoprophylactic drugs such as chloroquine, sulfadoxine/pyrimethamine (Fansidar), proguanil, mefloquine, and doxycycline continues to increase, with many of these agents now becoming clinically useless. Other antimalarial agents like quinine, halofantrine, or the artimisinine derivatives are too toxic or have too short a half-life to be used for prophylaxis.

Perhaps the most common approach to chemoprophylaxis in travelers to areas with multidrug-resistant *P falciparum* is the use of doxycycline. However, this tetracycline derivative must be taken daily, and its use must be continued for 4 weeks after the patient has left the area. Potential side effects include diarrhea, upper gastrointestinal upset, and phototoxicity. Patients may also be predisposed to oral or vaginal candidiasis, and the drug cannot be given during pregnancy or to young children. Also, breakthrough can occur in individuals who have missed only a single dose.

Radical Cure

The radical cure approach to therapy eradicates all malarial organisms, both the liver and the RBC stages, from the body. Therapy is usually given to individuals who have returned from areas where malaria is endemic and will prevent relapses with *P vivax* or *P ovale* infection, although relapses with both *P vivax* and *P ovale* infections occasionally occur after treatment with primaquine.[16] The gametocytes are also eliminated, thus stopping the chain of transmission to the mosquito vector. The drugs used are primaquine and other 8-aminoquinolones. Treatment with primaquine is usually not necessary for malarial cases acquired by transfusion or contaminated needles, or passed from mother to child as a congenital infection.

An increase in the incidence of malaria caused by *P falciparum* is well recognized, and delays in diagnosis and subsequent therapy may result in complicated or fatal cases, particularly in the nonimmune host. Some of the complications of *P falciparum* malaria that have been discussed include cerebral malaria, renal failure, respiratory problems, disseminated intravascular coagulation, blackwater fever, and hepatic dysfunction. Death is directly related to the level of parasitemia and onset of complications, with significant mortality related to more than 5% parasitemia despite appropriate parenteral therapy and supportive care. In these situations, the role of exchange blood transfusion may be appropriate for the following reasons: (1) rapid reduction of the parasitemia, (2) decreased risk of severe intravascular hemolysis, (3) improved blood flow, and (4) improved oxygen-carrying capacity.[59,77]

Exposure to both placental malaria and maternal human immunodeficiency virus (HIV) infection increases postnatal mortality to a greater degree than does the independent risk associated with exposure to either maternal HIV or placental malaria infection alone. Therefore, malaria chemoprophylaxis during pregnancy could decrease the impact of HIV transmission from mother to infant.[78]

Overall Patient Care

It is important to remember that patients who present to a medical clinic, office, or the emergency room that does not have expertise in tropical medicine tend to receive suboptimal treatment. Malaria may not be recognized, and the diagnosis may be delayed until it is no longer possible to save the patient. Improvements in obtaining the patient history, symptom recognition, presumptive diagnosis development, and treatment of malaria are mandatory to prevent severe illness and death among travelers.

Prognosis and Outcomes

In cases of severe cerebral malaria, advances have been made in antiparasitic treatment, but the identification of a treatment to increase survival and reduce brain damage is still pending.[79] In general, patient prognosis depends on many factors, beginning with a timely and correct diagnosis. The use of appropriate therapeutic regimens, including adequate monitoring of parasitemia for evidence of drug resistance or tolerance, is critical for quality patient cure. The development of artemisinin-based combination treatments (ACTs) and other drugs, long-lasting insecticide-treated bed nets (with synthetic pyrethroids), and a search for nontoxic, long-lasting, afford-able insecticides for indoor residual spraying (IRS) will all impact the eventual outcomes of malaria.[80] Malaria vaccine development and testing continue to prog-ress, and a recombinant protein directed against the circumsporozoite protein will soon be in phase 3 trials. Support for malaria control, research, and advocacy through the Global Fund for HIV/AIDS, Tuberculosis and Malaria, the US President's Malaria Initiative, the Bill & Melinda Gates Foundation, World Health Organization, and other organizations continues to decrease morbidity and mortality in many endemic coun-tries. Sustainability of these programs, along with improved surveillance and research, will be required for malaria elimination.[80]

IMMUNITY AND REINFECTION

There are some genetic alterations in the RBCs that confer natural immunity to malaria. Changes in the RBC surface interfere with attachment and invasion of mero-zoites. Changes in hemoglobin or intracellular enzymes interfere with parasite growth and multiplication (**Table 7**).

Duffy antigen–negative RBCs lack surface receptors for *P vivax* invasion. Many West Africans and some American blacks are Duffy antigen negative, which may explain the low incidence of *P vivax* in West Africa. In other areas of Africa, *P vivax* is much more prevalent.

Partial resistance is seen in individuals with the sickle cell trait and in those with sickle cell anemia. Resistance is related to the sickling of hemoglobin S (HbS)-contain-ing RBCs. Other factors include the formation of deoxyhemoglobin aggregates within the cells, the loss of potassium from sickled cells, and the fact that the parasites actu-ally cause HbS cells to sickle.

Resistance to *P falciparum* is also seen in glucose-6-phosphate dehydrogenase–deficient cells. Partial immunity to malarial infection is seen in areas where malaria is endemic when HbC, HbE, β-thalassemia, and pyruvate kinase (PK) deficiencies exist.

Infants are also relatively immune to malarial infections during the first year of life as a result of the presence of a large percentage of HbF, passive immunity from maternal antibodies, and diets deficient in *p*-aminobenzoic acid.

Slowly eliminated antimalarial drugs suppress malaria reinfections for a period of time determined by the dose, the pharmacokinetic properties of the drug, and the susceptibility of the infecting parasites. This effect is called post-treatment prophy-laxis, and can last for a very short time to several months; obviously, drug resistance shortens this type of prophylaxis. The clinical benefits of preventing recrudescence (reflecting treatment efficacy) compared with preventing reinfection (reflecting post-treatment prophylaxis) need further assessment before any specific recommenda-tions are made.[81]

Immunity reduces the probability of an infection becoming patent. Immunity to malaria parasites is complex and poorly defined, but is generally unrelated to drug resistance. In malaria-endemic areas, therapeutic responses vary with age as young children have little or no immunity compared with older children and adults. Immunity results in better therapeutic responses for any level of resistance. Immunity inhibits parasite development and multiplication, and thereby augments the effects of antima-larial drugs. This fact explains the greater efficacy of failing antimalarial drugs in areas of moderate to high malaria transmission in older children and adults. Both cellular and humoral immunities play a part in protection. However, immunity is species specific and in some cases even strain specific. It has also been noted that acute malarial infections can cause immunosuppression. Actual impairment of immune responses to vaccination after acute malaria has been documented. Depending on many parasite and host factors, reinfection with *Plasmodium* spp (same/different species; different strains) is not only possible, but in certain situations probable.

REFERENCES

1. Lou J, Lucas R, Grau GE. Pathogenesis of cerebral malaria: recent experimental data and possible applications for humans. Clin Microbiol Rev 2001;14:810–20.
2. Jongwutiwes S, Putaporntip C, Iwasaki T, et al. Naturally acquired *Plasmodium knowlesi* malaria in human, Thailand. Emerg Infect Dis 2004;10:2211–3.
3. Singh B, Kim Sung L, Matusop A, et al. A large focus of naturally acquired *Plasmodium knowlesi* infections in human beings. Lancet 2004;363(9414): 1017–24.
4. Lee KS, Cox-Singh J, Singh B. Morphological features and differential counts of *Plasmodium knowlesi* parasites in naturally acquired human infections. Malar J 2009;8:73.
5. Eliades MJ, Shah S, Nguyen-Dinh P, et al. Malaria surveillance—United States, 2003. MMWR Surveill Summ 2005;54:25–40.
6. Lefere F, Besson C, Datry A, et al. Transmission of *Plasmodium falciparum* by allogeneic bone marrow transplantation. Bone Marrow Transplant 1996;18:473–4.
7. Odonnell J, Goldman JM, Wagner K, et al. Donor-derived *Plasmodium vivax* infection following volunteer unrelated bone marrow transplantation. Bone Marrow Transplant 1998;21:313–4.
8. Raina V, Sharma A, Gujral S, et al. *Plasmodium vivax* causing pancytopenia after allogeneic blood stem cell transplantation in CML. Bone Marrow Transplant 1998; 22:205–6.
9. Salutari P, Sica S, Chiusolo P, et al. *Plasmodium vivax* malaria after autologous bone marrow transplantation: an unusual complication. Bone Marrow Transplant 1996;18:805–6.
10. Tran VB, Tran VB, Lin KH. Malaria infection after allogeneic bone marrow transplantation in a child with thalassemia. Bone Marrow Transplant 1997;19:1259–60.
11. Turkmen A, Sever MS, Ecder T, et al. Posttransplant malaria. Transplantation 1997;62:1521–3.
12. Robert LL, Santos-Ciminera PD, Andre RG, et al. Plasmodium-infected anopheles mosquitoes collected in Virginia and Maryland following local transmission of *Plasmodium vivax* malaria in Loudoun County, Virginia. J Am Mosq Control Assoc 2005;21:187–93.
13. Petersen E. Malaria chemoprophylaxis: when should we use it and what are the options? Expert Rev Anti Infect Ther 2004;2:119–32.
14. Beier JC, Vanderberg JP. Sporogonic development in the mosquito. In: Sherman IW, editor. Malaria: parasite biology, pathogenesis, and protection. Washington, DC: ASM Press; 1998. p. 49–61.
15. Krotoski WA, Garnham PCC, Bray RS, et al. Observations on early and late post sporozoite tissue stages in primate malaria. 1. Discovery of a new latent form of *Plasmodium cynomolgi* (the hypnozoite), and failure to detect hepatic forms within the first 24 hours after infection. Am J Trop Med Hyg 1982;31:24–35.
16. Beaver PC, Jung RC, Cupp EW. Clinical parasitology. 9th edition. Philadelphia: Lea & Febiger; 1984.

17. Trigg PI, Kondrachine AV. The current global malaria situation. In: Sherman IW, editor. Malaria: parasite biology, pathogenesis, and protection. Washington, DC: ASM Press; 1998. p. 11–22.
18. Peterson AT. Shifting suitability for malaria vectors across Africa with warming climates. BMC Infect Dis 2009;9:59–63.
19. Ikemoto T. Tropical malaria does not mean hot environments. J Med Entomol 2008;45:963–9.
20. Dash AP, Valecha N, Anvikar AR, et al. Malaria in India: challenges and opportunities. J Biosci 2008;33:583–92.
21. Chin T, Welsby PD. Makaria in the UK: past, present, and future. Postgrad Med J 2004;80:663–6.
22. Reiter P. Global warming and malaria: knowing the horse before hitching the cart. Malar J 2008;7(Suppl 1):S3.
23. Lindblade KA, Eisele TP, Gimnig JE, et al. Sustainability of reductions in malaria transmission and infant mortality in western Kenya with use of insecticide-treated bednets: 4 to 6 years of follow-up. JAMA 2004;291:2639–41.
24. Shiff C. Integrated approach to malaria control. Clin Microbiol Rev 2002;15:278–93.
25. World Malaria Report, 2005. Available at: http://rbm.who.int/wmr2005/html/exsummary_en.htm. 2005. Accessed November 23, 2009.
26. Soto J, Medina F, Dember N, et al. Efficacy of permethrin-impregnated uniforms in the prevention of malaria and leishmaniasis in Colombian soldiers. Clin Infect Dis 1995;21:599–602.
27. Schmunis GA, Cruz JR. Safety of the blood supply in Latin America. Clin Microbiol Rev 2005;18:12–29.
28. Ballou WR, Arevalo-Herrera M, Carucci D, et al. Update on the clinical development of candidate malaria vaccines. Am J Trop Med Hyg 2004;71S:239–47.
29. Good MF. Genetically modified *Plasmodium* highlights the potential of whole parasite vaccine strategies. Trends Immunol 2005;26:295–7.
30. Good MF. Vaccine-induced immunity to malaria parasites and the need for novel strategies. Trends Parasitol 2005;21:29–34.
31. Heppner DG Jr, Kester KE, Ockenhouse CF, et al. Towards an RTS, S-based, multi-stage, multi-antigen vaccine against falciparum malaria: progress at the Walter Reed Army Institute for Research. Vaccine 2005;23:2243–50.
32. Kwiatkowski D, Marsh K. Development of a malaria vaccine. Lancet 1998;350:1696–701.
33. Todryk SM, Walther M. Building better T-cell-inducing malaria vaccines. Immunology 2005;115:163–9.
34. Baird JK. Resistance to therapies for infection by *Plasmodium vivax*. Clin Microbiol Rev 2009;22:508–34.
35. Kochar DK, Saxena V, Singh N, et al. *Plasmodium vivax* malaria. Emerg Infect Dis 2005;11:132–4.
36. Spudick JM, Garcia LS, Graham DM, et al. Diagnostic and therapeutic pitfalls associated with primaquine-tolerant *Plasmodium vivax*. J Clin Microbiol 2005;43:978–81.
37. Collins WE, Jeffery GM. Plasmodium ovale: parasite and disease. Clin Microbiol Rev 2005;18:570–81.
38. Win TT, Jalloh A, Tantular IS, et al. Molecular analysis of *Plasmodium ovale* variants. Emerg Infect Dis 2004;10:1235–40.
39. van Velthuysen MLF, Florquin S. Glomerulopathy associated with parasitic infections. Clin Microbiol Rev 2000;13:55–66.

40. Dondorp AM, Angus BJ, Chotivanich K, et al. Red blood cell deformability as a predictor of anemia in severe falciparum malaria. Am J Trop Med Hyg 1999; 60:733–7.
41. Kawai S, Kano S, Suzuki M. Rosette formation by *Plasmodium coatneyi*-infected erythrocytes of the Japanese macaque (*Macaca fuscata*). Am J Trop Med Hyg 1995;53:295–9.
42. Clark IA, Alleva LM, Mills AC, et al. Pathogenesis of malaria and clinically similar conditions. Clin Microbiol Rev 2004;17:509–39.
43. Guyatt HL, Snow RW. Impact of malaria during pregnancy on low birth weight in sub-Saharan Africa. Clin Microbiol Rev 2004;17:760–9.
44. Mayxay M, Pukrittayakamee S, Chotivanich K, et al. Identification of cryptic coinfection with *Plasmodium falciparum* in patients presenting with vivax malaria. Am J Trop Med Hyg 2001;65:588–92.
45. Purnomo A, Solihin E, Gomez-Saladin, et al. Rare quadruple malaria infection in Irian Jaya Indonesia. J Parasitol 1999;85:574–9.
46. White NJ. Malaria pathophysiology. In: Sherman IW, editor. Malaria: parasite biology, pathogenesis, and protection. Washington, DC: ASM Press; 1998. p. 371–85.
47. Bloland PB. Drug resistance in malaria. Geneva (Switzerland): World Health Organization; 2001. (WHO/CDS/CSR/DRS/2001.4).
48. Farooq U, Mahajan RC. Drug resistance in malaria. J Vector Borne Dis 2004;41: 45–53.
49. Hill AVS, Weatherall DJ. Host genetic factors in resistance to malaria. In: Sherman IW, editor. Malaria: parasite biology, pathogenesis, and protection. Washington, DC: ASM Press; 1998. p. 445–55.
50. Milhous WK, Kyle DE. Introduction to the modes of action of and mechanisms of resistance to antimalarials. In: Sherman IW, editor. Malaria: parasite biology, pathogenesis, and protection. Washington, DC: ASM Press; 1998. p. 303–16.
51. Talisuna AO, Bloland P, D'Alessandro U. History, dynamics, and public health importance of malaria parasite resistance. Clin Microbiol Rev 2004;17:235–54.
52. Yeung S, Pingtavornpinyo W, Hastings IM, et al. Antimalarial drug resistance, artemisinin-based combination therapy and the contribution of modeling to elucidating policy choices. Am J Trop Med Hyg 2004;71:179–86.
53. Garcia LS. Diagnostic medical parasitology. 5th edition. Washington, DC: ASM Press; 2007.
54. Garcia LS. Practical guide to diagnostic parasitology. 2nd edition. Washington, DC: ASM Press; 2009.
55. National Committee for Clinical Laboratory Standards. Laboratory diagnosis of blood-borne parasitic diseases. Approved guideline M15-A. Wayne (PA): National Committee for Clinical Laboratory Standards; 2000.
56. Lyke KE, Diallo DA, Dicko A, et al. Association of intraleukocytic *Plasmodium falciparum* malaria pigment with disease severity, Clinical manifestations, and prognosis in severe malaria. Am J Trop Med Hyg 2003;69:253–9.
57. Berger SA, David L. Pseudo-borreliosis in patients with malaria. Am J Trop Med Hyg 2005;73:207–9.
58. Palmer CJ, Bonilla JA, Bruckner DA, et al. Multicenter study to evaluate the OptiMAL test for rapid diagnosis of malaria in U.S. hospitals. J Clin Microbiol 2003;41:5178–82.
59. Wilkinson RJ, Brown JL, Pasvol G, et al. Severe falciparum malaria: predicting the effect of exchange transfusion. QJM 1994;87:553–7.
60. Winstanley P, Ward S, Snow R, et al. Therapy of falciparum malaria in sub-Saharan Africa: from molecule to policy. Clin Microbiol Rev 2004;17:612–37.

61. De Monbrison F, Gerome P, Chaulet JF, et al. Comparative diagnostic performance of two commercial rapid tests for malaria in a non-endemic area. Eur J Clin Microbiol Infect Dis 2004;10:784–6.
62. Forney JR, Wongsrichanalai C, Magill AJ, et al. Devices for rapid diagnosis of malaria: evaluation of prototype assays that detect *Plasmodium falciparum* histidine-rich protein 2 and a *Plasmodium vivax*-specific antigen. J Clin Microbiol 2003;41: 2358–66.
63. Grobusch MP, Hanscheid T, Gobels K, et al. Comparison of three antigen detection tests for diagnosis and follow-up of falciparum malaria in travelers returning to Berlin, Germany. Parasitol Res 2003;89:354–7.
64. Hanscheid T. Diagnosis of malaria: a review of alternatives to conventional microscopy. Clin Lab Haematol 1999;21:235–45.
65. Iqbal J, Khalid N, Hira PR. Comparison of two commercial assays with expert microscopy for confirmation of symptomatically diagnosed malaria. J Clin Microbiol 2002;40:4675–8.
66. Iqbal J, Muneer A, Khalid N, et al. Performance of the OptiMAL test for malaria diagnosis among suspected malaria patients at the rural health centers. Am J Trop Med Hyg 2003;68:624–8.
67. Iqbal J, Siddique A, Jameel M, et al. Persistent histidine-rich protein 2, parasite lactate dehydrogenase, and panmalarial antigen reactivity after clearance of *Plasmodium falciparum* monoinfection. J Clin Microbiol 2004;42:4237–41.
68. Moody A. Rapid diagnostic tests for malaria parasites. Clin Microbiol Rev 2002; 15:66–78.
69. Playford EG, Walker J. Evaluation of the ICT malaria P.f/P.v and the OptiMAL rapid diagnostic tests for malaria in febrile returned travelers. J Clin Microbiol 2002;40: 4166–71.
70. Berry A, Fabre R, Benoit-Vical F, et al. Contribution of PCR-based methods to diagnosis and management of imported malaria. Med Trop 2005;65:176–83.
71. Schneider P, Wolters L, Schoone G, et al. Real-time nucleic acid sequence-based amplification is more convenient than real-time PCR for quantification of *Plasmodium falciparum*. J Clin Microbiol 2005;43:402–5.
72. Garcia LS, Shimizu RY, Bruckner DA. Blood parasites: problems in diagnosis using automated differential instrumentation. Diagn Microbiol Infect Dis 1986;4: 173–6.
73. Wever PC, Henskens YMC, Kager PA, et al. Detection of imported malaria with the Cell-Dyn 4000 hematology analyzer. J Clin Microbiol 2002;40:4729–31.
74. Rosenblatt JE. Antiparasitic agents. Mayo Clin Proc 1999;74:1161–75.
75. Dondorp AM, Newton PN, Mayxay M, et al. Fake antimalarials in Southeast Asia are a major impediment to malaria control: multinational cross-sectional survey on the prevalence of fake antimalarials. Trop Med Int Health 2004;9:1241–6.
76. Baird JK. Chloroquine resistance in *Plasmodium vivax*. Antimicrobial Agents Chemother 2004;48:4075–83.
77. Powell VI, Grima K. Exchange transfusion for malaria and *Babesia* infection. Transfus Med Rev 2002;16:239–50.
78. Ayisi JG, van Eijk AM, Newman RD, et al. Maternal malaria and perinatal HIV transmission, western Kenya. Emerg Infect Dis 2004;10:643–52.
79. Chen Q, Schlichtherle M, Wahlgren M. Molecular aspects of severe malaria. Clin Microbiol Rev 2001;13:439–50.
80. Breman JG. Eradicating malaria. Sci Prog 2009;92:1–38.
81. White NJ. How antimalarial drug resistance affects post-treatment prophylaxis. Malar J 2008;11:7–9.

Human Metapneumovirus

Christina R. Hermos, MD[a], Sara O. Vargas, MD[b,c],
Alexander J. McAdam, MD, PhD[b,d,*]

KEYWORDS

- Metapneumovirus • Respiratory syncytial virus
- Respiratory infection • Bronchiolitis

Respiratory tract infections (RTI) are the leading cause of death in low-income countries and the second leading cause of death in children less than 5 years old worldwide, according to the World Health Organization. Most upper and lower RTI (URTI and LRTI) are viral, although in many cases a pathogen is never identified.[1,2] Advances in viral diagnostics and molecular virology have allowed identification of previously unknown pathogens. Human metapneumovirus (hMPV) was discovered in 2001 in routine viral cultures of respiratory specimens from children with RTI. hMPV has been implicated as a common cause of URTI and LRTI in children and adults and a cause of severe disease in immunocompromised hosts.

MICROBIOLOGY

hMPV phylogenic classification is illustrated by the method of its discovery. Van den Hoogen and colleagues[3] identified 28 viral isolates from cultures of nasal secretions of patients presenting with symptoms of RTI. All isolates caused cytopathic effects in tertiary monkey kidney cells that were morphologically indistinguishable from, though later than, those of respiratory syncytial virus (RSV). On electron microscopy, these investigators observed pleomorphic particles measuring 150 to 600 nm with short envelope projections and rare nucleocapsids, features that are characteristics of Paramyxoviridae. A representative electron micrograph of hMPV is shown in **Fig. 1**. Other results that were also consistent with inclusion of the new virus in the Paramyxoviridae

[a] Division of Infectious Diseases, Department of Medicine, Children's Hospital Boston, 300 Longwood Avenue, Boston, MA 02115, USA
[b] Department of Pathology, Harvard Medical School, 77 Avenue Louis Pasteur, Boston, MA 02115, USA
[c] Department of Pathology, Children's Hospital Boston, 300 Longwood Avenue, Boston, MA 02115, USA
[d] Infectious Diseases Diagnostic Division, Department of Laboratory Medicine, Children's Hospital Boston, 300 Longwood Avenue, Boston, MA 02115, USA
* Corresponding author. Infectious Diseases Diagnostic Division, Department of Laboratory Medicine, Children's Hospital Boston, 300 Longwood Avenue, Boston, MA 02115.
E-mail address: Alexander.McAdam@childrens.harvard.edu

Clin Lab Med 30 (2010) 131–148
doi:10.1016/j.cll.2009.10.002
0272-2712/10/$ – see front matter © 2010 Elsevier Inc. All rights reserved.

labmed.theclinics.com

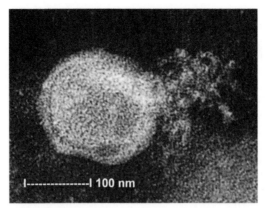

Fig. 1. Electron micrograph of hMPV grown in rhesus monkey kidney cells. The nucleocapsid is ruptured and the virion is spilling out. Note the pleomorphic viral shape and the envelope projections. (*From* Chan PKS, Tam JS, Lam C-W, Chan E, Wu A, Li C-K, et al. Human metapneumovirus detection in patients with severe acute respiratory syndrome. Emerg Infect Dis [serial online] 2003 Sept. Available from: URL: http://www.cdc.gov/ncidod/EID/vol9no9/03-0304.htm.)

included abrogation of infectivity by chloroform treatment, lack of hemagglutination of turkey, chicken, or guinea pig erythrocytes, and dependence on trypsin for replication in cell cultures.[3]

Members of the Paramyxoviridae family are enveloped viruses with single-stranded, nonsegmented, negative sense RNA. Paramyxoviridae include the subfamilies Paramyxovirinae and Pneumovirinae; the Pneumovirinae subfamily is further divided into the genera *Pneumovirus* and *Metapneumovirus*. RSV is an important human pathogen in the *Pneumovirus* genus. Metapneumoviruses differ from pneumoviruses by the absence of 2 nonstructural proteins, NS1 and NS2, and a difference in gene order.[3,4] Sequencing data from hMPV demonstrate an absence of NS1 and NS2 open reading frames (ORFs) and positioning of the F gene adjacent to the M gene, confirming its classification as a metapneumovirus.[4] The genomic organization of hMPV is 3-N-PM-F-M2-SH-G-L-5 with 2 ORFs of M2 coding for proteins M2-1 and M2-2. The other known member of the *Metapneumovirus* genus is avian pneumovirus.[3,5]

The sequence of the hMPV RNA suggests that hMPV makes 9 proteins. Three viral glycoproteins (attachment [G], fusion [F], and small hydrophobic [SH]) are believed to be inserted into the lipid envelope. The F protein contains an F1/F2 cleavage site in the hydrophobic region and has 2 heptad repeats in the extracellular domain, features distinctive for a viral protein that fuses viral and host cell membranes.[6,7] The G protein is a heavily glycosylated type II mucinlike protein, and its O glycosylation pattern, efficient export to the host cell surface, and type II membrane orientation suggest its role as an attachment protein.[8–11] The sequence of the G protein is highly variable between strains, similar to the RSV G protein, which suggests that there is serotypic variation of this protein (discussed later). A G-protein deficient mutant is able to replicate in vivo and in vitro, albeit less efficiently than wild-type hMPV, suggesting that G-protein is not absolutely required for viral replication.[12,13] The function of the SH protein remains unknown.

The helical nucleocapsid is believed to be composed of viral RNA and the nucleocapsid protein (N), phosphoprotein protein (P), large polymerase protein (L), and transcriptional enhancer protein (M2-1).[14] The 3 nucleocapsid proteins N, P, and L are likely involved with viral replication and transcription. M2-1 and M2-2 proteins of

Pneumovirinae are regulatory proteins, functioning as a transcriptional elongation factor (M2-1) and a promoter of viral assembly (M2-2) in RSV.[15] hMPV strains lacking M2-2 have more frequent point mutations and display upregulated transcription, supporting the role of M2-2 as a regulator of viral transcription.[16] The matrix protein (M) surrounds the nucleocapsid within the lipid envelope, and likely facilitates the connection of nucleocapsids with the viral lipid envelope.[14,15]

Van Den Hoogen separated hMPV into 2 lineages based on sequence homology. The distinct lineages, now called hMPV type A and B, have been identified in multiple phylogenic studies, and each type is further grouped into 2 subtypes, called A1, A2, B1, and B2.[9,17–20] Overall genetic identity between types is more than 80%, whereas amino acid sequence identity is more than 90%.[17,19,20] hMPV type A and B grouping is concordant based on sequence diversity between genes encoding for N, M, F, G, and L proteins, although the extent of sequence diversity varies.[17,19,21] Subtypes A1, A2, B1, and B2 are distinguished by diversity between gene sequences for the surface glycoproteins G and F. Identity of the F genes between subtypes within groups A and B is 94% to 96%, whereas identity between G gene sequences is 76% to 83%.[17,19]

EPIDEMIOLOGY

Humans are the only known natural host for hMPV. The virus is presumably spread from person to person by respiratory droplets similar to other paramyxoviruses, although this has not been definitively determined.[22] hMPV infection has been detected worldwide, with reports from North and South America, Europe, Asia, Africa, and Australia.[20,23–41] Serologic studies of stored specimens indicate that hMPV has infected humans for at least 5 decades.[3]

hMPV infection is seasonal, with winter epidemics occurring from December to April in the northern hemisphere, simultaneous with or slightly later than RSV epidemics (**Fig. 2**).[26,39,41–43] All 4 subtypes of hMPV usually circulate in the same season, and the predominant serotype may alternate in consecutive years in the same location.[20,42,44,45] Whereas Agapov and colleagues[21] found a shift in predominance

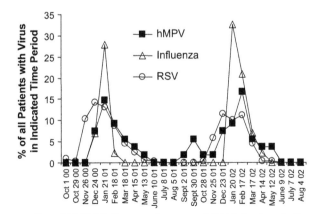

Fig. 2. The seasonality of hMPV, influenza viruses, and RSV infections in Boston, MA, USA. Each curve shows the percentage of patients with the indicated virus during the indicated 4-week period. (*From* McAdam AJ, Hasenbein ME, Feldman HA, et al. Human metapneumovirus in children tested at a tertiary-care hospital. J Infec Dis 2004;190(1):21–6; with permission.)

(>80% of isolates) from type B to type A in St Louis, Missouri, USA, Mackay and colleagues[46] detected a shift in predominant subtype (>50% of isolates) from A1 to A2 in Queensland, Australia in sequential years.

hMPV is most commonly a disease of young children, causing approximately 5% to 10% of LRTI in infants, and in some studies it is the second leading cause of bronchiolitis after RSV.[35,41,47–49] Multiple methods of evaluating seroprevalence have shown that more than 90% of children have evidence of prior hMPV infection by the age of 5 years.[3,50–52] The peak age of hMPV infection ranges from 5 to 22 months, typically older than that of RSV, younger than that of influenza, and with a more even distribution among age groups.[41,42,45,47,53–55] In 1 study of potential risk factors for viral infection, hMPV and coronavirus showed a stronger association to childcare attendance than RSV, picornaviruses, influenza viruses, adenovirus, and parainfluenza viruses.[39]

Young healthy adults have a higher yearly hMPV infection rate, ranging from 4% to 15%, than do elderly or high-risk adults, perhaps because of more frequent contact with children.[56] Yearly seroconversion rates in patients more than 65 years old living in long-term care facilities (LTCFs) is up to 12%, and in 1 hMPV outbreak among elderly patients in an LTCF the mortality in confirmed cases was 50%.[57,58] hMPV seroprevalence was found to be 83% among adults with underlying chronic obstructive pulmonary disease (COPD).[59]

CLINICAL PRESENTATION

hMPV is a respiratory pathogen known to cause LRTI and URTI. It is detected only rarely from asymptomatic hosts.[42,57] hMPV has been implicated in the cause of childhood bronchiolitis, pneumonia, asthma exacerbation, and croup, and it also plays a role in exacerbation of COPD in adults and severe disease in the immunocompromised host.

LRTI

hMPV has been isolated from respiratory specimens from children and adults with pneumonia.[33,42,60,61] Williams and colleagues[42] retrospectively identified hMPV in 20% of frozen respiratory samples that were collected for 20 years from children with LRTI. These samples had previously tested negative for other viruses. The hMPV rate in samples previously found to be positive for another virus (coinfection rate) was 4%, demonstrating that hMPV is most often found as sole pathogen. Diagnoses in this cohort included bronchiolitis in 59%, croup in 18%, pneumonia in 8%, and asthma exacerbation in 14%. Children presenting with hMPV LRTI commonly have a preceding URTI (83%), fever (52%–100%), dyspnea (80%–83%), cough (68%–90%), and coryza (88%). Signs of hMPV infection include rhinitis (64%–77%), wheezing/stridor (50%–56%), tachypnea (77%), abnormal tympanic membrane (51%), pharyngitis (39%), rhonchi (20%), rales (8%), and hypoxia of less than 90% (31%–38%).[26,29,42,45,53,60] In an analysis of 132 patients presenting with acute wheeze, hMPV accounted for 10 of 116 cases (9%) in which a pathogen was detected.[43]

Chest radiographs (CXRs) of patients with hMPV LRTI are abnormal in about half of patients, with findings that include diffuse perihilar infiltrates, peribronchial cuffing, lobar infiltrates, or hyperaeration (**Fig. 3**).[29,42,45,60] White blood cell counts and C-reactive protein levels are typically normal during acute hMPV infection with a range of 6.3 to 16.4×10^9/L (mean of 9.5–10.5) and 9 mg/L, respectively.[43,60]

It is not clear whether the severity of hMPV LRTI differs from that of other respiratory viruses. Williams and colleagues[42] found no difference in rates of abnormal CXRs, hospitalization, or emergency room visits when comparing the severity of disease caused by hMPV and other respiratory viruses (influenza, RSV, parainfluenza, and

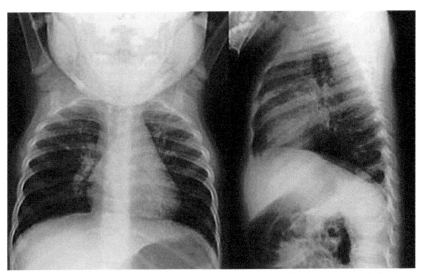

Fig. 3. CXR from a 6-month-old child with bronchiolitis caused by hMPV. Hyperinflation and diffuse infiltrates are seen. (*From* Williams JV, Harris PA, Tollefson SJ, et al. Human metapneumovirus and lower respiratory tract disease in children. N Engl J Med 2004;350:443; with permission.)

adenovirus). A smaller study from Thailand found longer mean hospitalizations (6.8 vs 3.5 days) for children with hMPV compared with RSV LRTI, although other studies showed no difference in rates of outpatient treatment and inpatient or intensive care unit (ICU) admissions between hMPV and RSV.[55,60]

Williams and colleagues[42] reported no clinical differences between infections caused by hMPV types A and B. However, Vicente and colleagues[62] suggest that infection with hMPV type A is more severe than infection with type B. They found that children with type A were more likely to present with pneumonia and had a higher mean severity score based on oxygen saturation of less than 90%, and admission to hospital or to an ICU.

Early studies suggested that coinfection with hMPV frequently occurs with severe RSV bronchiolitis in children. Greensill and colleagues[63] studied a cohort of infants with RSV-positive bronchiolitis admitted to the ICU and found that 70% overall and 90% of those without an underlying condition tested positive for hMPV. These investigators followed this observation with a larger retrospective study of children less than 2 years old with bronchitis and found that infants coinfected with hMPV and RSV were significantly more likely to be admitted to the ICU than infants infected with RSV only.[64] Williams and colleagues[42] later reported no epidemiologic or clinical differences between children infected with hMPV and children with hMPV coinfection with another respiratory virus. An additional study by van Woensel and colleagues [65] did not find hMPV coninfection in any of 30 children who required mechanical ventilation for RSV LRTI. Taken together, these studies suggest that hMPV coinfection is not required for, and is not particularly common with, severe manifestations of RSV bronchiolitis in young children.

URTI

Williams and colleagues[42] described children with hMPV URTI in a 20-year period during which 5% of specimens that were negative for other respiratory viruses tested positive for hMPV. Symptoms and signs most frequently included fever (54%), coryza (82%), cough (66%), rhinitis (79%), pharyngitis (63%), otalgia (31%), and abnormal tympanic membrane (63%). Other signs occurring in less than 10% of patients were hoarseness and conjunctivitis. hMPV was the most common pathogen isolated from another cohort of children tested for pertussis; 9.9% had hMPV versus 7.3% who tested positive for *Bordetella pertussis*, suggesting an overlap with the signs and symptoms of whooping cough.[66] As in LRTIs, hMPV serotype does not seem to affect URTI disease severity.[42]

The presence of otalgia and abnormal tympanic membranes suggests that hMPV is associated with acute otitis media in children.[42,67] In a prospective cohort of children aged 1 to 10 years presenting with acute otitis media, 13% were infected with hMPV.[68]

hMPV is a significant contributor to URTI in adults, accounting for 2% to 4.5% of URTIs in healthy adults and adults with cardiopulmonary diseases.[31,56,69,70] hMPV has also been implicated in COPD exacerbation and has been detected in up to 12% of patients with COPD exacerbations.[57,71] Another study documented that 4.2% of patients with COPD exacerbation seroconvert to hMPV.[59]

Immunocompromised and Vulnerable Hosts

hMPV causes URTI and LRTI in individuals infected with the human immunodeficiency virus (HIV). In South Africa, the hospitalization rates for hMPV pneumonia were more than 5-fold greater in children infected with HIV than in children who were HIV negative.[72] In a separate study, however, these investigators found no significant clinical differences between the HIV-negative and HIV-positive children hospitalized with hMPV infection, though HIV-infected children had a trend toward longer hospitalization (9 vs 2 days).[35] Clinical features of hMPV infection in this HIV-positive cohort include mean O_2 saturations of 92% on room air with 47% of children requiring supplemental oxygen. Half of these subjects had wheeze and 57% had rales; 50% received a diagnosis of bronchiolitis and 65% a diagnosis of pneumonia.[35]

hMPV can cause severe respiratory disease in immunocompromised hosts, as demonstrated by numerous case reports. Severe hMPV infections have been reported in patients with acute lymphoblastic leukemia (ALL), lymphoma, and lung cancer and patients following lung transplants and hematopoetic stem cell transplants (HSCT) (with and without concurrent neutropenia). In 2002, hMPV was identified at autopsy as the cause of a pneumonia-related death of a child being treated for ALL.[73] Of 2 hMPV-infected children younger than 5 years old with ALL on chemotherapy, 1 died of acquired respiratory distress syndrome; of 2 adults older than 65 years old with leukemia, neutropenia and hMPV, 1 died of pneumonitis.[53] In a prospective study of adult HSCT recipients with LRTI or URTI, 16 of 83 samples in which a pathogen was isolated tested positive for hMPV.[74] The yearly infection rate in these patients was 3% to 5%. Five patients had LRTI; significantly more patients with LRTI had had allogeneic transplants, and 2 patients died. In a separate series, 5 HSCT transplant patients who tested positive for hMPV progressed to hemorrhagic pneumonia, respiratory failure, and septic shock, and 4 of 5 patients died. In symptomatic patients who had had a lung transplant 4% to 14% of bronchoalveolar lavage (BAL) samples tested positive for hMPV; all patients clinically recovered, although in 1 series 60% of lung transplant patients infected with hMPV developed graft dysfunction.[44,66,75]

Similar to RSV, other high-risk conditions such as premature birth, congenital heart disease, and chronic lung disease increase the severity of disease and likelihood of hospitalization during hMPV infection.[26,35,62] Several cohorts of hMPV-infected children included more than 30% with an underlying condition such as prematurity, chronic lung disease, or congenital heart disease.[29,45,55,60] A 2-year prospective study followed 194 infants with prematurity or congenital heart disease and found that although just 2% of 567 RTI were caused by hMPV, 30% of those infections led to moderate or severe disease (only 15% of illnesses resulted in any positive viral diagnosis, suggesting an underdiagnosis of all pathogens in this study).[76]

PATHOGENESIS

Animal models used to study pathophysiology and immunogenicity of hMPV infection include the cotton rat, the BALB/c mouse, and cynomolgus macaques. Intranasal challenge of BALB/c mice and cotton rats with hMPV results in peak viral titer in nasal turbinates on day 2 and in lung homogenates on day 4 to 5 post infection.[77–79] Most small animal models show viral clearance from the respiratory tract by day 21, although BALB/c mice have prolonged infection with biphasic viral replication with hMPV serotype B.[80] Although mice show weight loss and breathing problems on days 5 to 7 post infection, rats seem to be asymptomatic.[78,81] In macaques, viral load in respiratory secretions peaks on day 4 then decreases to zero by day 10 post infection, and some macaques display rhinorrhea after nasal inoculation with hMPV.[82] In rodents and nonhuman primates, hMPV is detectable throughout the respiratory tract, but does not spread to any other internal organ.[79,82]

Histopathologic changes of the lung during hMPV infection have been studied in rodents, nonhuman primates, and humans. At the peak of infection with hMPV, the rat lungs show peribronchial lymphoplasmocytic infiltrates and edema of the bronchial submucosa.[79] Small and medium bronchi show hypersecretory epithelium. Mononuclear infiltrates cause alveolar interstitial expansion. Bronchial lumens contain sloughed epithelium, neutrophils, macrophages, and other debris. BALB/c mice develop parenchymal pneumonia and neutrophilic infiltrates during hMPV infection; they seem to have less severe peribronchiolitis than cotton rats, although increased histopathologic scores persist for 21 days compared with just 1 week in rats.[77,78] In macaques, histopathologic studies show a similar loss of ciliated epithelium, neutrophil transmigration, interstitial edema, and intraluminal sloughed epithelial cells and debris.[82] Six BAL samples and 3 lung biopsies from children with hMPV infection, obtained between 2 months before and 2 months after the positive hMPV specimen, were reported. BAL samples show epithelial cell degeneration or necrosis with ciliocytophthoria and round red cytoplasmic inclusions, hemosiderin-laden macrophages, frequent neutrophils and mucus (**Fig. 4**).[83] In acute disease, lung biopsies can show eosinophilic nuclear and cytoplasmic inclusions (**Fig. 5**). In more longstanding disease, chronic airway inflammation and intra-alveolar foamy and hemosiderin-laden macrophages have been observed.

Immunohistochemistry provides insight into the location and extent of viral replication in the respiratory tract. In cotton rats and macaques, hMPV antigen is detected at the luminal surfaces of epithelial cells from nasal tissue to bronchioles.[79] In macaques, individual or groups of ciliated cells are affected, often in morphologically normal tissue.[82] Goblet and basal cells are spared. Occasional positive hMPV staining is identified in alveoli, including type 1 pneumocytes, adjacent alveolar macrophages, and intraluminal debris, although giant cells are spared. It was unclear whether hMPV in intraluminal macrophages is from infection of macrophages or from phagocytosis of infected material.

hMPV infection of the respiratory tract leads to increased levels of chemokines and cytokines in respiratory secretions of animals and humans. Levels of macrophage inflammatory protein 1α (MIP-1α), regulation on activation of normal T cells expressed

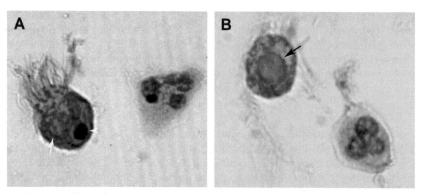

Fig. 4. Hematoxylin and eosin-stained BAL specimen from a 14-year-old girl who underwent lung transplantation, showing (*A*) a glassy red cytoplasmic inclusion within a ciliated respiratory epithelial cell with a degenerating (pyknotic) nucleus (*arrowhead*) and (*B*) a glassy pink inclusion within a ciliated respiratory epithelial cell without a visible nucleus. Original magnification, ×1000. (*From* Vargas SO, Kozakewich HPW, Perez-Atayde AP, et al. Pathology of human metapneumovirus infection: insights into the pathogenesis of a newly identified respiratory virus. Pediatr Dev Pathol 2004;7(5):478–86; with permission.)

and secreted (RANTES), interferon γ (IFN-γ), interleukin 4 (IL-4) and monocyte chemotactic protein 1 (MCP-1) all increase in the lungs of hMPV-infected mice.[78] Levels of mRNA for these cytokines in the lung (except IL-4, which was not measured) and IL-2 are also increased by hMPV infection in the cotton rat.[78] The kinetics with which the levels of these proteins increase and decrease parallel the kinetics of the inflammatory response within the rodent lung, and all decrease to baseline levels by 12 to 21 days after infection. In an analysis of respiratory specimens from infants with hMPV and RSV infection of similar clinical severity, hMPV elicited 2- to 6-fold lower production of IL-12, TNF-α, IL-6, IL-1β, IL-8, and IL-10.[84] These investigators suggest that mechanisms other than innate immunity must be elicited in human hMPV infection

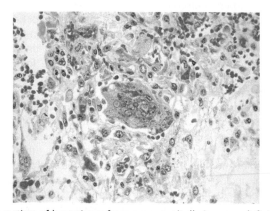

Fig. 5. Histologic section of lung tissue from a congenitally immunodeficient 15-month-old infant dying with culture-positive hMPV pneumonia. A giant cell (center) shows round smudgy pale pink intranuclear inclusions with a surrounding halo and globular dark pink intracytoplasmic inclusions (hemotoxylin and eosin; original magnification, ×400). (*Courtesy of* Milton J. Finegold, MD, Houston, TX, USA.)

to account for its clinical severity. These mechanisms might include direct epithelial damage, Th2 polarization leading to pulmonary airway hyperreactivity or chemokine-mediated inflammation.[84] Evidence for Th2 polarization in hMPV infection includes significantly lower IFN-γ/IL-4 ratios in secretions from infants infected with hMPV compared with influenza and RSV, suggesting a Th2 bias in the T-helper cell response to this pathogen.[85] These investigators also report that compared with influenza, hMPV and RSV infection result in lower levels of IFN-γ, IL-4, and IL-2 and that levels of cytokine production are not related to severity of illness for any of these viruses. These studies suggest that despite structures and clinical sequelae that are similar to other pathogens, innate immunity and inflammatory responses to hMPV are unique and not fully understood.

DIAGNOSIS
Culture

As discussed earlier, hMPV was discovered by culture of respiratory samples with tertiary monkey kidney cells. Cytopathic effects appear after 14 days (later than those typically caused by RSV), and they include cellular rounding without syncytia formation (**Fig. 6**).[3,86] The virus grows most efficiently in rhesus monkey kidney cell lines (LLC-MK2) with exogenous trypsin.[18,53,87] hMPV grows poorly in Vero and A-549 (human lung adenocarcinoma) cell lines and slowly in MDCK and MCR-5 cell lines.[3,18,53,67] More recently, it has been shown that hMPV replicates well without trypsin in a human bronchiolar cell line 16HBE140.[88] Despite improvements, culture

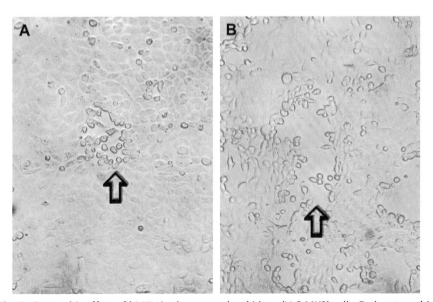

Fig. 6. Cytopathic effect of hMPV in rhesus monkey kidney (LLC-MK2) cells. Early cytopathic effect (*I*) shows a single focus of infected cells with refractile rounding is indicated by an arrow whereas late cytopathic effect (*B*) shows a larger focus and also shows detachment of cells from the monolayer. Original magnification ×100. (*From* Chan PKS, Tam JS, Lam C-W, Chan E, Wu A, Li C-K, et al. Human metapneumovirus detection in patients with severe acute respiratory syndrome. Emerg Infect Dis [serial online] 2003 Sept. Available from: URL: http://www.cdc.gov/ncidod/EID/vol9no9/03-0304.htm.)

is generally insensitive for detection of hMPV and this, along with the slow replication of the virus in culture, makes this an uncommon method for diagnosis of hMPV.

Immunofluorescent staining of shell vial centrifugation culture (SVCC) has been used successfully for a more rapid detection of respiratory viruses.[89] SVCC allows detection of viral antigen after a culture time of just 2 days. A monoclonal antibody (MAb-8) specific to hMPV is not useful for immunofluorescence assay (IFA) directly on patient specimens, but it can be used to detect hMPV when used with SVCC with several cell lines.[89] Subsequent studies have found the LLC-MK2 cell line is the most sensitive for SVCC of hMPV and that an incubation time of 3 to 5 days increases culture sensitivity.[90]

Immunoassays

Immunofluorescent staining for hMPV in respiratory secretions has moderate sensitivity and high specificity. Using an anti-hMPV mouse monoclonal IgG antibody, which recognizes both subgroups of hMPV A and B, Ebihara and colleagues[27] compared IFA to reverse transcriptase-polymerase chain reaction (RT-PCR) of posterior nasal samples. IFA was positive in 11 of 15 symptomatic patients who tested positive for hMPV by RT-PCR. In addition, 1 of 33 RT-PCR negative patients tested positive by IFA. The sensitivity and specificity of IFA compared with RT-PCR was found to be 73% and 97%, respectively. Similar results were obtained for direct fluorescent antibody staining of respiratory specimens with a pool of MAbs (sensitivity 72.7%, specificity 94.4%).[91]

Given its ease and objectivity, there is likely a clinical role for enzyme immunoassay (EIA) to detect antigen rapidly from nasopharyngeal aspirates. A commercial immunoassay for hMPV has been produced by Biotrin Ltd (Mount Merrion, Co. Dublin, Ireland), but it does not have approval by the US Food and Drug Administration (FDA) for clinical use. A combination of MAbs and matrix and fusion proteins is used as capture antibodies. Using culture and RT-PCR as gold standard, EIA was found to have a sensitivity and specificity of 81% and 100%, respectively.[92] A high proportion of samples gave equivocal results in this assay (8.3%) and, after performing discrepant analysis, the investigators counted these results as positive results, so more careful statistical evaluation of this test is needed. Despite their lower sensitivity than PCR, the ease, rapidity, and lower cost of IFA and EIA make them clinical diagnostics that could be feasibly offered by most microbiology laboratories.

PCR

PCR has been found to have higher sensitivity than culture and IFA.[27,93] Sensitive and specific RT-PCR techniques have been developed for the detection of hMPV from nasopharyngeal aspirates and bronchoalveolar lavage specimens. Primers chosen to amplify a segment of the N gene sequence have been shown to be the most sensitive when compared with primers directed at L, M, P, and F genes with sensitivities of 100%, 90%, 75%, 60%, and 55%, respectively.[94] When PCR amplification product is subjected to an enzyme-linked amplicon hybridization assay (ELAHA) the technique yields a 512-fold increased sensitivity compared with routine electrophoresis.[93] Real-time RT-PCR using the same primers as those used for PCR-ELAHA increases sensitivity, and reduces turn-around time and the risk for contamination to the assay. A nucleic acid sequence-based amplification (NASBA) assay targeting the M gene was found to be slightly less sensitive in pediatric patients compared with RT-PCR of the N gene.[66] These investigators also found RT-PCR and NASBA to be slightly less sensitive for the detection of hMPV serotype B than A. Real time RT-PCR for hMPV is available in 2 assays that have been approved by the FDA. The xTAG Respiratory Viral Panel (Luminex, Austin, TX, USA) is a multiplex PCR assay for several respiratory viruses in which PCR products are detected by hybridization to oligonucle-otides on fluorescent beads, which are then analyzed by flow cytometry. It is reported to have a sensitivity and specificity of 96% and 98.6%, respectively, for hMPV.[95] The second real time RT-PCR approved by the FDA for hMPV is the pro hMVP+ assay (Gen-Probe Prodesse, Waukesha, WI, USA). The package insert for this assay claims a sensitivity of 95.5% and a specificity of 99.3%.

Serology

Enzyme-linked immunosorbent assays (ELISAs) were first developed using hMPV-in-fected cells as antigen to detect hMPV antibody in sera.[3,28,50,52,53,56] To increase sensitivity and specificity, a recombinant N protein was developed as capture antigen.[96] The N protein was selected as antigen because it is highly conserved between hMPV types A and B.[19] An ELISA using recombinant N-A or N-B protein can reliably detect seroconversion in recently infected individuals, although there is significant cross-reactivity between the 2 types caused by antibody recognition of conserved epitopes.[96] An ELISA has also been developed using a recombinant F protein as antigen, also showing 100% cross-reactivity between hMPV serotypes A and B.[51] By developing recombinant G-proteins from each of the 4 hMPV subgroups, Endo and colleagues[97] were able to detect subtype specific antibody in all convales-cent samples from hMPV-infected children.

DIFFERENTIAL DIAGNOSIS

The clinical presentation for hMPV, including URTI and LRTI, is most similar to that of RSV. The differential diagnosis for hMPV includes other respiratory viruses such as influenza A and B, RSV, parainfluenza viruses, rhinoviruses, coronaviruses, and para-influenza viruses. In addition, bacterial causes of community-acquired pneumonia must also be considered. In patients with underlying asthma and COPD, acute hMPV infection may mimic exacerbations of these conditions. The differential diag-nosis for hMPV is summarized in **Table 1**.

TREATMENT, PROGNOSIS, AND LONG-TERM OUTCOME

There is currently no approved, specific therapy for hMPV infection, and treatment is supportive. Several agents have been evaluated for their effect on hMPV repli-cation in vitro or in animal models. Ribavirin and pooled human immunoglobulin inhibit hMPV and RSV replication equally in cell culture.[98] Ribavarin also reduces

Table 1
Differential diagnosis for syndromes resembling hMPV infection

Viruses	RSV
	Influenza A and B viruses
	Parainfluenza viruses
	Coronaviruses
	Picornaviruses (eg, rhinovirus)
	Adenovirus
Bacterial infections	*Mycoplasma pneumoniae*
	Chlamydia pneumoniae
	Bordatella pertussis
Noninfectious causes	Asthma
	COPD

the level of hMPV and inflammation in infected BALB/c mice.[99] Palivizumab and other chemotherapeutics directed at the F protein of RSV are not active against hMPV.[98] NMSO3, a sulfated sialyl lipid known to inhibit RSV replication in cell culture and in the cotton rat model, has also been shown to inhibit hMPV replication, syncytia formation, and cell-to-cell virus spread in culture.[100] None of these compounds have been systematically tested in humans for the treatment of hMPV infection, although a case report describes apparently successful treatment with ribavirin of a patient who had undergone lung transplant and had severe hMPV infection.[101]

Novel experimental therapeutics for hMPV have been evaluated in model systems, but not in humans. Two potent small interfering RNAs targeting the nucleoprotein and phosphoprotein mRNA inhibit 50% of hMPV replication in vitro at subnanomolar concentrations.[102] Another strategy for therapy targets a coiled-coil structure formed by multimers of the F-protein during fusion of the viral and host-cell membranes.[103] Treatment of hMPV-infected mice with a peptide (HRA2) that mimics the hydrophobic F-protein heptad repeats, protects mice from lethal hMPV infection if the peptide is given at the time of initial infection, but not if it is given a day later.[103] Administration of HRA2 at the time of hMPV infection also prevented infection associated airway obstruction and reduced production of inflammatory markers (RANTES, MCP-1 and IFN-γ) in the mouse lung.[103]

IMMUNITY AND REINFECTION

It is controversial whether the 2 hMPV genetic lineages, A and B, are different serotypes. Van den Hoogen and colleagues[17] studied in vitro neutralization of hMPV infectivity with antisera raised in ferrets infected with type A or B hMPV. They found reduced neutralization capacity by antisera raised to the heterologous hMPV lineage and preserved neutralization of hMPV strains within the same lineage, suggesting that lineages A and B represent distinct serotypes. However, Skiadopoulos and colleagues[81] measured the cross-protective efficacy between types A and B hMPV in the hamster and nonhuman primate models and found that the hMPV types A and B are highly antigenically related and conferred significant cross-protection measured by viral replication in the respiratory tract, indicating that they do not represent distinct serotypes. Whether there is cross-protection in humans between the hMPV types remains to be fully explored.

Human adult populations typically show 100% seroprevalence of stable neutralizing antibodies against hMPV. Reinfection rates in adults are between 1% and 9% yearly. It is thought that such frequent reinfection throughout life explains the ubiquitous presence of anti-hMPV antibody in the adult population.[53,56,104] The high frequency of seropositivity in children, and frequent infection and seroconversion in adults, suggests that immunity to hMPV is short lived and probably provides only incomplete protection.

Reinfection with hMPV has also been well documented in children. Williams and colleagues[42] describe several patients who presented with distinct hMPV clinical episodes from homologous and heterologous hMPV lineages. Recurrent infection in HIV-1-infected children caused by homologous and heterologous strains has also been reported.[72] Consistent with reports of recurrent infections in humans in subsequent seasons, cynomolgus macaques infected with 3 consecutive doses of wild-type hMPV were not protected against challenge infection after 8 months. Such a finding suggests that vaccine candidates would require enhanced immunogenicity to confer long-term protection.[105]

REFERENCES

1. Ruiz M, Ewig S, Marcos MA, et al. Etiology of community-acquired pneumonia: impact of age, comorbidity, and severity. Am J Respir Crit Care Med 1999; 160(2):397–405.
2. Cevey-Macherel M, Galetto-Lacour A, Gervaix A, et al. Etiology of community-acquired pneumonia in hospitalized children based on WHO clinical guidelines. Eur J Pediatr 2009. [Epub ahead of print].
3. van den Hoogen BG, de Jong JC, Groen J, et al. A newly discovered human pneumovirus isolated from young children with respiratory tract disease. Nat Med 2001;7(6):719–24.
4. van den Hoogen BG, Bestebroer TM, Osterhaus AD, et al. Analysis of the genomic sequence of a human metapneumovirus. Virology 2002;295(1): 119–32.
5. Njenga MK, Lwamba HM, Seal BS. Metapneumoviruses in birds and humans. Virus Res 2003;91(2):163–9.
6. Collins PL, Mottet G. Oligomerization and post-translational processing of glyco-protein G of human respiratory syncytial virus: altered O-glycosylation in the presence of brefeldin A. J Gen Virol 1992;73(Pt 4):849–63.
7. Broor S, Bharaj P, Chahar HS. Human metapneumovirus: a new respiratory pathogen. J Biosci 2008;33(4):483–93.
8. Bastien N, Liu L, Ward D, et al. Genetic variability of the G glycoprotein gene of human metapneumovirus. J Clin Microbiol 2004;42(8):3532–7.
9. Bastien N, Normand S, Taylor T, et al. Sequence analysis of the N, P, M and F genes of Canadian human metapneumovirus strains. Virus Res 2003;93(1): 51–62.
10. Peret TC, Abed Y, Anderson LJ, et al. Sequence polymorphism of the predicted human metapneumovirus G glycoprotein. J Gen Virol 2004;85(Pt 3):679–86.
11. Liu L, Bastien N, Li Y. Intracellular processing, glycosylation, and cell surface expression of human metapneumovirus attachment glycoprotein. J Virol 2007; 81(24):13435–43.
12. Biacchesi S, Skiadopoulos MH, Yang L, et al. Recombinant human metapneu-movirus lacking the small hydrophobic SH and/or attachment G glycoprotein: deletion of G yields a promising vaccine candidate. J Virol 2004;78(23): 12877–87.
13. Biacchesi S, Pham QN, Skiadopoulos MH, et al. Infection of nonhuman primates with recombinant human metapneumovirus lacking the SH, G, or M2-2 protein categorizes each as a nonessential accessory protein and identifies vaccine candidates. J Virol 2005;79(19):12608–13.
14. Crowe JE Jr. Human metapneumovirus as a major cause of human respiratory tract disease. Pediatr Infect Dis J 2004;23(Suppl 11):S215–21.
15. Easton AJ, Domachowske JB, Rosenberg HF. Animal pneumoviruses: molecular genetics and pathogenesis. Clin Microbiol Rev 2004;17(2):390–412.
16. Schickli JH, Kaur J, Macphail M, et al. Deletion of human metapneumovirus M2-2 increases mutation frequency and attenuates growth in hamsters. Virol J 2008;5:69.
17. van den Hoogen BG, Herfst S, Sprong L, et al. Antigenic and genetic variability of human metapneumoviruses. Emerg Infect Dis 2004;10(4):658–66.
18. Peret TC, Boivin G, Li Y, et al. Characterization of human metapneumoviruses isolated from patients in North America. J Infect Dis 2002;185(11):1660–3.
19. Biacchesi S, Skiadopoulos MH, Boivin G, et al. Genetic diversity between human metapneumovirus subgroups. Virology 2003;315(1):1–9.

20. Boivin G, Mackay I, Sloots TP, et al. Global genetic diversity of human meta-pneumovirus fusion gene. Emerg Infect Dis 2004;10(6):1154–7.
21. Agapov E, Sumino KC, Gaudreault-Keener M, et al. Genetic variability of human metapneumovirus infection: evidence of a shift in viral genotype without a change in illness. J Infect Dis 2006;193(3):396–403.
22. Hall CB, Douglas RG Jr. Modes of transmission of respiratory syncytial virus. J Pediatr 1981;99(1):100–3.
23. Al-Sonboli N, Hart CA, Al-Aeryani A, et al. Respiratory syncytial virus and human metapneumovirus in children with acute respiratory infections in Yemen. Pediatr Infect Dis J 2005;24(8):734–6.
24. Bastien N, Ward D, Van Caeseele P, et al. Human metapneumovirus infection in the Canadian population. J Clin Microbiol 2003;41(10):4642–6.
25. Cuevas LE, Nasser AM, Dove W, et al. Human metapneumovirus and respiratory syncytial virus, Brazil. Emerg Infect Dis 2003;9(12):1626–8.
26. Dollner H, Risnes K, Radtke A, et al. Outbreak of human metapneumovirus infection in Norwegian children. Pediatr Infect Dis J 2004;23(5):436–40.
27. Ebihara T, Endo R, Kikuta H, et al. Human metapneumovirus infection in Japanese children. J Clin Microbiol 2004;42(1):126–32.
28. Ebihara T, Endo R, Kikuta H, et al. Seroprevalence of human metapneumovirus in Japan. J Med Virol 2003;70(2):281–3.
29. Esper F, Boucher D, Weibel C, et al. Human metapneumovirus infection in the United States: clinical manifestations associated with a newly emerging respiratory infection in children. Pediatrics 2003;111(6 Pt 1):1407–10.
30. Garcia-Garcia ML, Calvo C, Perez-Brena P, et al. Prevalence and clinical characteristics of human metapneumovirus infections in hospitalized infants in Spain. Pediatr Pulmonol 2006;41(9):863–71.
31. Gray GC, Capuano AW, Setterquist SF, et al. Multi-year study of human metapneumovirus infection at a large US Midwestern Medical Referral Center. J Clin Virol 2006;37(4):269–76.
32. Gray GC, Capuano AW, Setterquist SF, et al. Human metapneumovirus, Peru. Emerg Infect Dis 2006;12(2):347–50.
33. Kim YK, Lee HJ. Human metapneumovirus-associated lower respiratory tract infections in Korean infants and young children. Pediatr Infect Dis J 2005;24(12):1111–2.
34. Ludewick HP, Abed Y, van Niekerk N, et al. Human metapneumovirus genetic variability, South Africa. Emerg Infect Dis 2005;11(7):1074–8.
35. Madhi SA, Ludewick H, Abed Y, et al. Human metapneumovirus-associated lower respiratory tract infections among hospitalized human immunodeficiency virus type 1 (HIV-1)-infected and HIV-1-uninfected African infants. Clin Infect Dis 2003;37(12):1705–10.
36. Maggi F, Pifferi M, Vatteroni M, et al. Human metapneumovirus associated with respiratory tract infections in a 3-year study of nasal swabs from infants in Italy. J Clin Microbiol 2003;41(7):2987–91.
37. Peiris JS, Tang WH, Chan KH, et al. Children with respiratory disease associated with metapneumovirus in Hong Kong. Emerg Infect Dis 2003;9(6):628–33.
38. Nissen MD, Siebert DJ, Mackay IM, et al. Evidence of human metapneumovirus in Australian children. Med J Aust 2002;176(4):188.
39. Lambert SB, Allen KM, Druce JD, et al. Community epidemiology of human metapneumovirus, human coronavirus NL63, and other respiratory viruses in healthy preschool-aged children using parent-collected specimens. Pediatrics 2007;120(4):e929–37.

40. Rao BL, Gandhe SS, Pawar SD, et al. First detection of human metapneumovirus in children with acute respiratory infection in India: a preliminary report. J Clin Microbiol 2004;42(12):5961–2.
41. McAdam AJ, Hasenbein ME, Feldman HA, et al. Human metapneumovirus in children tested at a tertiary-care hospital. J Infect Dis 2004;190(1):20–6.
42. Williams JV, Harris PA, Tollefson SJ, et al. Human metapneumovirus and lower respiratory tract disease in otherwise healthy infants and children. N Engl J Med 2004;350(5):443–50.
43. Jartti T, van den Hoogen B, Garofalo RP, et al. Metapneumovirus and acute wheezing in children. Lancet 2002;360(9343):1393–4.
44. Hopkins MJ, Redmond C, Shaw JM, et al. Detection and characterisation of human metapneumovirus from children with acute respiratory symptoms in north-west England, UK. J Clin Virol 2008;42(3):273–9.
45. Esper F, Martinello RA, Boucher D, et al. A 1-year experience with human metapneumovirus in children aged <5 years. J Infect Dis 2004;189(8):1388–96.
46. Mackay IM, Bialasiewicz S, Jacob KC, et al. Genetic diversity of human metapneumovirus over 4 consecutive years in Australia. J Infect Dis 2006;193(12): 1630–3.
47. Xepapadaki P, Psarras S, Bossios A, et al. Human metapneumovirus as a causative agent of acute bronchiolitis in infants. J Clin Virol 2004;30(3):267–70.
48. Freymouth F, Vabret A, Legrand L, et al. Presence of the new human metapneumovirus in French children with bronchiolitis. Pediatr Infect Dis J 2003;22(1):92–4.
49. Mansbach JM, Emond JA, Camargo CA Jr. Bronchiolitis in US emergency departments 1992 to 2000: epidemiology and practice variation. Pediatr Emerg Care 2005;21(4):242–7.
50. Ebihara T, Endo R, Kikuta H, et al. Comparison of the seroprevalence of human metapneumovirus and human respiratory syncytial virus. J Med Virol 2004; 72(2):304–6.
51. Leung J, Esper F, Weibel C, et al. Seroepidemiology of human metapneumovirus (hMPV) on the basis of a novel enzyme-linked immunosorbent assay utilizing hMPV fusion protein expressed in recombinant vesicular stomatitis virus. J Clin Microbiol 2005;43(3):1213–9.
52. Wolf DG, Zakay-Rones Z, Fadeela A, et al. High seroprevalence of human metapneumovirus among young children in Israel. J Infect Dis 2003;188(12):1865–7.
53. Boivin G, Abed Y, Pelletier G, et al. Virological features and clinical manifestations associated with human metapneumovirus: a new paramyxovirus responsible for acute respiratory-tract infections in all age groups. J Infect Dis 2002; 186(9):1330–4.
54. Caracciolo S, Minini C, Colombrita D, et al. Human metapneumovirus infection in young children hospitalized with acute respiratory tract disease: virologic and clinical features. Pediatr Infect Dis J 2008;27(5):406–12.
55. Martin ET, Kuypers J, Heugel J, et al. Clinical disease and viral load in children infected with respiratory syncytial virus or human metapneumovirus. Diagn Microbiol Infect Dis 2008;62(4):382–8.
56. Falsey AR, Erdman D, Anderson LJ, et al. Human metapneumovirus infections in young and elderly adults. J Infect Dis 2003;187(5):785–90.
57. Falsey AR. Human metapneumovirus infection in adults. Pediatr Infect Dis J 2008;27(Suppl 10):S80–3.
58. Boivin G, De Serres G, Hamelin ME, et al. An outbreak of severe respiratory tract infection due to human metapneumovirus in a long-term care facility. Clin Infect Dis 2007;44(9):1152–8.

59. Hamelin ME, Cote S, Laforge J, et al. Human metapneumovirus infection in adults with community-acquired pneumonia and exacerbation of chronic obstructive pulmonary disease. Clin Infect Dis 2005;41(4):498–502.
60. Samransamruajkit R, Thanasugarn W, Prapphal N, et al. Human metapneumovirus in infants and young children in Thailand with lower respiratory tract infections; molecular characteristics and clinical presentations. J Infect 2006;52(4): 254–63.
61. Vicente D, Cilla G, Montes M, et al. Human metapneumovirus and community-acquired respiratory illness in children. Emerg Infect Dis 2003;9(5):602–3.
62. Vicente D, Montes M, Cilla G, et al. Differences in clinical severity between genotype A and genotype B human metapneumovirus infection in children. Clin Infect Dis 2006;42(12):e111–3.
63. Greensill J, McNamara PS, Dove W, et al. Human metapneumovirus in severe respiratory syncytial virus bronchiolitis. Emerg Infect Dis 2003;9(3):372–5.
64. Semple MG, Cowell A, Dove W, et al. Dual infection of infants by human metapneumovirus and human respiratory syncytial virus is strongly associated with severe bronchiolitis. J Infect Dis 2005;191(3):382–6.
65. van Woensel JB, Bos AP, Lutter R, et al. Absence of human metapneumovirus co-infection in cases of severe respiratory syncytial virus infection. Pediatr Pulmonol 2006;41(9):872–4.
66. Dare R, Sanghavi S, Bullotta A, et al. Diagnosis of human metapneumovirus infection in immunosuppressed lung transplant recipients and children evaluated for pertussis. J Clin Microbiol 2007;45(2):548–52.
67. Boivin G, De Serres G, Cote S, et al. Human metapneumovirus infections in hospitalized children. Emerg Infect Dis 2003;9(6):634–40.
68. Schildgen O, Geikowski T, Glatzel T, et al. Frequency of human metapneumovirus in the upper respiratory tract of children with symptoms of an acute otitis media. Eur J Pediatr 2005;164(6):400–1.
69. Stockton J, Stephenson I, Fleming D, et al. Human metapneumovirus as a cause of community-acquired respiratory illness. Emerg Infect Dis 2002;8(9):897–901.
70. van den Hoogen BG, Osterhaus DM, Fouchier RA. Clinical impact and diagnosis of human metapneumovirus infection. Pediatr Infect Dis J 2004;23(Suppl 1):S25–32.
71. Martinello RA, Esper F, Weibel C, et al. Human metapneumovirus and exacerbations of chronic obstructive pulmonary disease. J Infect 2006;53(4):248–54.
72. Madhi SA, Ludewick H, Kuwanda L, et al. Seasonality, incidence, and repeat human metapneumovirus lower respiratory tract infections in an area with a high prevalence of human immunodeficiency virus type-1 infection. Pediatr Infect Dis J 2007;26(8):693–9.
73. Pelletier G, Dery P, Abed Y, et al. Respiratory tract reinfections by the new human metapneumovirus in an immunocompromised child. Emerg Infect Dis 2002;8(9):976–8.
74. Martino R, Porras RP, Rabella N, et al. Prospective study of the incidence, clinical features, and outcome of symptomatic upper and lower respiratory tract infections by respiratory viruses in adult recipients of hematopoietic stem cell transplants for hematologic malignancies. Biol Blood Marrow Transplant 2005; 11(10):781–96.
75. Gerna G, Campanini G, Rovida F, et al. Changing circulation rate of human metapneumovirus strains and types among hospitalized pediatric patients during three consecutive winter-spring seasons. Brief report. Arch Virol 2005; 150(11):2365–75.

76. Klein MI, Coviello S, Bauer G, et al. The impact of infection with human metapneumovirus and other respiratory viruses in young infants and children at high risk for severe pulmonary disease. J Infect Dis 2006;193(11):1544–51.

77. Darniot M, Petrella T, Aho S, et al. Immune response and alteration of pulmonary function after primary human metapneumovirus (hMPV) infection of BALB/c mice. Vaccine 2005;23(36):4473–80.

78. Hamelin ME, Yim K, Kuhn KH, et al. Pathogenesis of human metapneumovirus lung infection in BALB/c mice and cotton rats. J Virol 2005;79(14):8894–903.

79. Williams JV, Tollefson SJ, Johnson JE, et al. The cotton rat (Sigmodon hispidus) is a permissive small animal model of human metapneumovirus infection, pathogenesis, and protective immunity. J Virol 2005;79(17):10944–51.

80. Alvarez R, Tripp RA. The immune response to human metapneumovirus is associated with aberrant immunity and impaired virus clearance in BALB/c mice. J Virol 2005;79(10):5971–8.

81. Skiadopoulos MH, Biacchesi S, Buchholz UJ, et al. The two major human metapneumovirus genetic lineages are highly related antigenically, and the fusion (F) protein is a major contributor to this antigenic relatedness. J Virol 2004;78(13): 6927–37.

82. Kuiken T, van den Hoogen BG, van Riel DA, et al. Experimental human metapneumovirus infection of cynomolgus macaques (Macaca fascicularis) results in virus replication in ciliated epithelial cells and pneumocytes with associated lesions throughout the respiratory tract. Am J Pathol 2004;164(6):1893–900.

83. Vargas SO, Kozakewich HP, Perez-Atayde AR, et al. Pathology of human metapneumovirus infection: insights into the pathogenesis of a newly identified respiratory virus. Pediatr Dev Pathol 2004;7(5):478–86 [discussion: 421].

84. Laham FR, Israele V, Casellas JM, et al. Differential production of inflammatory cytokines in primary infection with human metapneumovirus and with other common respiratory viruses of infancy. J Infect Dis 2004;189(11): 2047–56.

85. Melendi GA, Laham FR, Monsalvo AC, et al. Cytokine profiles in the respiratory tract during primary infection with human metapneumovirus, respiratory syncytial virus, or influenza virus in infants. Pediatrics 2007;120(2):e410–5.

86. Chan PK, Tam JS, Lam CW, et al. Human metapneumovirus detection in patients with severe acute respiratory syndrome. Emerg Infect Dis 2003;9(9):1058–63.

87. Biacchesi S, Skiadopoulos MH, Tran KC, et al. Recovery of human metapneumovirus from cDNA: optimization of growth in vitro and expression of additional genes. Virology 2004;321(2):247–59.

88. Ingram RE, Fenwick F, McGuckin R, et al. Detection of human metapneumovirus in respiratory secretions by reverse-transcriptase polymerase chain reaction, indirect immunofluorescence, and virus isolation in human bronchial epithelial cells. J Med Virol 2006;78(9):1223–31.

89. Landry ML, Ferguson D, Cohen S, et al. Detection of human metapneumovirus in clinical samples by immunofluorescence staining of shell vial centrifugation cultures prepared from three different cell lines. J Clin Microbiol 2005;43(4): 1950–2.

90. Reina J, Ferres F, Alcoceba E, et al. Comparison of different cell lines and incubation times in the isolation by the shell vial culture of human metapneumovirus from pediatric respiratory samples. J Clin Virol 2007;40(1):46–9.

91. Percivalle E, Sarasini A, Visai L, et al. Rapid detection of human metapneumovirus strains in nasopharyngeal aspirates and shell vial cultures by monoclonal antibodies. J Clin Microbiol 2005;43(7):3443–6.

92. Kukavica-Ibrulj I, Boivin G. Detection of human metapneumovirus antigens in nasopharyngeal aspirates using an enzyme immunoassay. J Clin Virol 2009; 44(1):88–90.

93. Mackay IM, Jacob KC, Woolhouse D, et al. Molecular assays for detection of human metapneumovirus. J Clin Microbiol 2003;41(1):100–5.

94. Cote S, Abed Y, Boivin G. Comparative evaluation of real-time PCR assays for detection of the human metapneumovirus. J Clin Microbiol 2003;41(8):3631–5.

95. Mahony JB. Detection of respiratory viruses by molecular methods. Clin Microbiol Rev 2008;21(4):716–47.

96. Hamelin ME, Boivin G. Development and validation of an enzyme-linked immunosorbent assay for human metapneumovirus serology based on a recombinant viral protein. Clin Diagn Lab Immunol 2005;12(2):249–53.

97. Endo R, Ebihara T, Ishiguro N, et al. Detection of four genetic subgroup-specific antibodies to human metapneumovirus attachment (G) protein in human serum. J Gen Virol 2008;89(Pt 8):1970–7.

98. Wyde PR, Chetty SN, Jewell AM, et al. Comparison of the inhibition of human metapneumovirus and respiratory syncytial virus by ribavirin and immune serum globulin in vitro. Antiviral Res 2003;60(1):51–9.

99. Hamelin ME, Prince GA, Boivin G. Effect of ribavirin and glucocorticoid treatment in a mouse model of human metapneumovirus infection. Antimicrob Agents Chemother 2006;50(2):774–7.

100. Wyde PR, Moylett EH, Chetty SN, et al. Comparison of the inhibition of human metapneumovirus and respiratory syncytial virus by NMSO3 in tissue culture assays. Antiviral Res 2004;63(1):51–9.

101. Raza K, Ismailjee SB, Crespo M, et al. Successful outcome of human metapneumovirus (hMPV) pneumonia in a lung transplant recipient treated with intravenous ribavirin. J Heart Lung Transplant 2007;26(8):862–4.

102. Deffrasnes C, Cavanagh MH, Goyette N, et al. Inhibition of human metapneumovirus replication by small interfering RNA. Antivir Ther 2008;13(6):821–32.

103. Deffrasnes C, Hamelin ME, Prince GA, et al. Identification and evaluation of a highly effective fusion inhibitor for human metapneumovirus. Antimicrob Agents Chemother 2008;52(1):279–87.

104. Hamelin ME, Abed Y, Boivin G. Human metapneumovirus: a new player among respiratory viruses. Clin Infect Dis 2004;38(7):983–90.

105. van den Hoogen BG, Herfst S, de Graaf M, et al. Experimental infection of macaques with human metapneumovirus induces transient protective immunity. J Gen Virol 2007;88(Pt 4):1251–9.

Dengue Virus

Ted M. Ross, PhD

KEYWORDS
- Dengue virus • Flavivirus • Infection• Clinical diagnosis
- Vaccines

OVERVIEW

Dengue fever (DF), the most prevalent arthropod-borne viral illness in humans, is caused by the dengue virus (DENV). The 4 serotypes of DENV (DENV 1-4) are transmitted to humans primarily by the *Aedes aegypti* mosquito (**Fig. 1**).

DENV is a member of the Flaviviridae family and is related to the viruses that cause yellow fever and the Japanese, St. Louis, and West Nile encephalitides.[1] Infection by DENV causes a spectrum of clinical diseases that range from an acute debilitating, self-limited febrile illness, DF, to a life-threatening hemorrhagic and capillary leak syndrome of dengue hemorrhagic fever/dengue shock syndrome (DHF/DSS). DENV causes an estimated 25 to 100 million cases of DF and 250,000 cases of DHF per year worldwide, with 2.5 billion people at risk of infection.[2,3] At present, no approved antiviral treatment or vaccine is in use, and therapy is supportive in nature (**Fig. 2**).

Epidemic DHF was first recognized in the 1950s in Southeast Asia, and by 1975 it had become a leading cause of hospitalization and death among children in many countries in that region. In the 1980s, DHF began a second expansion into Asia, and in countries where DHF is endemic, the epidemics have become progressively larger over the last 15 years (**Box 1**). In 1980, the first indigenous transmission of dengue in the United States in more than 40 years occurred. Later, infections also occurred in Texas. In 2001 to 2002, a dengue outbreak occurred in Hawaii spread by *Aedes albopictus* mosquitoes.

The Americas have seen the most dramatic rise in the emergence of dengue cases (**Fig. 3**). The mosquito vector for dengue was eradicated in most of the region as part of the Pan American Health Organization's yellow fever eradication campaign in the 1950s and 1960s. The *A aegypti* eradication program was officially discontinued in the United States and other Western Hemisphere regions, leading to reinfestation of the mosquito vector in most countries during the 1980s and 1990s. By 1997, the geographic distribution of *A aegypti* was wider than its distribution before the eradication program. Dengue is now endemic in much of the Western Hemisphere.

Funding Support: TMR is supported by research awards, W81XWH-BAA-06-1 and W81XWH-BAA-06-2, from the United States Department of Defense.
Department of Microbiology and Molecular Genetics, Center for Vaccine Research, University of Pittsburgh, 9047 BST3, 3501 Fifth Avenue, Pittsburgh, PA 15261, USA
E-mail address: tmr15@pitt.edu

Clin Lab Med 30 (2010) 149–160
doi:10.1016/j.cll.2009.10.007
0272-2712/10/$ – see front matter © 2010 Elsevier Inc. All rights reserved.

labmed.theclinics.com

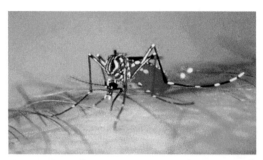

Fig. 1. The *A aegypti* mosquito is the most common epidemic vector for spread of dengue virus. It can be identified by the white bands or scale patterns on its legs and thorax. (*Courtesy of* Centers for Disease Control and Prevention (CDC), http://www.cdc.gov/ncidod/dvbid/dengue.)

Hyperendemicity, the presence of multiple circulating serotypes, is widespread in most countries and epidemics caused by multiple serotypes are more frequent.

VIROLOGY

DENV is an enveloped virus with a single-stranded, positive-sense 10.7 kilobase RNA genome,[4] which is translated as a single polyprotein and then cleaved into 3 structural proteins (capsid [C], premembrane/membrane [prM/M], and envelope [E]) and 7 nonstructural (NS) proteins by virus- and host-encoded proteases. The 3 structural components are required for capsid formation (C) and assembly into viral particles (prM and E). The NS proteins contain a serine protease and ATP-dependent helicase (NS3), which is required for virus polyprotein processing, a methyltransferase and RNA-dependent RNA polymerase (NS5), and a cofactor for the NS3 protease (NS2B). NS4B has been implicated in blocking the interferon (IFN) response. NS1, NS2A, and NS4A have either unknown or incompletely understood functions. All the NS proteins appear to be necessary for efficient replication.

In primary DENV infection, the virus enters target cells after the E protein adheres to cell surface receptors, such as dendritic cell-specific intercellular adhesion molecule-3-grabbing non-integrin (DC-SIGN) on dendritic cells.[5] Viral uptake occurs by receptor-mediated endocytosis. Endosomal acidification induces a conformational change in the E protein, resulting in fusion of the viral and endosomal membranes and nucleocapsid release into the cytoplasm.[6,7] Virus genome replication occurs in discrete domains within the endoplasmic reticulum (ER). Virus assembly occurs at the ER, and virions are exocytosed via Golgi-derived secretory vesicles.[8]

EPIDEMIOLOGY

Following the bite of a mosquito, usually *A aegypti* or *A albopictus*,[2] DENV can cause a range of mild-to-severe illnesses. The mosquito eradication program, which was officially discontinued in the United States in 1970, gradually weakened elsewhere, and the mosquito began to reinfest countries from which it had been eradicated. Consequently, the geographic distribution of *A aegypti* in 2002 was much wider than that before the eradication program and there was a corresponding increase in dengue infections. There are 4 distinct serotypes of DENV. Primary infection with one DENV serotype provides lifelong immunity to that specific serotype. However, when an individual is infected with a different serotype of DENV, there is an increased

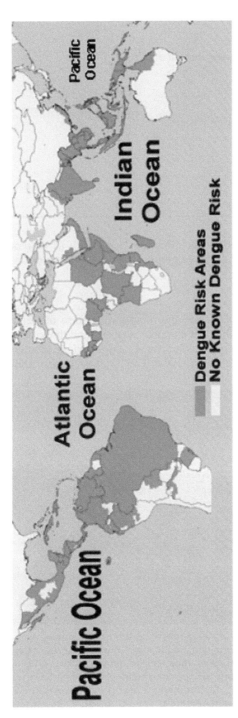

Fig. 2. World map indicating regions with known risks of dengue infection. (*Courtesy of CDC, available at:* http://www.cdc.gov/ncidod/dvbid/dengue.)

Box 1
Recent dengue virus infections in the United States

Texas:

    1980: 23 cases, first locally acquired since 1945

    1986: 9 cases

    1995: 7 cases

    1997: 3 cases

    1998: 1 case

    1999: 18 cases

    2005: 25 cases

Hawaii:

    2001 to 2002: 122 cases (first since 1944)

risk of severe dengue disease.[9] This can occur with all 4 serotypes; therefore, in regions with multiple endemic serotypes, the risk of severe disease is higher.

PATHOGENESIS

The pathogenesis of DHF/DSS, the most severe form of DENV infection, reflects a complex interplay of the host immune response and the viral determinants of virulence.[2,10,11] Epidemiologic studies have suggested an immune system linkage, because there is an increased risk of DHF with secondary DENV infection and in

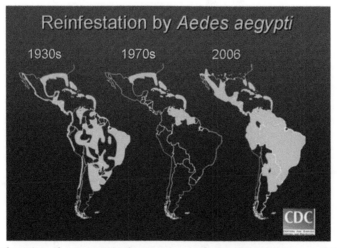

Fig. 3. Reinfestation of *A aegypti* in the Americas Unfortunately, the success of the eradication campaign was not sustained. Beginning in the early 1970s, it began to be disbanded, and many countries channeled their limited resources into other areas. Consequently, *A aegypti* began to reinfest the countries from which it had been eradicated. Comparing the 1970 and 2006 maps, the mosquito is seen reestablishing itself throughout Central America and most of South America. As the mosquito has spread, the number and frequency of dengue epidemics have increased, as has dengue hemorrhagic fever activity in the Americas. (*Courtesy of* CDC, available at: http://www.cdc.gov/ncidod/dvbid/dengue.)

children within the first year of life born to DENV-immune mothers.[12–15] From these observations, the hypothesis of antibody-dependent immune enhancement (ADE) of infection emerged. In support of the ADE pathogenesis concept, antibody enhancement of DENV infection in monocytes in vitro correlated with increased risk of DHF,[15,16] and peak viremia was increased in patients with severe secondary DENV infection.[17,18] Differences in specific genetic determinants among viral isolates[19–21] may also affect virulence, because some DENV strains fail to cause severe disease.[22,23] Finally, a pathologic cytokine response that occurs after extensive T-cell activation may contribute to the capillary leak syndrome associated with DHF.[11] Elevated levels of cytokines, including IFN-γ, tumor necrosis factor (TNF)-γ, and interleukin (IL)-10, to some extent correlate with severe disease[24–28]; and disease severity has been associated with activation of CD8$^+$ T cells and the expansion of serotype-reactive low-affinity DENV-specific T cells that produce high levels of vasoactive cytokines.[29–33]

CLINICAL PRESENTATIONS

Dengue fever may present in many forms: as an undifferentiated febrile illness with a maculopapular rash, particularly in children, as flulike symptoms, or as classic Dengue with 2 or more symptoms, such as fever, headache, bone or joint pain, muscular pain, rash, pain behind the eyes, and petechial hemorrhaging. Often, there is prolonged fatigue and depression. During dengue epidemics, hemorrhagic complications may also appear, such as bleeding from the gums, nosebleeds, and bruising. Case fatalities due to DF are low, whereas DHF mortality is fairly high. There is no specific treatment for dengue fever except for symptomatic treatment, rest, and rehydration. Recognizing the warning signs and symptoms of dengue infection are critical for appropriate diagnosis and treatment (**Fig. 4**).

DHF is characterized by spontaneous bleeding, plasma leakage, fever, and thrombocytopenia. Four clinical manifestations need to be observed to be classified as DHF. These include (1) fever; (2) hemorrhagic episodes with the presence of at least one of the following: a positive tourniquet test result (also called a capillary fragility test: a clinical diagnostic method to determine a patient's hemorrhagic tendency and assess fragility of capillary walls); petechiae, ecchymoses, or purpura; or bleeding from mucosa, gastrointestinal tract, injection sites, or others; (3) plasma leakage due to increased capillary permeability; and (4) thrombocytopenia (100,000/mm^3 or less).

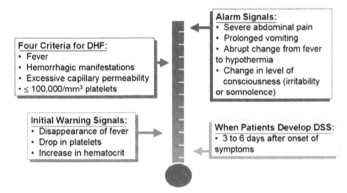

Fig. 4. Warning signs of dengue infection. (*Courtesy of* CDC, available at: http://www.cdc.gov/ncidod/dvbid/dengue.)

Moderate-to-marked thrombocytopenia with concurrent hemoconcentration is a distinctive clinical laboratory finding of DHF. However, to distinguish DHF from DF, an observation of plasma leakage manifested by a rising hematocrit value (ie, hemoconcentration) must be observed (**Fig. 5**).

The normal course of DHF lasts between 7 to 10 days, and with appropriate intensive maintenance of the circulating fluid volume, mortality may be reduced to less than 1%. Only severe DF and DHF cases should be hospitalized. Serologic tests are necessary to confirm cases of dengue. However, these tests may take several days.[34,35] Developing countries may not have the resources to perform these expensive confirmatory assays, and therefore, many suspected cases of dengue are not fully diagnosed. In severe cases of DHF, the patient's condition may suddenly deteriorate after a few days of fever; the temperature drops, followed by signs of circulatory failure; and the patient may rapidly go into a critical state of shock (dengue shock syndrome), dying within 12 to 24 hours or quickly recovering following appropriate volume replacement therapy **Box 2**.

DSS is the most severe form of DHF and is characterized by the presence of all 4 DHF clinical manifestations and circulatory failure. All 3 manifestations of circulatory failure must be present: rapid and weak pulse; narrow pulse pressure or hypotension for the patient's age; and cold, clammy skin and altered mental state.

DIAGNOSIS

Establishing a laboratory diagnosis of dengue infection is critical for diagnosis of dengue. A major challenge for disease surveillance and case diagnosis is that the dengue viruses produce asymptomatic infections and a spectrum of clinical illness ranging from a mild, nonspecific febrile illness to fatal hemorrhagic disease. Important risk factors of DHF include the strain and serotype of the infecting virus and the age, immune status, and genetic predisposition of the patient. The most common method of detecting the virus is to propagate virus from serum in cell culture or detect anti-dengue antibodies by serology. Virus can be cultured in vitro or by detection of viral RNA and specific dengue virus antigens. Countries that do not have access to sophisticated laboratory tests rely on identification of early clinical or simple laboratory indicators that can provide a reliable diagnosis of dengue before hospitalization. Early distinction between dengue and other febrile illnesses could help identify patients that should be monitored for signs of DHF.

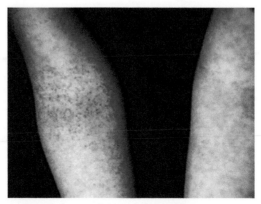

Fig. 5. Petechial hemorrhages from a dengue infected patient. (*Courtesy of* CDC, available at: http://www.cdc.gov/ncidod/dvbid/dengue.)

<table>
<tr><td>

Box 2
Grades of DHF

All 4 grades must be met for a diagnosis of DHF.

Grade 1: Fever and nonspecific constitutional symptoms and positive tourniquet test result

Grade 2: Grade 1 manifestations plus spontaneous bleeding.

Grade 3[a]: Incipient shock with signs of circulatory failure.

Grade 4[a]: Profound shock with undetectable pulse and blood pressure.

[a] Grades 3 and 4 are Dengue Shock Syndrome.

</td></tr>
</table>

DIFFERENTIAL DIAGNOSIS

Febrile illnesses, such as measles, typhoid fever, leptospirosis, and severe acute respiratory syndrome (SARS), can produce symptoms similar to DF.[36–41] At presentation, these illnesses may share similar clinical features, including headache, myalgia, and rash **Box 3**.

TREATMENT AND LONG-TERM OUTCOMES

There are no specific antivirals that can eliminate the virus from an infected individual. However, supportive care and treatment can be effective in treating DF. Paracetamol and other antipyretics can be used to treat fever. Bone pain should be treated by analgesics or painkilling tablets. During episodes of DHF/DSS, the mortality rate in the absence of hospitalization can be as high as 50%. With proper treatment, such as intravenous fluid replacement, the mortality rate is greatly reduced.

VACCINES AND IMMUNITY

Multiple correlates of protection have been described for dengue. However, the primary correlate seems to be long-term homotypic protection.[42,43] Most protective antibodies are directed at the surface E glycoprotein.[44,45] However, antibodies to

<table>
<tr><td>

Box 3
Differential diagnosis of dengue infection

Influenza

Measles

Rubella

Malaria

Typhoid fever

Leptospirosis

Meningococcemia

Rickettsial infections

Bacterial sepsis

Other viral hemorrhagic fevers

</td></tr>
</table>

the M and NS1 proteins show some protective efficacy.[46] Passively transferring antibodies from seroconverted animals results in decreased infection and disease following challenge.[44,46] In addition, maternal antibodies decrease disease in infants.[15,47] Using in vitro neutralization assays, antibodies directed against the E protein prevent virus infection.[48] Antibodies that block viral attachment or prevent fusion to target cells neutralize virus infection.[49,50] In addition to neutralization, antibodies that mediate cell-mediated cytotoxicity reduce virus infection in complement-independent[51,52] and complement-dependent mechanisms.[53] Cellular immune responses are generally weakly protective.[54] However, these responses are critical for viral clearance.[55,56] Innate immune responses directed against NS proteins, such as NS4B (a putative IFN antagonist), seem to mediate viral escape.[57]

Currently, no DENV vaccine is approved by the US Food and Drug Administration (FDA). Four related but serologically distinct DENVs can cause disease. Non-neutralizing, cross-reactive antibodies may contribute to DHF pathogenesis via antibody-dependent enhancement. Therefore, an effective vaccine must induce high-titer neutralizing antibodies against all 4 strains[58,59]; failure to do so could increase the risk of severe disease on natural challenge. To circumvent this problem, tetravalent live-attenuated candidate vaccines are in varying stages of development.[60–64] In clinical trials, tetravalent serologic responses were observed in some individuals, but

Table 1
Experimental dengue virus vaccines

Type	Sponsor	Stage of Development
Live attenuated		
Tetravalent	Mahidol University/Sanofi Pasteur	Phase I
Tetravalent	WRAIR/GSK	Phase II
Chimeric		
ChimeriVax (17D YF)	Acambis/Sanofi Pasteur	Phase I
DENV-2/4d30 (all serotypes)	NIAID, NIH	Phase I/II
DENV-1	US FDA	Phase I
DENV-2 (16,681, PDK53)	CDC/Inviragen	Preclinical
DNA		
Several approaches	Various	
(ie, Domain III, prM/E, NS1)	NMRC/University of Pittsburgh	Phase I/Preclinical
Inactivated		
Several approaches	WRAIR	Preclinical
Subvirion particles/viruslike particles		
Drosophila cells	Hawaii Biotech	Phase I
Baculovirus (E, NS1)	Various	Preclinical
Replication-defective AV (E)	RepliVax-UTMB/Acambis	Preclinical
Yeast (C/prM/E, E-IIBsAg)	Various	Preclinical
Escherichia coli (E, E-NS1)	Various	Preclinical
DNA	University of Pittsburgh	Preclinical
Subunit/recombinant	Various	Preclinical

Abbreviations: AV, adenovirus; CDC, Centers for Disease Control and Prevention; GSK, GlaxoSmithKline; NIAID, National Institute of Allergy and Infectious Diseases; NIH, National Institutes of Health; UTMB, University of Texas Medical Branch; WRAIR, Walter Reed Army Institute of Research; YF, yellow fever.

many do not develop high titer neutralizing antibodies despite multiple immunizations.[65,66] Additionally, each part of the tetravalent vaccine does not elicit high titer immune response leading to immunodominance. Subunit-based vaccines, as purified proteins or DNA plasmid, are alternative vaccine strategies. Repeated immunization of purified recombinant DENV domain III of the E protein (DIII) or DIII-encoding plasmids induced protective antibodies in mice, albeit at fairly low neutralizing titers.[67–71]

Live attenuated vaccines and nonreplicating vaccines, such as inactivated virus vaccines, viruslike particles, and DNA vaccines, have been developed for dengue (**Table 1**). These vaccines elicit protective neutralizing antibodies. These vaccines can elicit long-lasting immunity against the specific serotype of DENV. However, they are poorly cross-reactive against infection with another subtype of DENV.

REFERENCES

1. Burke DS, Monath TP. Flaviviruses. In: Knipe DM, Howley PM, editors. Fields virology. Philadelphia: Lippincott Williams & Wilkins; 2001. p. 1043–125.
2. Halstead SB. Pathogenesis of dengue: challenges to molecular biology. Science 1988;239:476–81.
3. Monath TP. Dengue: the risk to developed and developing countries. Proc Natl Acad Sci U S A 1994;91:2395–400.
4. Chambers TJ, Hahn CS, Galler R, et al. Flavivirus genome organization, expression, and replication. Annu Rev Microbiol 1990;44:649–88.
5. Tassaneetrithep B, Burgess T, Granelli-Piperno A, et al. DC-SIGN (CD209) mediates dengue virus infection of human dendritic cells. J Exp Med 2003;197(7): 823–9.
6. Heinz F, Auer G, Stiasny K, et al. The interactions of the flavivirus envelope proteins: implications for virus entry and release. Arch Virol 1994;9(S):339–48.
7. Heinz F, Stiasny K, Puschner-Auer G, et al. Structural changes and functional control of the tick-borne encephalitis virus glycoprotein E by the heterodimeric association with the protein prM. Virology 1994;198:109–17.
8. Mackenzie JM, Jones MK, Westaway EG. Markers for trans-Golgi membranes and the intermediate compartment localize to induced membranes with distinct replication functions in flavivirus-infected cells. J Virol 1999;73:9555–67.
9. Solomon T, Mallewa M. Dengue and other emerging flaviviruses. J Infect 2001;42: 104–15.
10. Rothman AL. Dengue: defining protective versus pathologic immunity. J Clin Invest 2004;113:946–51.
11. Rothman AL, Ennis FA. Immunopathogenesis of Dengue hemorrhagic fever. Virology 1999;257:1–6.
12. Halstead SB, Simasthien P. Observations related to the pathogenesis of dengue hemorrhagic fever. II. Antigenic and biologic properties of dengue viruses and their association with disease response in the host. Yale J Biol Med 1970;42: 276–92.
13. Halstead SB, Nimmannitya S, Cohen SN. Observations related to pathogenesis of dengue hemorrhagic fever. IV. Relation of disease severity to antibody response and virus recovered. Yale J Biol Med 1970;42:311–28.
14. Halstead SB. Global epidemiology of dengue hemorrhagic fever. Southeast Asian J Trop Med Public Health 1990;21:636–41.
15. Kliks SC, Nimmanitya S, Nisalak A, et al. Evidence that maternal dengue antibodies are important in the development of dengue hemorrhagic fever in infants. Am J Trop Med Hyg 1988;38:411–9.

16. Kliks SC, Nisalak A, Brandt WE, et al. Antibody-dependent enhancement of dengue virus growth in human monocytes as a risk factor for dengue hemorrhagic fever. Am J Trop Med Hyg 1989;40:444–51.
17. Libraty DH, Endy TP, Houng HS, et al. Differing influences of virus burden and immune activation on disease severity in secondary dengue-3 virus infections. J Infect Dis 2002;185:1213–21.
18. Vaughn DW, Green S, Kalayanarooj S, et al. Dengue viremia titer, antibody response pattern, and virus serotype correlate with disease severity. J Infect Dis 2000;181:2–9.
19. Leitmeyer KC, Vaughn DW, Watts DM, et al. Dengue virus structural differences that correlate with pathogenesis. J Virol 1999;73:4738–47.
20. Cologna R, Rico-Hesse R. American genotype structures decrease dengue virus output from human monocytes and dendritic cells. J Virol 2003;77:3929–38.
21. Pryor MJ, Carr JM, Hocking H, et al. Replication of dengue virus type 2 in human monocyte-derived macrophages: comparisons of isolates and recombinant viruses with substitutions at amino acid 390 in the envelope glycoprotein. Am J Trop Med Hyg 2001;65:427–34.
22. Watts DM, Porter KR, Putvatana P, et al. Failure of secondary infection with American genotype dengue 2 to cause dengue haemorrhagic fever. Lancet 1999;354:1431–4.
23. Messer WB, Vitarana UT, Sivananthan K, et al. Epidemiology of dengue in Sri Lanka before and after the emergence of epidemic dengue hemorrhagic fever. Am J Trop Med Hyg 2002;66:765–73.
24. Green S, Vaughn DW, Kalayanarooj S, et al. Early immune activation in acute dengue illness is related to development of plasma leakage and disease severity. J Infect Dis 1999;179:755–62.
25. Hober D, Poli L, Roblin B, et al. Serum levels of tumor necrosis factor-alpha (TNF-alpha), interleukin-6 (IL-6), and interleukin-1 beta (IL-1 beta) in dengue-infected patients. Am J Trop Med Hyg 1993;48:324–31.
26. Hober D, Nguyen TL, Shen L, et al. Tumor necrosis factor alpha levels in plasma and whole-blood culture in dengue-infected patients: relationship between virus detection and pre- existing specific antibodies. J Med Virol 1998;54:210–8.
27. Hober D, Delannoy AS, Benyoucef S, et al. High levels of sTNFR p75 and TNF alpha in dengue-infected patients. Microbiol Immunol 1996;40:569–73.
28. Bethell DB, Flobbe K, Cao XT, et al. Pathophysiologic and prognostic role of cytokines in dengue hemorrhagic fever. J Infect Dis 1998;177:778–82.
29. Mongkolsapaya J, Duangchinda T, Dejnirattisai W, et al. T cell responses in dengue hemorrhagic fever: are cross-reactive T cells suboptimal? J Immunol 2006;176:3821–9.
30. Mongkolsapaya J, Dejnirattisai W, Xu XN, et al. Original antigenic sin and apoptosis in the pathogenesis of dengue hemorrhagic fever. Nat Med 2003;9:921–7.
31. Green S, Pichyangkul S, Vaughn DW, et al. Early CD69 expression on peripheral blood lymphocytes from children with dengue hemorrhagic fever. J Infect Dis 1999;180:1429–35.
32. Zivna I, Green S, Vaughn DW, et al. T cell responses to an HLA-B*07-restricted epitope on the dengue NS3 protein correlate with disease severity. J Immunol 2002;168:5959–65.
33. Bashyam HS, Green S, Rothman AL. Dengue virus-reactive CD8+ T cells display quantitative and qualitative differences in their response to variant epitopes of heterologous viral serotypes. J Immunol 2006;176:2817–24.

34. Schwartz E, Mileguir F, Grossman Z, et al. Evaluation of ELISA-based sero-diag-nosis of dengue fever in travelers. J Clin Virol 2000;19:169–73.
35. Schwartz E, Moskovitz A, Potasman I, et al. Changing epidemiology of dengue fever in travelers to Thailand. Eur J Clin Microbiol Infect Dis 2000;19:784–6.
36. Flannery B, Pereira MM, Velloso LDF, et al. Referral pattern of leptospirosis cases during a large urban epidemic of dengue. Am J Trop Med Hyg 2001; 65:657–63.
37. Watt G, Jongsakul K, Chouriyagune C, et al. Differentiating dengue virus infection from scrub typhus in Thai adults with fever. Am J Trop Med Hyg 2003;68:536–8.
38. Karande S, Gandhi D, Kulkarni M, et al. Concurrent outbreak of leptospirosis and dengue in Mumbai, India, 2002. J Trop Pediatr 2005;51:174–81.
39. Dietz VJ, Nieburg P, Gubler DJ, et al. Diagnosis of measles by clinical case defi-nition in dengue-endemic areas: implications for measles surveillance and control. Bull World Health Organ 1992;70:745–50.
40. Wilder-Smith A, Earnest A, Paton NI. Use of simple laboratory features to distin-guish the early stage of severe acute respiratory syndrome from dengue fever. Clin Infect Dis 2004;39:1818–23.
41. Wilder-Smith A, Foo W, Earnest A, et al. Seroepidemiology of dengue in the adult population of Singapore. Trop Med Int Health 2004;9:305–8.
42. Sabin AB. Research on dengue during World War II. Am J Trop Med Hyg 1952;1: 30–50.
43. Halstead SB. Etiologies of the experimental dengues of Siler and Simmons. Am J Trop Med Hyg 1974;23:974–82.
44. Kaufman BM, Summers PL, Dubois DR, et al. Monoclonal antibodies against dengue 2 virus E-glycoprotein protect mice against lethal dengue infection. Am J Trop Med Hyg 1987;36:427–34.
45. Bray M, Zhao BT, Markoff L, et al. Mice immunized with recombinant vaccinia virus expressing dengue 4 virus structural proteins with or without nonstructural protein NS1 are protected against fatal dengue virus encephalitis. J Virol 1989; 63:2853–6.
46. Kaufman BM, Summers PL, Dubois DR, et al. Monoclonal antibodies for dengue virus prM glycoprotein protect mice against lethal dengue infection. Am J Trop Med Hyg 1989;41:576–80.
47. Pengsaa K, Luxemburger C, Sabchareon A, et al. Dengue virus infections in the first 2 years of life and the kinetics of transplacentally transferred dengue neutral-izing antibodies in thai children. J Infect Dis 2006;194:1570–6.
48. Russell PK, Nisalak A, Sukhavachana P, et al. A plaque reduction test for dengue virus neutralizing antibodies. J Immunol 1967;99:285–90.
49. Crill WD, Roehrig JT. Monoclonal antibodies that bind to domain III of dengue virus E glycoprotein are the most efficient blockers of virus adsorption to Vero cells. J Virol 2001;75:7769–73.
50. Roehrig JT, Bolin RA, Kelly RG. Monoclonal antibody mapping of the envelope glycoprotein of the dengue 2 virus, Jamaica. Virology 1998;246:317–28.
51. Garcia G, Arango M, Perez AB, et al. Antibodies from patients with dengue viral infection mediate cellular cytotoxicity. J Clin Virol 2006;37:53–7.
52. Laoprasopwattana K, Libraty DH, Endy TP, et al. Dengue Virus (DV) enhancing antibody activity in preillness plasma does not predict subsequent disease severity or viremia in secondary DV infection. J Infect Dis 2005;192:510–9.
53. Falgout B, Bray M, Schlesinger JJ, et al. Immunization of mice with recombinant vaccinia virus expressing authentic dengue virus nonstructural protein NS1 protects against lethal dengue virus encephalitis. J Virol 1990;64:4356–63.

54. Calvert AE, Huang CY, Kinney RM, et al. Non-structural proteins of dengue 2 virus offer limited protection to interferon-deficient mice after dengue 2 virus challenge. J Gen Virol 2006;87:339–46.
55. Bukowski JF, Kurane I, Lai CJ, et al. Dengue virus-specific cross-reactive CD8+ human cytotoxic T lymphocytes. J Virol 1989;63:5086–91.
56. Kurane I, Meager A, Ennis FA. Dengue virus-specific human T cell clones. Serotype crossreactive proliferation, interferon gamma production, and cytotoxic activity. J Exp Med 1989;170:763–75.
57. Munoz-Jordan JL, Laurent-Rolle M, Ashour J, et al. Inhibition of alpha/beta interferon signaling by the NS4B protein of flaviviruses. J Virol 2005;79:8004–13.
58. Barrett AD. Current status of flavivirus vaccines. Ann N Y Acad Sci 2001;951:262–71.
59. Halstead SB, Deen J. The future of dengue vaccines. Lancet 2002;360:1243–5.
60. Guirakhoo F, Arroyo J, Pugachev KV, et al. Construction, safety, and immunogenicity in nonhuman primates of a chimeric yellow fever-dengue virus tetravalent vaccine. J Virol 2001;75:7290–304.
61. Huang CY, Butrapet S, Pierro DJ, et al. Chimeric dengue type 2 (vaccine strain PDK-53)/dengue type 1 virus as a potential candidate dengue type 1 virus vaccine. J Virol 2000;74:3020–8.
62. Durbin AP, Karron RA, Sun W, et al. Attenuation and immunogenicity in humans of a live dengue virus type-4 vaccine candidate with a 30 nucleotide deletion in its 3'-untranslated region. Am J Trop Med Hyg 2001;65:405–13.
63. Markoff L, Pang X, Houng Hs HS, et al. Derivation and characterization of a dengue type 1 host range-restricted mutant virus that is attenuated and highly immunogenic in monkeys. J Virol 2002;76:3318–28.
64. Bhamarapravati N, Sutee Y. Live attenuated tetravalent dengue vaccine. Vaccine 2000;18(Suppl 2):44–7.
65. Edelman R, Wasserman SS, Bodison SA, et al. Phase I trial of 16 formulations of a tetravalent live-attenuated dengue vaccine. Am J Trop Med Hyg 2003;69:48–60.
66. Sun W, Edelman R, Kanesa-thasan N, et al. Vaccination of human volunteers with monovalent and tetravalent live-attenuated dengue vaccine candidates. Am J Trop Med Hyg 2003;69:24–31.
67. Khanam S, Etemad B, Khanna N, et al. Induction of neutralizing antibodies specific to dengue virus serotypes 2 and 4 by a bivalent antigen composed of linked envelope domains III of these two serotypes. Am J Trop Med Hyg 2006;74:266–77.
68. Mota J, Acosta M, Argotte R, et al. Induction of protective antibodies against dengue virus by tetravalent DNA immunization of mice with domain III of the envelope protein. Vaccine 2005;23:3469–76.
69. Hermida L, Rodriguez R, Lazo L, et al. A dengue-2 Envelope fragment inserted within the structure of the P64k meningococcal protein carrier enables a functional immune response against the virus in mice. J Virol Methods 2004;115:41–9.
70. Simmons M, Nelson WM, Wu SJ, et al. Evaluation of the protective efficacy of a recombinant dengue envelope B domain fusion protein against dengue 2 virus infection in mice. Am J Trop Med Hyg 1998;58:655–62.
71. Simmons M, Murphy GS, Hayes CG. Short report: Antibody responses of mice immunized with a tetravalent dengue recombinant protein subunit vaccine. Am J Trop Med Hyg 2001;65:159–61.

Ebola and Marburg Hemorrhagic Fever

Amy L. Hartman, PhD[a,b,*], Jonathan S. Towner, PhD[c],
Stuart T. Nichol, PhD[c]

KEYWORDS
- Ebola • Marburg • Filovirus • Hemorrhagic fever

Ebola and Marburg viruses are the causative agents of severe viral hemorrhagic fever that occurs in sporadic outbreaks on the continent of Africa. Patients presenting in the United States with a history of travel to Africa and symptoms including high fever, hemorrhage, and myalgia may be considered suspect cases of viral hemorrhagic fever. This article provides an overview of the microbiology, epidemiology, clinical presentation, and pathogenesis of Ebola and Marburg virus infections.

MICROBIOLOGY

Ebola and Marburg viruses belong to the *Filoviridae* family of RNA viruses (**Table 1**). The *Filoviridae* family is classified within the order Mononegavirales, which also includes members of the *Bornaviridae*, *Rhadoviridae*, and *Paramyxoviridae* families. The genome of all viruses within Mononegavirales consists of a linear, nonsegmented single-stranded RNA molecule that is of a negative polarity.[1] The organization of a representative filovirus genome is shown in **Fig. 1**.

Filovirus virions have a uniform diameter (80 nm) but are variable in length. They have been visualized by electron microscopy as long filamentous particles, short bacillus-like particles, U-shaped, and even circular (**Fig. 2**). The name Filovirus (fílum meaning "thread" in Latin) is derived from this unique morphology.

The *Filoviridae* family consists of two genera: *Ebolavirus* (EBOV) and *Marburgvirus* (MARV), which likely diverged from a common genetic ancestor several thousand years ago.[2] A phylogenetic tree showing the genetic relationships between members of the *Filoviridae* family is shown in **Fig. 3**. There is only one known species of MARV

[a] University of Pittsburgh, Regional Biocontainment Laboratory, Center for Vaccine Research, 9015 Biomedical Science Tower 3, 3501 5th Avenue, Pittsburgh, PA 15261, USA
[b] Department of Infectious Diseases and Microbiology, University of Pittsburgh Graduate School of Public Health, 130 DeSoto Street, Pittsburgh, PA 15261, USA
[c] Special Pathogens Branch, Division of Viral and Rickettsial Diseases, Centers for Disease Control and Prevention, MS G-14, 1600 Clifton Road, NE, Atlanta, GA 30333, USA
* Corresponding author. University of Pittsburgh, Regional Biocontainment Laboratory, Center for Vaccine Research, 9015 Biomedical Science Tower 3, 3501 5th Avenue, Pittsburgh, PA 15261.
E-mail address: hartman2@pitt.edu

Clin Lab Med 30 (2010) 161–177
doi:10.1016/j.cll.2009.12.001   labmed.theclinics.com
0272-2712/10/$ – see front matter © 2010 Elsevier Inc. All rights reserved.

Table 1
Taxonomy of the *Filoviridae* family

Genus	Species	Abbreviation
Ebolavirus	*Zaire ebolavirus*	EBOV-Z
	Sudan ebolavirus	EBOV-S
	Reston ebolavirus	EBOV-R
	Cote d'Ivoire ebolavirus	EBOV-IC
	Bundibugyo ebolavirus	EBOV-B
Marburgvirus	*Lake Victoria marburgvirus*	MARV

and five identified species of EBOV (see **Table 1**), with 30% to 40% nucleotide sequence divergence between the five known species of EBOV.[3] A new species of EBOV (termed "Bundibugyo") was recently identified in Uganda.[3]

EPIDEMIOLOGY

EBOV and MARV cause severe viral hemorrhagic fever in humans, referred to as "filoviral hemorrhagic fever" (FHF). A summary of all known filovirus outbreaks can be found in **Table 2**, and a map of recent filovirus outbreaks is shown in **Fig. 4**. The first filovirus disease identified was MARV, which broke out in Marburg and Frankfurt, Germany, and Yugoslavia after laboratory workers contracted the unusual disease by working with infected primates that had been imported from Uganda. A total of 31 cases were eventually identified, and the mortality among these cases was 23% (see **Table 2**). The newly discovered virus was named Marburg after the original outbreak location. Outbreaks of MARV have occurred sporadically since the 1967 discovery. The largest known MARV outbreak occurred in northeastern Angola in

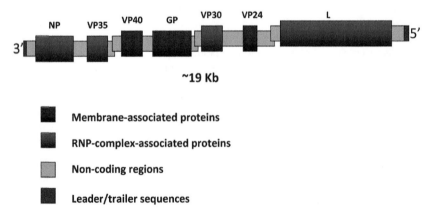

Fig. 1. Genomic organization of a representative member of the *Filoviridae* family of viruses. A schematic diagram of the genome of *Zaire ebolavirus* is shown. The genome of most filoviruses codes for at least seven proteins and is approximately 19 kb in length. Four proteins (shown in red: NP, VP35, VP30, and L polymerase) are involved in formation of the viral ribonucleoprotein complexes, which represent the basic unit for viral replication. Three other proteins (shown in purple: VP40, GP, and VP24) are membrane-associated proteins and form the matrix and envelope glycoproteins. All members of the *Filoviridae* have conserved leader and trailer sequences and noncoding regions between genes. The genome is transcribed into seven monocistronic mRNA species.

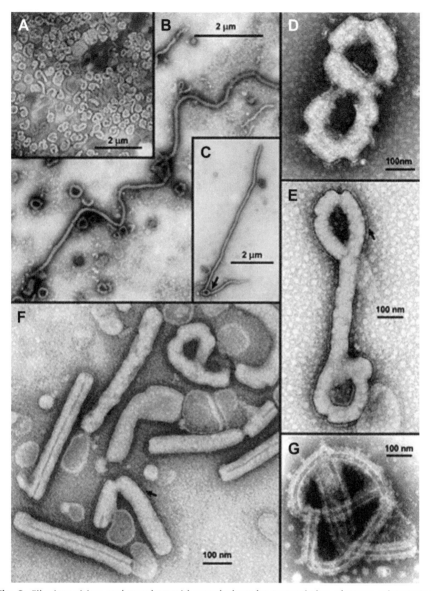

Fig. 2. Filovirus virion and nucelocapsid morphology by transmission electron microscopy. (*A*) MARV. (*B*) EBOV-S. (*C*) MARV (*arrow* indicates a branch point in filamentous particle). (*D*) EBOV-Z. (*E*) EBOV-Z (*arrow* indicates glycoprotein peplomers on virion surface). (*F*) MARV (*arrow* indicates glycoprotein peplomers on virion surface). (*G*) EBOV-S nucleocapsids obtained from infected Vero E6 cell culture medium. (*From* Sanchez A, Geisbert TW, Feldmann H. Filoviridae: Marburg and Ebola viruses. In: Knipe BM, Howley PM, Griffen DE, et al, editors. Fields virology. 5th edition. Philadelphia: Lippincott-Raven; 2007. p. 1409–48; with permission.)

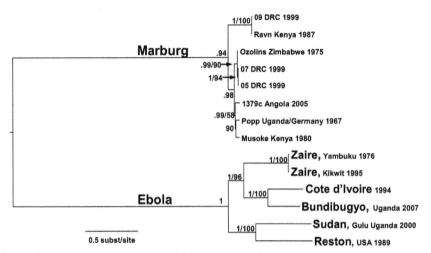

Fig. 3. Phylogenetic tree of the *Filoviridae* family of viruses. Phylogenetic tree comparing full-length genomes of EBOV and MARV by Bayesian analysis.[3] Posterior probabilities greater than 0.5 and maximum likelihood bootstrap values greater than 50 are indicated at the nodes. (*Courtesy of* Serena A. Carroll, Centers for Disease Control and Prevention, Atlanta, GA.)

the spring of 2005, with over 250 cases identified. In contrast to the original MARV outbreak in primate facilities in Europe, very high case fatalities (83%–90%) were seen in the two largest MARV outbreaks, in rural Democratic Republic of the Congo (formerly known as Zaire, 1998–2000) and Angola (2005).

EBOV disease was first identified in two separate large outbreaks occurring simultaneously in 1976, one in the Democratic Republic of the Congo and the other in Sudan. EBOV derives its name from the Ebola River located in northwestern Democratic Republic of the Congo where the outbreak occurred. These two initial outbreaks resulted in identification of the *Zaire ebolavirus* and *Sudan ebolavirus* species. Later studies confirmed that the two species of virus are distinct (see **Fig. 3**). The *Zaire* and *Sudan* species of Ebola have been responsible for most Ebola outbreaks since 1976 (see **Table 2**). The largest filovirus outbreak recorded to date was that of *Sudan ebolavirus* in Uganda during 2000 to 2001. A total of 425 cases were identified with a fatality of 53%.

The remaining three species of EBOV (*Cote d'Ivoire*, *Reston*, and *Bundibugyo ebolavirus*) have occurred less frequently. The *Cote d'Ivoire ebolavirus* species is genetically distinct from the other EBOV species and has only been known to cause a single nonfatal infection acquired during the necropsy of a dead chimpanzee.[4] The newly identified and genetically distinct *Bundibugyo ebolavirus* species was responsible for an outbreak in 2007 to 2008 in Uganda[3] resulting in over 100 cases with a fatality of 42%.

The *Reston ebolavirus* species was discovered during an investigation of hemorrhagic fever deaths in primates in a quarantine facility in Reston, Virginia, in 1989. Primates imported from a single export facility in the Philippines were responsible for this and several subsequent outbreaks in primate facilities in the United States and Italy. Nine workers in the affected United States and Philippines facilities were identified as having been infected with the virus, but none were associated with disease, suggesting that *Reston ebolavirus* may be nonpathogenic in humans, or at least less virulent than the other viruses in the genus. *Reston ebolavirus* has recently been detected in pigs on commercial pig farms in the Philippines. It is currently unclear

Table 2 List of Filovirus outbreaks			
Date	Location	Cases	Fatality (%)
Marburgvirus			
1967	Germany/Yugoslavia from Uganda	31	23
1975	South Africa from Zimbabwe	3	33
1980	Kenya	2	50
1987	Kenya	1	100
1998–2000	Democratic Republic of the Congo	154	83
2005	Angola	252	90
2007	Uganda	4	25
2007	Uganda	1	0
2008	Uganda	1	100
Zaire ebolavirus			
1976	Democratic Republic of the Congo	318	88
1977	Democratic Republic of the Congo	1	100
1994	Gabon	49	65
1995	Democratic Republic of the Congo	315	88
1996 spring	Gabon	37	57
1996 autumn	Gabon	60	75
2001–2002	Gabon and Republic of Congo	123	79
2003 spring	Republic of Congo	90	143
2003 autumn	Republic of Congo	35	83
2005	Republic of Congo	12	75
2007	Democratic Republic of the Congo	264	71
2008	Democratic Republic of the Congo	32	47
Sudan ebolavirus			
1976	Sudan	284	53
1979	Sudan	34	65
2000–2001	Uganda	425	53
2004	Sudan	17	42
Reston ebolavirus			
1989–1990	United States	4	0
1992	Italy	0	0
1996	United States	0	0
2008	Philippines	6	0
Ivory Coast ebolavirus			
1994	Ivory Coast	1	0
Bundibugyo ebolavirus			
2007–2008	Uganda	102	42

whether the virus causes disease in pigs. Again, some Filipino abbatoir workers were found to be virus antibody–positive but without history of hemorrhagic fever illness.[5]

Filovirus outbreaks continue to occur sporadically mostly within the continent of Africa, and increased surveillance and detection methods have led to the identification of new species and strains. Recent filovirus outbreaks from the last decade are shown

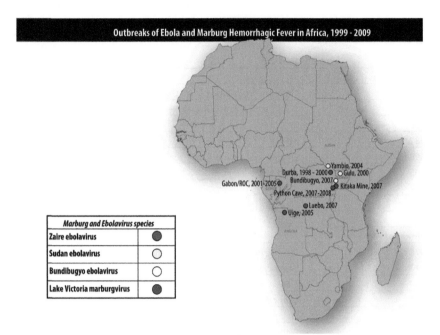

Fig. 4. Map of recent filovirus disease outbreaks in Africa. The EBOV and MARV outbreaks over the last decade are shown and color-coded according to virus species. For each outbreak location, the corresponding town and year of outbreak is shown, which corresponds with the outbreaks listed in **Table 2**. (*Courtesy of* Craig Manning, Centers for Disease Control and Prevention, Atlanta, GA.)

geographically in **Fig 4**. Increased air travel makes the spread of deadly filovirus infections outside of Africa a real possibility, as evidenced by the recent exportation of two MARV-infected tourists from Uganda, one into the United States in late 2007[6] and another into the Netherlands in 2008 (see **Table 2**).[7]

Filoviruses are classified as Biosafety Level 4 (BSL-4) pathogens because they cause a rapid, severe disease with high mortality for which there is no effective treatment or licensed vaccine.[8] BSL-4 provides the highest protection for the laboratory worker and the environment. There are a limited number of laboratories in the United States that are capable of handling filovirus specimens, which makes positive identification of samples difficult.

CLINICAL PRESENTATION AND LABORATORY FINDINGS

Because filovirus outbreaks occur infrequently and sporadically and because national and international health organizations are usually not present at the outbreak location at the beginning of outbreaks, definitive clinical data from filovirus outbreaks are spotty at best and difficult to obtain. The data collected from a limited number of human outbreaks of EBOV and MARV suggest the incubation period (asymptomatic period) can be as short as 2 days or as long as 21 days.[9] FHF disease manifests abruptly with nonspecific flulike symptoms (chills, fever, myalgia, general malaise). Subsequent symptoms often include lethargy, nausea, vomiting, abdominal pain, anorexia, diarrhea, coughing, headache, and hypotension (**Fig. 5**). Hemorrhagic manifestations do not occur in all cases, vary in severity, and generally develop during the

Early → Late

General	Gastrointestinal	Respiratory	Vascular	Neurologic	Hemorrhagic	Late Stage	Convalescence
fever	nausea	non-productive cough	hypotension	headache	petechiae	shock	myalgia
chills	vomiting	shortness of breath	conjunctival injection	confusion	rash (trunk and shoulders)	convulsions	arthralgia
myalgia	diarrhea	chest pain	edema	seizure	erythema and desquamation	delirium	muscle weakness
general malaise	abdominal pain			coma	bruising	coma	hepatitis
lethargy					bleeding from venipuncture sites	diffuse coagulopathy	ocular disease
fatigue					nosebleeds	increased respiration rate	myelitis
					mucosal hemorrhage, esp. GI/GU	anuria	hearing loss
					visceral hemorrhagic effusions	metabolic abnormalities	psychosis

Fig. 5. Signs and symptoms of disease caused by Ebola and Marburg viruses.

time of peak illness.[10] These include a rash; easy bruising; frequent nosebleeds; bleeding from venipuncture sites; and bleeding from mucosal sites, especially the gastrointestinal and genitourinary tracts. Examples of hemorrhagic manifestations in nonhuman primates infected with EBOV and MARV are shown in **Fig. 6**.

Early symptoms are similar between survivors and nonsurvivors. Testing of blood samples from infected patients has shown a dramatic difference in the levels of virus in the blood in patients who die versus patients who survive.[11,12] Nonsurvivors have 100- to 1000-fold higher levels of viremia than survivors. Survivors also have higher levels of virus-specific antibodies compared with fatal cases, which have little or no detectable antibody responses. Fatal cases progress to more severe symptoms by days 7 to 14 after the onset of disease; death is generally imminent shortly after the onset of coma and shock. Tachypnea (rapid respiration rate) is one characteristic of late-stage disease that differentiates fatal from nonfatal cases.[13]

Pathology performed on patients with EBOV and MARV infection all reveal extensive necrosis in a variety of organs including the liver, spleen, kidney, thymus, lymph nodes, and reproductive organs.[14] In the liver, hepatocellular necrosis is widespread and an exceedingly large number of virus particles are present (**Fig. 7**). Inclusion bodies are often visible in intact cells.

Survivors of FHF experience a prolonged convalescence and can be characterized by myalgia, arthralgia, muscle weakness, hepatitis, ocular disease, myelitis, hearing loss, and even psychosis (see **Fig. 5**). During early convalescence, virus can be

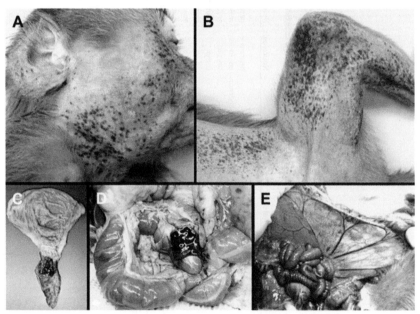

Fig. 6. Hemorrhagic symptoms in nonhuman primates infected with EBOV and MARV. Petechiae on the head and neck of a rhesus macaque infected with MARV (A) and on the trunk and leg of a cynomolgous macaque infected with EBOV-S (B). A gastroduodenal lesion (C) and hemorrhage in the ileum (D) of a cynomolgous macaque infected with EBOV-S. (E) Hemorrhaging within mesenteric blood vessels of a rhesus monkey infected with EBOV-Z. (From Sanchez A, Geisbert TW, Feldmann H. Filoviridae: Marburg and Ebola viruses. In: Knipe BM, Howley PM, Griffen DE, et al, editors. Fields virology. 5th edition. Philadelphia: Lippincott-Raven; 2007. p. 1409–48; with permission.)

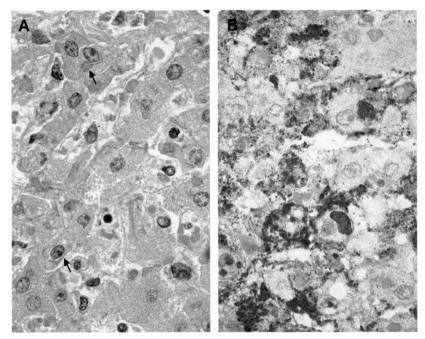

Fig. 7. Liver pathology in EBOV-infected humans. (*A*) Hepatocytes illustrating hepatocellular necrosis and viral inclusions (*arrows*) (hematoxylin-eosin, original magnification ×100). (*B*) Immunohistochemistry results demonstrating extensive EBOV antigen distribution in the liver. Viral inclusions within hepatocytes are shown and abundant antigens in sinusoids and sinusoidal lining cells (hematoxylin-eosin, original magnification ×250). (*Courtesy of Sherif Zaki, Centers for Disease Control and Prevention, Atlanta, GA.*)

detectable in immunologically protected sites of the body, particularly the uveal and seminal tracts. Although long-term viral shedding is not thought to occur in FHF patients, infectious virus can be detected in genital secretions for up to 80 days postonset of illness.[15–17] Recovering patients should be counseled to take adequate precautions to prevent inadvertent sexual transmission to close contacts during this time period.

PATHOGENESIS

The severe disease caused by EBOV and MARV infections can be attributed to three main factors: (1) rapid viral replication, (2) host immune suppression induced by the virus, and (3) vascular dysfunction. Recent data suggest that the central player in the pathogenesis of filovirus infections may be the infected macrophage.[18–20]

Filoviruses are pantropic, meaning that they can infect a wide variety of cell types. The cellular receptor for filoviruses is currently not known, but is likely a lectin or other ubiquitously expressed protein. The lectins DC-SIGN, DC-SIGNR, and L-SIGN all increase the binding of filoviruses to target cells.[21] Macrophages and dendritic cells (DCs) are highly susceptible to infection by EBOV and MARV and are likely the primary cellular targets at the site of infection (eg, a mucosal surface).[19] Infected macrophages and DCs play a pivotal role in virus dissemination by trafficking the virus to draining lymph nodes, where there is a larger pool of susceptible cells. Virus gains easy access to the blood, where it travels to the liver and spleen, two key infected organs in FHF patients. Macrophages residing in the liver and spleen secrete soluble factors that recruit more macrophages.[18,19] The macrophages, DCs, and surrounding parenchymal cells become virus factories and cause extensive focal necrosis. Fatal cases of FHF can have greater than 10^8 copies of viral RNA per milliliter of blood.[12] Elevated liver enzymes, hepatocellular degeneration, and necrosis are prominent in many FHF cases.[14] Decreased liver function may result in decreased synthesis of coagulation factors, which may contribute to the vascular and coagulation dysfunction.

Early studies of filovirus patients noted the fact that survivors have demonstrable levels of virus-specific antibody responses, whereas fatal cases have little to no detectable humoral immune responses.[11,12,22] Immunosuppression is a hallmark of fatal filovirus infections, and there seems to be several potential explanations for the lack of adequate immune response in fatal cases. Abnormal responses of macrophages and DCs to viral infection may result in immune dysregulation. Infected macrophages secrete high levels of inflammatory cytokines, which may lead to recruitment of more susceptible cells and uncontrolled inflammation.[21,23] Conversely, infected DCs fail to mature correctly, thereby failing to provide costimulation of T cells.[24,25] Lymphocytes are not directly infected by the virus, but a massive decrease in lymphocytes occurs in infected patients, possibly caused by bystander apoptosis.[22,26] Filoviruses also inhibit the Type I Interferon system through a number of mechanisms involving the VP35 and VP24 proteins.[27–30] The interferon response is responsible for the early control of virus replication; by impairing this cellular mechanism, EBOV can replicate unchecked during the critical early stages of infection.

Vascular impairment is another hallmark of filovirus pathogenesis. At end-stage disease, there is a significant loss of vascular integrity resulting in bleeding and leakage of fluid into tissue spaces. Virus infection of macrophages results in expression of tissue factor on the surface of the cells.[20] Tissue factor initiates the coagulation cascade leading to microthrombosis and disseminated intravascular coagulation (DIC).[31] DIC is activation of the coagulation system resulting in development of microthrombi (locally or systemically) that then hamper blood supply leading to multiple organ failure. During DIC, platelets and clotting factors are consumed, leading to hemorrhage elsewhere in the body. The vascular impairment seen in filovirus patients may be the result of direct infection and death of hepatocytes. Macrophages seem to play a key role in the pathogenesis of filoviral infections because they support high levels of virus replication, initiate virus dissemination, secrete high levels of inflammatory cytokines resulting in immune dysregulation, and express tissue factor leading to DIC and vascular impairment.[31]

DIAGNOSIS

Because local hospitals and health departments in the United States do not have the technology or resources to routinely test for filovirus infections, the clinical assessment is critical for the initial diagnosis of a filovirus infection. Local and state health departments should be notified of suspected FHF cases, but diagnostic confirmation can only be obtained by sending samples to the Centers for Disease Control and Prevention (CDC) in Atlanta. Information for sample submission in the United States can be found at the following website: http://www.cdc.gov/ncidod/dvrd/spb/mnpages/specimen.htm. Samples from suspected FHF patients should be handled minimally and with the utmost caution. A class II biosafety cabinet should be used to process clinical specimens and BSL-3 practices should be used. This includes use of barrier gowns, two pairs of gloves, eye protection, and a mask or N95 respirator.

Routine laboratory tests include enzyme-linked immunosorbent assays (ELISAs) to detect levels of viral antigen or the presence of antibodies, virus isolation, and reverse transcriptase–polymerase chain reaction (RT-PCR). Filovirus-specific IgM and IgG antibodies can often be detected by ELISA in serum of convalescent patients. Filovirus infection in deceased patients can be diagnosed by immunohistochemistry, antigen detection, virus isolation, or RT-PCR. **Table 3** summarizes the assays used to diagnose suspected filovirus specimens and lists the advantages and disadvantages of each method. Blood and serum are the samples most preferred for diagnostic testing; however, recent data indicate that high levels of viral nucleic acid can be detected in oral and nasal swabs from patients in the end-stage of disease.[32,33]

National and international reference laboratories have a range of assays available for testing and identification of filovirus samples (see **Table 3**). During large outbreaks, mobile laboratories have been deployed to provide on-site testing of patient samples. Antigen ELISA and q-RT-PCR are the methods most often used in a field setting for acute case diagnosis because a combination of both assays provides the most rapid and sensitive testing with the fewest resources. Antigen-capture ELISAs are broadly reactive and can generally detect all of the different EBOV species.[11] The MARV antigen-capture ELISA proved less sensitive than q-RT-PCR, however, in the 2005 outbreak in Angola.[32] Quantitative Taqman RT-PCR assays are ideal for detecting low quantities of viral nucleic acids in a rapid time frame.[32,33] The q-RT-PCR assays have the ability to detect all known strains of MARV,[32] but have the potential for false-negatives if the strain sequence differs significantly enough so that the primers and probe no longer detect the target sequence, as illustrated in the recent *Bundibugyo ebolavirus* outbreak.[3] A combination of ELISAs for viral antigen, IgG, and IgM along with q-RT-PCR have in recent years proved to be a suitable set of assays for diagnosing suspected Ebola hemorrhagic fever and Marburg hemorrhagic fever patient samples from all stages of disease.

DIFFERENTIAL DIAGNOSIS

The differential diagnosis for filovirus infections is challenging because of the generalized early symptoms. Febrile patients with either a recent travel history to areas of ongoing filovirus activity, contact with a person or animal known to be infected with a filovirus, or other known exposure (eg, laboratory worker) should be considered likely cases of FHF.[34] Febrile individuals with a history of travel to endemic areas of Africa who also display symptoms listed in **Fig. 5** should be considered as possible FHF cases. Malaria, shigellosis, and typhoid fever are the most common causes of acute febrile illness in the areas of sub-Saharan Africa where filoviruses are endemic. Other diagnoses to consider include yellow fever, Chickungunya fever, fulminant viral hepatitis, plague, typhus, leptospirosis, and meningococcal septicemia.

TREATMENT, PROGNOSIS, AND LONG-TERM OUTCOME

Filoviruses spread through the human population by close contact with acutely infected patients. Virus-containing bodily fluids include blood, vomitus, saliva, stool, semen, breast milk, and tears.[35] Virus transmission has only been documented between patients exhibiting symptoms of the disease and does not likely occur during the incubation period.[34] Transmission of filoviruses from human to human requires close proximity, such as fomites or direct contact with blood or bodily fluids leading

Table 3
Diagnostic assays used to detect Filovirus infection in humans

Test	Target	Source	Advantages	Disadvantages	Useful in Field Laboratory?
IFA	Antiviral antibodies	Serum	Rapid and easy	Nonspecific positives; subjective	N
ELISA	Antiviral antibodies	Serum	Rapid, specific, sensitive, high throughput	Slower than IFA	Y
Immunoblot	Antiviral antibodies	Serum	Protein specific	Interpretation sometimes difficult	N
Antigen detection ELISA	Viral antigen	Blood, serum, tissues, oral/nasal washes, breast milk	Rapid, sensitive, high throughput	None	Y
Immunohistochemistry	Viral antigen	Tissue	Shows histologic location of viral antigen	Slow, requires formalin fixation of	N
PCR	Viral nucleic acid	Blood, serum, tissues, oral/nasal washes, breast milk	Rapid, sensitive, can distinguish between strains	Requires specialized equipment	Y
Electron microscopy	Viral particle	Blood, tissues	Distinguishes unique morphology	Insensitive; requires specialized equipment	N
Virus isolation	Viral particle	Blood, tissues	Isolate is available for study	Slow (~1 wk)	N

Abbreviations: ELISA, enzyme-linked immunosorbent assay; IFA, indirect immunofluorescence assay; PCR, polymerase chain reaction.
Adapted from Sanchez A, Geisbert TW, Feldmann H. Filoviridae: Marburg and Ebola viruses. In: Knipe BM, Howley PM, Griffen DE, et al, editors. Fields virology. 5th edition. Philadelphia: Lippincott-Raven; 2007. p. 1409–48.

to mucous membrane exposure.[36] No true aerosol transmission between humans has been documented.

EBOV and MARV are easily transmitted to health care workers in Africa because of deficient barrier nursing practices, poor sanitary conditions, and frequent reuse of needles. Nosocomial transmission of EBOV and MARV have contributed significantly to the spread of filovirus outbreaks.[37-39] In addition, traditional healers are the preferred and often only source of health services in remote areas of Africa and have been implicated in the spread of EBOV in Gabon[40] and MARV in Angola in 2005[41] through the use of unsterilized blades or needles. To prevent spread of filoviruses in a health care setting, barrier nursing and isolation of patients is critical. Barrier nursing techniques should include the proper use and disinfection of protective clothing, gloves, facemasks, and eye protection or face shield.

There are currently no licensed vaccines or therapeutic treatments available for filovirus infections. Until an effective vaccine or postexposure therapy is licensed, the prognosis for patients infected with MARV or EBOV (*Zaire*, *Sudan*, or *Bundibugyo* species) is grim. Based on the known outbreaks, the case fatality ratios range from 42% to 90%, depending on the viral species (see **Table 2**). Filovirus-infected patients should be managed with supportive therapy to maintain blood volume and electrolyte balance.

Strategies for treating EBOV- and MARV-infected patients in an outbreak setting have proved unsuccessful to date.[42] Treatment of patients with convalescent sera and passive immunotherapy in animal studies has not been effective.[43-47] Other therapies that have been evaluated in animal models include ribavirin,[48] recombinant interferon-α,[49] siRNA,[50] recombinant anticoagulant (rNAPC2),[51] S-adenosylhomocysteine hydrolase inhibitor,[52,53] and activated protein C.[54] Some of these potential therapies were promising when given before or immediately after exposure to virus, including the use of live-attenuated vaccines within 24 hours of exposure (discussed later).[55] In animal models, however, no therapy has been able to reverse the fatal outcome once disease has begun.

Recent research studies have identified a number of potential filovirus vaccine candidates.[56] Inactivated vaccines (either by formalin or γ-irradiation) have not shown consistent protection of nonhuman primates from EBOV or MARV.[57,58] New-generation DNA and vector-based vaccine candidates have been extensively evaluated in rodents and nonhuman primates. Vector-based vaccines have relied on the idea that a live virus vector expressing a foreign gene of interest may illicit a stronger immune response than inactivated vaccines. Live-attenuated and replication-defective vectors have been tested as candidates for filovirus vaccines[42,56] and include replication-defective Venezuelan equine encephalomyelitis, replication-defective adenovirus, live attenuated vesicular stomatitis virus (VSV), recombinant vaccinia virus, and recombinant human parainfluenza virus 3. Various levels of protection have been seen in animal models. However, a live-attenuated or replication-deficient virus vector presents concerns that include safety and, in the case of adenovirus vectors, interference by pre-existing immunity.

Virus-like particles (VLPs) consist of viral proteins presented in a native conformation. VLPs are generally considered safer than live attenuated or replication-defective vectors. EBOV and MARV VLPs are generated by coexpression of glycoprotein and VP40 in cell culture; the VLPs seem identical to authentic particles by electron microsopy.[59] VLPs have been able to protect mice, guinea pigs, and nonhuman primates from homologous challenge with wild type virus.[60-62]

Evaluation of vaccine and therapeutic candidates in rodents and nonhuman primates is an important component of the Food and Drug Administration's "animal rule."

Adequate human clinical trials for EBOV and MARV vaccine and therapeutic candidates are not possible given the sporadic nature of filovirus outbreaks. The information learned from the nonhuman primate studies is critical, however, toward identifying an effective vaccine and treatment option for filovirus-infected patients because rodent models are not considered to be predictive of primate responses. As an example, a laboratory worker in Germany recently suffered a needlestick injury with a mouse-adapted Ebola virus. The patient was immediately given an experimental vaccine comprised of a live-attenuated VSV expressing the EBOV glycoprotein. This vaccine had recently been shown to protect nonhuman primates from disease when given as a postexposure treatment.[55] The patient never displayed symptoms of EBOV infection. It has yet to be determined whether this can be attributed to the experimental vaccine or simply that the patient was never infected, but it does illustrate a potential use of this vaccine.

SUMMARY

EBOV and MARV cause some of the most severe viral hemorrhagic fever diseases known to humans. Unfortunately, there is no licensed vaccine or therapy for filovirus-infected patients. Although outbreaks of EBOV and MARV generally occur sporadically in Africa, there is the potential for filoviruses to spread to other continents. Although rare, clinicians in the United States should be aware of the symptoms of EBOV and MARV infection in humans and know the appropriate procedures for contacting local and state health departments and the CDC in the event of a suspected case of FHF.

REFERENCES

1. Regnery RL, Johnson KM, Kiley MP. Virion nucleic acid of Ebola virus. J Virol 1980;36(2):465–9.
2. Suzuki Y, Gojobori T. The origin and evolution of Ebola and Marburg viruses. Mol Biol Evol 1997;14(8):800–6.
3. Towner JS, Sealy TK, Khristova ML, et al. Newly discovered Ebola virus associated with hemorrhagic fever outbreak in Uganda. PLoS Pathog 2008;4(11): e1000212.
4. Formenty P, Hatz C, Le Guenno B, et al. Human infection due to Ebola virus, subtype Cote d'Ivoire: clinical and biologic presentation. J Infect Dis 1999; 179(Suppl 1):S48–53.
5. World Health Organization. Ebola Reston in pigs and humans in the Philippines: update. Available at: http://www.who.int/csr/don/2009_03_31/en/index.html. Accessed April 27, 2009.
6. Centers for Disease Control and Prevention. Marburg hemorrhagic fever, imported case—United States. Available at: http://www.cdc.gov/ncidod/dvrd/spb/outbreaks/index.htm. Accessed June 20, 2009.
7. World Health Organization. Epidemic and pandemic alert and response (EPR): case of Marburg haemorrhagic fever imported into the Netherlands from Uganda. Available at: http://www.who.int/csr/don/2008_07_10/en/index.html. Accessed June 20, 2009.
8. US Department of Health and Human Services. Biosafety in microbiological and biomedical laboratories. 5th edition. Washington, DC: U.S. Government Printing Office; 2007.
9. Sanchez A, Geisbert TW, Feldmann H. Filoviridae: Marburg and Ebola viruses. In: Knipe BM, Howley PM, Griffen DE, et al, editors. Fields virology. 5th edition. Philadelphia: Lippincott-Raven; 2007. p. 1409–48.

10. Colebunders R, Tshomba A, Van Kerkhove MD, et al. Marburg hemorrhagic fever in Durba and Watsa, Democratic Republic of the Congo: clinical documentation, features of illness, and treatment. J Infect Dis 2007;196(Suppl 2):S148–53.
11. Ksiazek TG, Rollin PE, Williams AJ, et al. Clinical virology of Ebola hemorrhagic fever (EHF): virus, virus antigen, and IgG and IgM antibody findings among EHF patients in Kikwit, Democratic Republic of the Congo, 1995. J Infect Dis 1999;179(Suppl 1):S177–87.
12. Towner JS, Rollin PE, Bausch DG, et al. Rapid diagnosis of Ebola hemorrhagic fever by reverse transcription-PCR in an outbreak setting and assessment of patient viral load as a predictor of outcome. J Virol 2004;78(8):4330–41.
13. Bwaka MA, Bonnet MJ, Calain P, et al. Ebola hemorrhagic fever in Kikwit, Democratic Republic of the Congo: clinical observations in 103 patients. J Infect Dis 1999;179(Suppl 1):S1–7.
14. Zaki SR, Goldsmith CS. Pathologic features of filovirus infections in humans. Curr Top Microbiol Immunol 1999;235:97–116.
15. Smith DH, Johnson BK, Isaacson M, et al. Marburg-virus disease in Kenya. Lancet 1982;1(8276):816–20.
16. Emond RT, Evans B, Bowen ET, et al. A case of Ebola virus infection. Br Med J 1977;2(6086):541–4.
17. Rowe AK, Bertolli J, Khan AS, et al. Clinical, virologic, and immunologic follow-up of convalescent Ebola hemorrhagic fever patients and their household contacts, Kikwit, Democratic Republic of the Congo. Commission de Lutte contre les Epidemies a Kikwit. J Infect Dis 1999;179(Suppl 1):S28–35.
18. Bray M, Geisbert TW. Ebola virus: the role of macrophages and dendritic cells in the pathogenesis of Ebola hemorrhagic fever. Int J Biochem Cell Biol 2005;37(8): 1560–6.
19. Geisbert TW, Hensley LE, Larsen T, et al. Pathogenesis of Ebola hemorrhagic fever in cynomolgus macaques: evidence that dendritic cells are early and sustained targets of infection. Am J Pathol 2003;163(6):2347–70.
20. Geisbert TW, Young HA, Jahrling PB, et al. Mechanisms underlying coagulation abnormalities in Ebola hemorrhagic fever: overexpression of tissue factor in primate monocytes/macrophages is a key event. J Infect Dis 2003;188(11): 1618–29.
21. Simmons G, Reeves JD, Grogan CC, et al. DC-SIGN and DC-SIGNR bind Ebola glycoproteins and enhance infection of macrophages and endothelial cells. Virology 2003;305(1):115–23.
22. Baize S, Leroy EM, Georges-Courbot MC, et al. Defective humoral responses and extensive intravascular apoptosis are associated with fatal outcome in Ebola virus-infected patients. Nat Med 1999;5(4):423–6.
23. Gupta M, Mahanty S, Ahmed R, et al. Monocyte-derived human macrophages and peripheral blood mononuclear cells infected with Ebola virus secrete MIP-1alpha and TNF-alpha and inhibit poly-IC-induced IFN-alpha in vitro. Virology 2001;284(1):20–5.
24. Bosio CM, Aman MJ, Grogan C, et al. Ebola and Marburg viruses replicate in monocyte-derived dendritic cells without inducing the production of cytokines and full maturation. J Infect Dis 2003;188(11):1630–8.
25. Mahanty S, Hutchinson K, Agarwal S, et al. Cutting edge: impairment of dendritic cells and adaptive immunity by Ebola and Lassa viruses. J Immunol 2003;170(6): 2797–801.
26. Geisbert TW, Hensley LE, Gibb TR, et al. Apoptosis induced in vitro and in vivo during infection by Ebola and Marburg viruses. Lab Invest 2000;80(2):171–86.

27. Harcourt BH, Sanchez A, Offermann MK. Ebola virus selectively inhibits responses to interferons, but not to interleukin-1beta, in endothelial cells. J Virol 1999;73(4):3491–6.

28. Hartman AL, Bird BH, Towner JS, et al. Inhibition of IRF-3 activation by VP35 is critical for the high virulence of Ebola virus. J Virol 2008;82(6):2699–704.

29. Hartman AL, Towner JS, Nichol ST. A C-terminal basic amino acid motif of Zaire ebolavirus VP35 is essential for type I interferon antagonism and displays high identity with the RNA-binding domain of another interferon antagonist, the NS1 protein of influenza A virus. Virology 2004;328(2):177–84.

30. Reid SP, Leung LW, Hartman AL, et al. Ebola virus VP24 binds karyopherin alpha1 and blocks STAT1 nuclear accumulation. J Virol 2006;80(11):5156–67.

31. Ruf W. Emerging roles of tissue factor in viral hemorrhagic fever. Trends Immunol 2004;25(9):461–4.

32. Towner JS, Khristova ML, Sealy TK, et al. Marburgvirus genomics and association with a large hemorrhagic fever outbreak in Angola. J Virol 2006;80(13):6497–516.

33. Towner JS, Sealy TK, Ksiazek TG, et al. High-throughput molecular detection of hemorrhagic fever virus threats with applications for outbreak settings. J Infect Dis 2007;196(Suppl 2):S205–12.

34. Centers for Disease Control and Prevention. Interim guidance for managing patients with suspected viral hemorrhagic fever in U.S. Hospitals. Available at: http://www.cdc.gov/ncidod/dhqp/bp_vhf_interimGuidance.html. Accessed June 5, 2009.

35. Bausch DG, Towner JS, Dowell SF, et al. Assessment of the risk of Ebola virus transmission from bodily fluids and fomites. J Infect Dis 2007;196(Suppl 2):S142–7.

36. Peters CJ, Jahrling PB, Khan AS. Patients infected with high-hazard viruses: scientific basis for infection control. Arch Virol Suppl 1996;11:141–68.

37. Francesconi P, Yoti Z, Declich S, et al. Ebola hemorrhagic fever transmission and risk factors of contacts, Uganda. Emerg Infect Dis 2003;9(11):1430–7.

38. Baron RC, McCormick JB, Zubeir OA. Ebola virus disease in southern Sudan: hospital dissemination and intrafamilial spread. Bull World Health Organ 1983; 61(6):997–1003.

39. Kerstiens B, Matthys F. Interventions to control virus transmission during an outbreak of Ebola hemorrhagic fever: experience from Kikwit, Democratic Republic of the Congo, 1995. J Infect Dis 1999;179(Suppl 1):S263–7.

40. Georges AJ, Leroy EM, Renaut AA, et al. Ebola hemorrhagic fever outbreaks in Gabon, 1994-1997: epidemiologic and health control issues. J Infect Dis 1999; 179(Suppl 1):S65–75.

41. World Health Organization. Marburg hemmorrhagic fever in Angola-Update 26. Available at: http://www.who.int/csr/don/2005_11_07a/en/index.html. Accessed June 7, 2009.

42. Bausch DG, Sprecher AG, Jeffs B, et al. Treatment of Marburg and Ebola hemorrhagic fevers: a strategy for testing new drugs and vaccines under outbreak conditions. Antiviral Res 2008;78(1):150–61.

43. Takada A, Ebihara H, Jones S, et al. Protective efficacy of neutralizing antibodies against Ebola virus infection. Vaccine 2007;25(6):993–9.

44. Mupapa K, Massamba M, Kibadi K, et al. Treatment of Ebola hemorrhagic fever with blood transfusions from convalescent patients. International Scientific and Technical Committee. J Infect Dis 1999;179(Suppl 1):S18–23.

45. Jahrling PB, Geisbert J, Swearengen JR, et al. Passive immunization of Ebola virus-infected cynomolgus monkeys with immunoglobulin from hyperimmune horses. Arch Virol Suppl 1996;11:135–40.

46. Jahrling PB, Geisbert JB, Swearengen JR, et al. Ebola hemorrhagic fever: evaluation of passive immunotherapy in nonhuman primates. J Infect Dis 2007; 196(Suppl 2):S400–3.
47. Oswald WB, Geisbert TW, Davis KJ, et al. Neutralizing antibody fails to impact the course of Ebola virus infection in monkeys. PLoS Pathog 2007;3(1):e9.
48. Huggins JW. Prospects for treatment of viral hemorrhagic fevers with ribavirin, a broad-spectrum antiviral drug. Rev Infect Dis 1989;11(Suppl 4):S750–61.
49. Jahrling PB, Geisbert TW, Geisbert JB, et al. Evaluation of immune globulin and recombinant interferon-alpha2b for treatment of experimental Ebola virus infections. J Infect Dis 1999;179(Suppl 1):S224–34.
50. Geisbert TW, Hensley LE, Kagan E, et al. Postexposure protection of guinea pigs against a lethal Ebola virus challenge is conferred by RNA interference. J Infect Dis 2006;193(12):1650–7.
51. Geisbert TW, Hensley LE, Jahrling PB, et al. Treatment of Ebola virus infection with a recombinant inhibitor of factor VIIa/tissue factor: a study in rhesus monkeys. Lancet 2003;362(9400):1953–8.
52. Bray M, Raymond JL, Geisbert T, et al. 3-deazaneplanocin A induces massively increased interferon-alpha production in Ebola virus-infected mice. Antiviral Res 2002;55(1):151–9.
53. Bray M, Driscoll J, Huggins JW. Treatment of lethal Ebola virus infection in mice with a single dose of an S-adenosyl-L-homocysteine hydrolase inhibitor. Antiviral Res 2000;45(2):135–47.
54. Hensley LE, Stevens EL, Yan SB, et al. Recombinant human activated protein C for the postexposure treatment of Ebola hemorrhagic fever. J Infect Dis 2007; 196(Suppl 2):S390–9.
55. Feldmann H, Jones SM, Daddario-DiCaprio KM, et al. Effective post-exposure treatment of Ebola infection. PLoS Pathog 2007;3(1):e2.
56. Reed DS, Mohamadzadeh M. Status and challenges of filovirus vaccines. Vaccine 2007;25(11):1923–34.
57. Geisbert TW, Pushko P, Anderson K, et al. Evaluation in nonhuman primates of vaccines against Ebola virus. Emerg Infect Dis 2002;8(5):503–7.
58. Ignatyev GM, Agafonov AP, Streltsova MA, et al. Inactivated Marburg virus elicits a nonprotective immune response in Rhesus monkeys. J Biotechnol 1996; 44(1–3):111–8.
59. Swenson DL, Warfield KL, Kuehl K, et al. Generation of Marburg virus-like particles by co-expression of glycoprotein and matrix protein. FEMS Immunol Med Microbiol 2004;40(1):27–31.
60. Warfield KL, Swenson DL, Olinger GG, et al. Ebola virus-like particle-based vaccine protects nonhuman primates against lethal Ebola virus challenge. J Infect Dis 2007;196(Suppl 2):S430–7.
61. Swenson DL, Warfield KL, Negley DL, et al. Virus-like particles exhibit potential as a pan-filovirus vaccine for both Ebola and Marburg viral infections. Vaccine 2005; 23(23):3033–42.
62. Swenson DL, Warfield KL, Larsen T, et al. Monovalent virus-like particle vaccine protects guinea pigs and nonhuman primates against infection with multiple Marburg viruses. Expert Rev Vaccines 2008;7(4):417–29.

Staphylococcus aureus: An Old Pathogen with New Weapons

Yi-Wei Tang, MD, PhD[a,b,]*, Charles W. Stratton, MD[a]

KEYWORDS

- *Staphylococcus aureus* • Necrotizing fasciitis
- Methicillin-resistant *S aureus* (MRSA)
- Community-associated MRSA • Panton-Valentine leukocidin

MICROBIOLOGY

S aureus is tentatively considered a member of the *Macrococcus* genus rather than a member of the *Micrococcus* genus.[1,2] Microscopically, *S aureus* is a gram-positive coccus that occurs in grape-like clusters. Because of its ability to divide in two planes, the tetrad is often considered characteristic for staphylococci on Gram stain and other stains (**Fig. 1**). *S aureus* is an aerobic, nonmotile organism that grows readily on sheep blood agar (SBA) characterized by a golden color of the colonies, which is produced by carotinoid pigments[3] and is responsible for the species name, *aureus*. The staphylococcal golden pigment seems to impair polymorphonuclear granulocyte killing and thus promotes virulence through its antioxidant activity.[4] In addition, *S aureus* generally produces beta hemolysis on SBA. Identification of *S aureus* is generally done by phenotypic methods, which include coagulase tests and agglutination tests that detect the presence of surface determinants, such as coagulase, clumping factor, protein A, and polysaccharides.[2] Other biochemical tests may be used on occasion. For example, mannitol fermentation may be used to screen for the presence of *S aureus*,[5] and the presence of thermostable deoxyribonuclease may be used for a more rapid identification of *S aureus* from blood cultures.[6] Finally, multiplex polymerase chain reaction (PCR) methods have been described; these offer the ability to rapidly identify resistance mechanisms and virulence factors from *S aureus* isolated

[a] Department of Pathology and Medicine, Vanderbilt University School of Medicine, 1161 21 st Avenue South, Nashville, TN 37232, USA
[b] Molecular Infectious Disease Laboratory, Vanderbilt University Hospital, 4605 TVC, Nashville, TN 37232-5310, USA
* Corresponding author. Molecular Infectious Disease Laboratory, Vanderbilt University Hospital, 4605 TVC, Nashville, TN 37232-5310.
E-mail address: yiwei.tang@vanderbilt.edu.

Clin Lab Med 30 (2010) 179–208
doi:10.1016/j.cll.2010.01.005
0272-2712/10/$ – see front matter © 2010 Elsevier Inc. All rights reserved.

labmed.theclinics.com

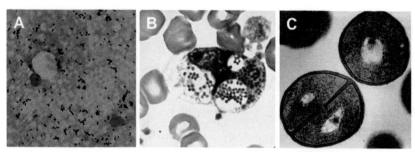

Fig. 1. *S aureus* under the microscope. (*A*) Gram stain from tissue with CA-MRSA infection. Note the absence of polymorphonuclear granulocytes. (*B*) Wright stain of blood smear showing intracellular *S aureus*. (*C*) Transmitted electron micrograph of *S aureus*.

from blood cultures.[7,8] Such DNA methods are likely to become increasingly important in the near future as a means of reducing the morbidity and mortality of *S aureus* infections.

Methicillin resistance in *S aureus* is mediated by the production of a low-affinity penicillin-binding protein 2a that is encoded by the *mecA* gene.[9,10] The gene is located on a mobile element, the staphylococcal chromosomal cassette *mec* (SCC*mec*).[11–13] Several different SCC*mec* elements have been identified in methicillin-resistant *S aureus* (MRSA). The SCC*mec* typing provides strong evidence for the independent deviation of health care-associated (HA)–MRSA and community-associated (CA)–MRSA clones.[13] The SCC*mec* types I, II, and III are predominantly found in HA-MRSA strains, whereas the SCC*mec* types IV and V are mainly observed in CA-MRSA isolates circulating worldwide.[12,14–16] The authors conducted a large-scale investigation of antimicrobial susceptibility patterns, Panton-Valentine leukocidin (PVL) occurrence, and SCC*mec* types in MRSA isolates from middle Tennessee. Among 1315 MRSA isolates, 34.1% were SCC*mec*-II and 64.4% were SCC*mec*-IV.[17] There were significant differences regarding isolation sites between HA- and CA-MRSA isolates. HA-MRSA strains were recovered more frequently from the respiratory tract among children than adults indicating that more respiratory site infections are caused by

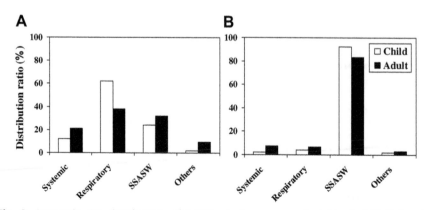

Fig. 2. Anatomic site distribution of MRSA strains recovered at Vanderbilt University Medical Center. (*A*) HA-MRSA; (*B*) CA-MRSA. SSASW, skin and soft tissues, abscess, and surgical wounds.

CA-MRSA strains in children (**Fig. 2**).[15,17] Antimicrobial susceptibility results in MRSA strains were consistent with previous findings in that most HA-MRSA isolates remain susceptible to tetracycline/minocycline, clindamycin, gentamicin, rifampin, and trimethoprim-sulfamethoxazole (**Fig. 3**).[17,18]

EPIDEMIOLOGY

S aureus has been recognized as an important human pathogen for more than 100 years.[19–21] The epidemiology of infections caused by *S aureus* must begin with the habitat of this microorganism, which is the skin and mucous membranes of mammals and birds. In humans, *S aureus* is most consistently isolated from the nares, although it can be isolated from many skin sites, including the axillae and inguinal regions as well as from the perianal area.[22] *S aureus* is present in the nares of approximately 30% of healthy humans although carriage rates up to 50% can be seen in certain populations, such as injection drug users, persons with insulin-dependent diabetes, patients with long-term indwelling catheters, patients with dermatologic conditions, and health care workers.[1] The nares are considered the most important colonization site in humans because elimination of *S aureus* from the nares results in the subsequent disappearance of this pathogen from other areas of the body and the reduction of postsurgical staphylococcal infections.[1,22] The prevalence of *S aureus* as a colonizer of human nares, however, in no way diminishes the importance of colonization of other sites or the potential for carriage and transmission on the hands of health care workers.[23,24]

Colonization is an important step in the pathogenesis of *S aureus* infection and is instrumental in the nosocomial epidemiology of these bacteria. Nasal carriage is a risk factor for acquiring nosocomial infection.[1] It has been shown that 80% of nosocomial *S aureus* bacteremia episodes in carriers of this bacteria were attributed to an endogenous source.[25] Nosocomial *S aureus* bacteremia was three times more frequent in *S aureus* carriers than in noncarriers.[26] Many studies of *S aureus* nasal carriage have been performed in various geographic regions in the United States and The Netherlands.[27–34] Cross section surveys of nasal carriage prevalence and transmission mechanisms in special healthy populations are beneficial in assessing risk factors associated with *S aureus* infections.[27–34] Military facilities provide unique opportunities for studying *S aureus* nasal

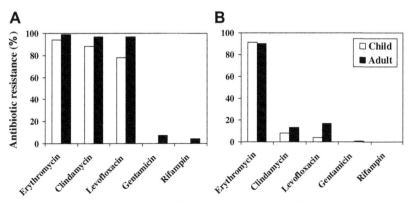

Fig. 3. Antimicrobial susceptibilities of MRSA strains recovered at Vanderbilt University Medical Center. (*A*) HA-MRSA; (*B*) CA-MRSA.

colonization and transmission.[35–37] In a cross-sectional observational study, the authors assessed the prevalence and risk factors of S aureus nasal colonization among Chinese military volunteers in two camps in the Beijing area. The data indicated that methicillin-sensitive S aureus (MSSA), not MRSA, nasal colonization, and clonal transmission occur in healthy military volunteers in Beijing. Younger, female, nonsmoking, volunteers with higher education and no social event participations, who served a shorter time, were at a higher risk for nasal MSSA carriage.[38] Previous studies reported several risk factors associated with MSSA colonization, including young age, female gender, chronic sinusitis, not taking antibiotics, hospital stay time, less education, and drug use.[27,28,35,37,39,40] The results confirmed that risk factors that attract MSSA and MRSA colonization were oppositely different, suggesting that competition by MSSA colonization may prevent the host from further MRSA nasal colonization.[38]

As one of the natural habitats of S aureus is the skin and mucous membranes of humans, the initial epidemiology of staphylococcal infections focused on the type of infection and whether or not there was an associated septicemia. The clinical occurrence of staphylococcal septicemia was recognized early, and the increased morbidity and mortality of such septicemia were noted.[19,41] For example, Skinner and Keefer[42] in 1941 found a mortality of 82% in 122 patients treated at Boston City Hospital for S aureus septicemia. The epidemiologic significance of staphylococcal septicemia was reduced with the introduction of penicillin for the therapy of serious staphylococcus bacteremias such as endocarditis.[43] Resistance to this wonder drug soon followed, however.[44] The epidemiology was then characterized by penicillin resistance, which was caused by a plasmid-borne β-lactamase gene.[45] This was the beginning of the molecular epidemiology of S aureus resistance mechanisms[46,47] as well as the beginning of molecular epidemiology.[48] The importance of gene transfer in the hospital environment was also recognized at this time[49] as the epidemiology of S aureus infections began to focus on resistance mechanisms and on acquisition of the staphylococcal infection in hospitals. The recognition of MRSA in 1961[50] and its association with hospital-acquired infections[51] resulted in the recognition that nosocomial MRSA infections[52] played a major role in the epidemiology of S aureus infections. This association of resistant strains of S aureus, in particular MRSA, with HA-MRSA was to remain the predominant focus for the epidemiology of S aureus infections until recently,[53] when genetic changes in S aureus resulted in the recognition of a new CA-MRSA.[54]

Currently, the epidemiology of S aureus infections, although changing, can be grouped into community-acquired and hospital-acquired infections with further subgrouping based on resistance traits. Community-acquired S aureus infections have always been an important aspect of the epidemiology of staphylococcal infections. Humans, due to their colonization/carriage of S aureus, are mostly at risk for community-acquired skin and soft tissue infections as a result of inoculation of their own staphylococci into cuts or wounds or via other alterations of the skin, such as atopy.[55] These community-acquired skin and soft tissue infections can be caused by MSSA or CA-MRSA.[56] In contrast, HA-MRSA rarely causes community-acquired skin and soft tissue infections.[57] Skin and soft tissue infections by either of these strains of S aureus (ie, infection caused by a methicillin-sensitive strain or by a methicillin-resistant stain) can be complicated by deeper invasion, abscess formation, or S aureus bacteremia, which may then result acutely in septicemia[58] or in endocarditits.[59] CA-MRSA skin and soft tissue infections seem to most likely result in more invasive disease with bacteremia.[58,60,61] This is most likely due to virulence factors in these CA-MRSA stains; these virulence factors are discussed at length in the pathogenesis section.

Hospital-acquired *S aureus* infections are another important epidemiologic aspect of staphylococcal infections. *S aureus* has long been a recognized cause of hospital-acquired infections[62] and, in particular, is associated with postoperative wound infections.[63] In addition to postoperative wound infections, nosocomial infections caused by *S aureus* include blood stream infections (often associated with intravenous lines) and respiratory tract infections (often associated with ventilators).[64] As the prevalence of MRSA in the United States increased,[53] the number of nosocomial MRSA infections increased.[52] These infections were most often seen in large, tertiary hospitals associated with medical schools, and the possible role of interhospital spread of MRSA by the transfer of infected patients and house staff from similar hospitals was raised.[65] In addition, these nosocomial MRSA infections were centered in critical care units with infected and colonized inpatients being the major institutional reservoir.[66] Transient carriage on the hands of hospital personnel seemed to be the most important mechanism of patient-to-patient transmission. There remains some debate, however, over the exact role of hospital personnel in the transmission of MRSA, with the characterization of hospital personnel ranging from victims[67] to superspreaders.[68] Finally, as would be predicted, nursing home patients who were hospitalized quickly became colonized/infected with MRSA.[69] These MRSA-colonized patients were sent back to the nursing homes, and soon nursing homes became another reservoir for MRSA.[70]

As discussed previously, the introduction of CA-MRSA is changing the epidemiology of *S aureus*. The reasons for this are addressed later. At this time, it is already clear that CA-MRSA is an emerging threat[71] that has become an important cause of community-acquired skin and soft-tissue infections[72] as well as community-acquired pneumonia[73] and is increasingly becoming recognized as a source of nosocomial staphylococcal infections.[74,75] It seems likely that the virulence traits associated with these CA-MRSA strains[76,77] result in an increased number of skin and soft-tissue infections as well as an increased number of more serious infections, such as septic arthritis[78] or osteomyelitis,[79] or a higher rate of staphylococcal bacteremia, but this remains to be determined as the epidemiology of these CA-MRSA infections unfolds. Individual case reports of unusual staphylococcal infections, such as one describing a case of xanthogranulomatous pyelonephritis,[80] suggest that CA-MRSA strains are causing an expanding spectrum of illness. Staphylococcal virulence factors, such as superantigens,[81,82] that can result in necrotizing fasciitis[83] also are associated with CA-MRSA infections. Another virulence factor, PVL,[84] is associated with the development of deep-seated follicular infection[85] and necrotizing pneumonitis.[86,87] Finally, staphylococcal bacteremia is recognized as an important factor in the morbidity and mortality of staphylococcal infections.[88–90] Staphylococcal bacteremia caused by HA-MRSA stains previously was associated with an increased morbidity and mortality[91]; CA-MRSA strains causing bacteremia seem to be associated with a morbidity and mortality that is increased even above that of HA-MRSA.[92] As the epidemiology of CA-MRSA infections evolves, the importance and role of this unique combination of resistance traits and virulence factors is becoming more apparent.

Another evolving subgrouping for the epidemiology of *S aureus* infections involves staphylococcal small colony variants (SCVs). SCVs of *S aureus* were described before the antimicrobial era,[93] yet the exact role of these staphylococcal variants in human infections remains unclear (**Fig. 4**). *S aureus* SVCs are a naturally occurring subpopulation of *S aureus* that grow slowly and have many atypical characteristics beleived due to defective electron transport.[94,95] Among the atypical characteristics seen are slow growth, impaired cell separation, absence of pigmentation, an unusual carbohydrate use, reduced hemolytic capability, low coagulase activity, and reduced toxin

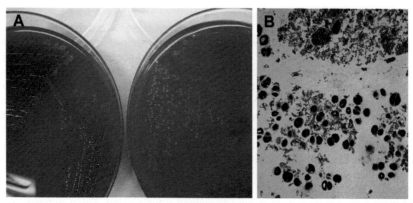

Fig. 4. SCVs of *S aureus*. (*A*) Colony characteristics of normal growth of *S aureus* (*left*) and SCVs (*right*). (*B*) Transmitted electron micrograph of *S aureus* in a heart valve. Note that most of these cocci exhibit the impaired cell separation characteristics of SCVs.

production.[95] SCVs seem particularly prone to invading mammalian cells and to persist in these cells, which may be a factor in the association of these forms with persistent, recurrent, and multiorgan infections.[96,97] The reduced production of alpha-toxin may, in part, allow survival in endothelial cells.[98] In addition, SCVs are less susceptible to antimicrobial agents than are strains from their parent population.[99] In part, the slow growth and impaired cell separation is responsible for this decreased susceptibility; resistance traits, such as the *mecA* gene, may also be present and responsible for part of the resistance.[100] In clinical stains of SCVs, the most frequent mutations that affect electron transport are in the operons encoding menaquinone or heme biosynthesis.[95] Moreover, stable mutants in electron transport have been generated by interrupting one of the heme biosynthetic genes, *hemB*.[98] These induced mutants have similar characteristics to clinical isolates of SCVs. Several different SCV mutants are described. Some mutants have a lower transmembrane potential that is believed to impede the uptake of aminoglycosides. Other SCV mutants have a mutation in their thymidylate synthase gene (*thyA*), and thus are dependent on exogenous thymidine to grow.[101,102]

The epidemiology of SCVs is becoming better defined. Although SCVs are seen in acute invasive staphylococcal infections, such as sternoclavicular joint septic arthritis,[103] these pathogens are more often seen in persistent device-related infections, such as those with prosthetic joints.[104] Such infections are difficult to diagnose and difficult to treat.[97,105,106] SCVs also are described in recurrent ventriculoperitoneal shunt infections[107] and pacemaker-related infection.[108] Finally, persistent infection with SCVs are reported in patients with cystic fibrosis.[101,109] All of these persistent infections caused by SCVs seem to involve biofilm, which is a recognized virulence factor for *S aureus*.[110] It is possible that SCVs represent a staphylococcal stringent response[111] related to reduced nutrients in biofilm. Such a stringent response is seen with *Pseudomonas aeruginosa* colonizing biofilms of cystic fibrosis patients.[112] Further elucidation of the role of SCVs in biofilm-related staphylococcal infections remains to be determined.

CLINICAL PRESENTATION

The clinical presentation of *S aureus* infections is varied and depends on the site of infection as well as the virulence factors produced by the staphylococcal stain causing infection. *S aureus* can colonize or infect the skin[113]; it therefore is appropriate to start with these skin infections when discussing the clinical presentation of staphylococcal infections. These skin infections may be minor and easily treated in the outpatient setting, or they may be serious and require hospitalization. Staphylococcal skin infections (**Fig. 5**) commonly encountered in the community setting include impetigo, bullous impetigo, folliculitis/furunculosis, simple abscesses, and complicated abscesses, including pyomyositis (**Fig. 6**)[114] and necrotizing fasciitis (**Fig. 7**).[115,116] In the hospital setting, staphylococcal skin infections are most often encountered postoperatively as surgical site infections.[117,118]

Pain at the site of staphylococcal skin and soft tissue infections is a frequent and important clinical clue that alerts patients and clinicians to the possibility of infection and allows localization of the infection. Sometimes these skin infections may not even be believed to be infections. For example, patients may confuse staphylococcal furunculosis with spider bites (see **Fig. 5**).[119] Some clinical syndromes associated with staphylococcal skin infections may be characteristic and, in part, defined by their anatomic distribution. Impetigo is a superficial staphylococcal surface infection of the skin involving only the epidermis in which toxins can lead to lifting of the stratum corneum resulting in the commonly seen bullous effect. Folliculitis is staphylococcal infection of the hair follicle. Deeper and more extensive staphylococcal infection of the hair follicle is defined as a furuncle or a carbuncle. Other examples of such clinical syndromes include blepharitis[120] and hordeolum,[121] which are staphylococcal infections involving the eyelid.

In addition to pain at the site of infection, staphylococcal infections are characterized by purulence and the formation of abscesses.[122,123] Purulence alone is most

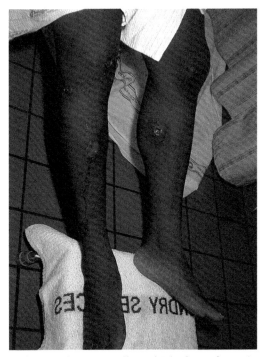

Fig. 5. CA-MRSA skin infections characterized by multiple abscess formation. (*Photograph courtesy of* Michael Gelfand, MD, University of Tennessee School of Medicine, Memphis, TN, USA.)

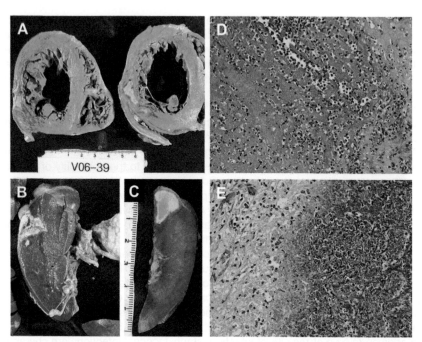

Fig. 6. Myocardial abscesses of heart (*A*), spleen (*B*), and kidney (*C*) in a patient with endocarditis caused by *S aureus*. Heart (*D*) and kidney (*E*) are hematoxylin-eosin stain stained infected tissue slides.

often seen in impetigo and bullous impetigo. Abscesses are usually seen in hair follicle–associated infections, such as folliculitis, furuncles, and carbuncles.[116,124] Drainage of such abscesses seems to be a critical aspect of the therapy of these soft tissue infections.[125,126]

Staphylococcal infections of the skin and soft tissues can have local and distant effects that are a result of the production of toxins (**Fig. 8**).[127] Exfoliative staphylococcal skin diseases, such as bullous impetigo[128] and staphylococcal scalded skin syndrome,[129] are well known examples of the ability of *S aureus* to produce toxin-mediated effects. Examples of exfoliative toxins produced by *S aureus* include toxins A, B, C, and D. Each of these toxins can cause the blisters seen in bullous impetigo as well as the more generalized exfoliation seen with scalded-skin syndrome. These toxins function as "molecular scissors" by producing cleavage of a single peptide bond in desmoglein, which is a desmosomal intercellular adhesion molecule.[130,131] Cleavage of desmoglein causes the loss of keratinocyte cell-cell adhesion in the superficial epidermis and produces a blistering skin disease. Cleavage only occurs in the epidermal stratum corneum. Mucosa is never involved; this, in part, differentiates staphylococcal scalded skin syndrome from toxic epidermal necrolysis. Toxic epidermal necrolysis is a potentially serious disease commonly associated with erythema multiforme major and drug reactions. Toxic epidermal necrolysis results in cleavage below the epidermis and the underlying dermis and typically involves mucosal tissues. In contrast to the cleavage seen with staphylococcal exfoliative processes, the epidermal stratum corneum is not involved.

Among the diverse clinical presentations of *S aureus* is food poisoning. This is not a direct effect caused by staphylococcal infection of the gastrointestinal tract but

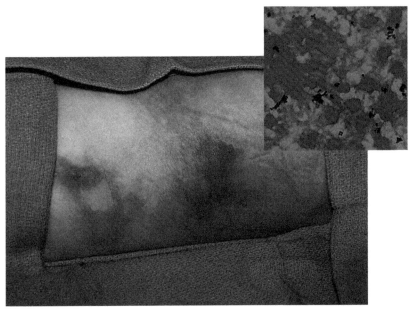

Fig. 7. Necrotizing fasciitis caused by CA-MRSA in an infant. Insert shows the Gram stain from this infection. Note the absence of polymorphonuclear granulocytes related to PVL.

instead is a distant effect caused by contamination of food or beverages by enterotoxins produced by S aureus. Staphylococcal enterotoxins are a family of heat-stable enterotoxins that are a leading cause of gastroenteritis.[132–134] Staphylococcal food poisoning is due to the ingestion of these heat-stable preformed enterotoxins. Cooking does not denature these toxins because they are heat stable. The association of food poisoning with S aureus was first described in 1935,[135] whereas the role of enterotoxins was not described until 35 years later.[136] Clinically, staphylococcal food poisoning is characterized by a short incubation period (hours) after the ingestion of the preformed toxin. This short incubation period usually allows the contaminated food to be identified. The clinical symptoms include the acute onset of nausea and vomiting rapidly followed by abdominal pain and diarrhea.[127] There is no fever associated with this food poisoning; the clinical course is usually short, lasting 6 to 12 hours.

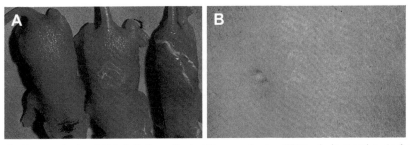

Fig. 8. S aureus toxins. (A) Exfoliative effect of S aureus toxins. (B) Staphylococcal toxic shock skin rash.

The clinical presentation of staphylococcal skin infections may reflect serious invasive infections. Deeper skin and soft tissue infections may lead to bacteremia with distant metastatic infection. Moreover, strains of S aureus that produce a superantigen, such as the toxic shock syndrome toxin-1 (TSST-1), can result in necrotizing fasciitis[137] or toxic-shock syndrome.[138] The clinical presentation of these severe staphylococcal infections can be different from that seen with minor skin and soft tissue infections. There is usually no question that the patient has a severe systemic infection of some sort. Severe staphylococcal infections are often accompanied by a high fever with associated rigors; these infections may have clinical features of sepsis, such as refractory hypotension.[139] An acute onset illness characterized by fever, rash, and refractory hypotension should suggest the possibility of staphylococcal toxic shock syndrome.[140]

Pain is also an important part of the clinical presentation of severe staphylococcal infections and may assist in the localization of these deeper infections. For example, fever and chest pain with cough suggest the possibility of staphylococcal pneumonia,[141] which in the era of CA-MRSA may be a rapidly fatal disease. Fever and back pain suggest the possibility of staphylococcal endocarditis (see **Fig. 6; Fig. 9**),[142] staphylococcal spondylodiscitis,[143] staphylococcal epidural abscess,[144] or staphylococcal pyogenic vertebral osteomyelitis.[145] Of these, epidural abscess is considered a medical emergency and requires urgent neurosurgical consultation/intervention. Janeway lesion can be seen in patients with staphylococcal endocarditis (**Fig. 10**). Fever with joint pain, swelling, and immobility suggest the possibility of staphylococcal septic arthritis.[146] Fever, headache, and stiff neck suggest staphylococcal meningitis.[147] Meningitis is also considered a medical emergency. Meningitis caused by S aureus is somewhat unusual unless a patient has had a recent neurosurgical procedure; in the absence of such a procedure, S aureus endocarditis with septic emboli to be CNS should be considered.

PATHOGENESIS

S aureus is an extraordinarily successful pathogen that has been able to adapt and evolve in terms of its resistance traits and virulence factors such that it continues to be among the most important causes of human infections in the twenty-first century.[30,148,149] The pathogenesis of S aureus infection begins with the attachment of this microbe to human skin and mucosal tissues. S aureus is able to bind to several

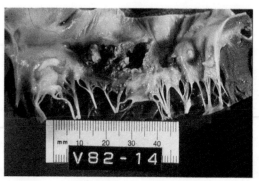

Fig. 9. Endocarditis caused by S aureus. Note the perforation of the valve leading to the need for a valve replacement.

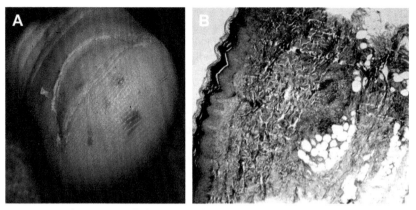

Fig. 10. Janeway lesion in staphylococcal endocarditis. (*A*) Foot Janeway lesions. (*B*) Brown-Brenn stain of Janeway lesion. Note the microabscesses.

sites in skin and mucosa. These sites include fibronectin-coated surfaces,[150] endothelial cells,[151] human nasal mucin,[152,153] and nasal epithelial cells.[154] Despite this ability to attach to skin and mucosal surfaces, *S aureus* seems not to grow readily on these surfaces, most likely due to the presence of resident flora, such as *S epidermidis*.[155] Thus, *S aureus* is often a transient colonizer of human skin and mucosal tissues. In some patients, this colonization seems to be long lasting (years). In colonized humans, an alteration of the normal host skin defenses may facilitate infection by *S aureus*. For example, hydration of the stratum corneum allows the growth of *S aureus*, which then produces toxins that enter the stratum corneum and produce an irritant reaction. This irritant reaction is followed by an inflammatory response in which polymorphonuclear granulocytes play a major role in containing this tissue invasion by *S aureus*. Alternatively, a simple break in the skin surface, such as that caused by a cut or an abrasion, allows direct tissue invasion by *S aureus*.

When circumstances allow or promote invasion of skin surfaces by *S aureus*, this pathogen is well equipped to evade the innate host defenses due to several virulence factors.[156,157] Virulence factors include biofilm, capsule, coagulase, lipase, hyaluronidase, protein A, fibronectin-binding protein, and multiple toxins.[158] For example, recent studies suggest that staphylococcal fibronectin-binding proteins also act as invasins and permit uptake of *S aureus* by nonphagocytic mammalian cells, such as epithelial cells and endothelial cells.[159,160] Invasion of such cells may provide a way for *S aureus* to evade normal host defenses. Moreover, *S aureus* is also able to survive engulfment by phagocytes, such as polymorphonuclear granulocytes, monocytes, and macrophages.[161] In particular, the ability of *S aureus* to survive phagocytosis by macrophages for several days without affecting the viability of these cells may prove to be a manner in which this pathogen may disseminate. CA-MRSA strains are able to evade the polymorphonuclear granulocyte response due to their production of PVL.[162] Evasion of the immune system allows *S aureus* the opportunity to reach local lymphatics and the blood stream where it can then reach distant tissues. Staphylococcal skin and soft tissue infections are well known for their ability to result in such metastatic infection. Septic emboli causing metastatic infection are often seen with staphylococcal endocarditis. Biopsies of Janeway lesions from endocarditis caused by *S aureus* demonstrate metastatic infections with suppuration and microabscesses as seen microscopically.[163]

In terms of its pathogenesis, S aureus is able to produce local effects at the site of infection or distant effects as a result of its ability to produce a wide variety of toxins. For example, PVL is an important virulence factor that causes leukocytolysis and tissue necrosis at the site of infection; the genetic element for this toxin is carried on a bacteriophage and thus is transmissible to other strains of S aureus.[164] In addition, there are additional toxins that can produce local and distant effects. These toxins include exfoliative toxins and enterotoxins. Staphylococcal enterotoxins are a family of nine major serologic types of heat-stable enterotoxins that are a major cause of gastroenteritis following ingestion of contaminated food.[132,134] Approximately 19 different enterotoxins and related toxins have been described to date. These enterotoxins are considered superantigens that activate T-cell subsets and elicit nonspecific T-cell proliferation after binding to major histocompatibility complex class II. Activated T cells vigorously proliferate and release proinflammatory cytokines and chemokines.

The genomics of S aureus have proved extremely important in understanding the pathogenesis of staphylococcal infections.[165] The availability of the complete genome sequencing of S aureus has revealed many new surface-attachment and secreted factors.[166] Moreover, S aureus harbors a wide variety of mobile genetic elements from exogenous origins.[167] These elements are horizontally transferred between strains of S aureus and can encode resistance determinants, such as the mecA gene, or virulence factors, such as PVL. These mobile genetic elements can be functionally characterized by whether or not they contain elements responsible for virulence or elements responsible for resistance. For example, superantigens are encoded by mobile genetic elements that are characterized by phage-related features and usually do not contain resistance determinants.[168] In contrast, resistance determinants are usually carried in a separate mobile genomic island known as the SCCmec.[11–13] The genetic plasticity achieved by such horizontal gene transfer in S aureus is, in part, responsible for the ongoing success of this pathogen.

DIAGNOSIS

Culture currently is the most commonly used method for the diagnosis of S aureus infection.[1] Rapid molecular identification in the clinical microbiology laboratory of these resistance and virulence factors expressed by S aureus promises in the near future to play an important role in decreasing the morbidity and mortality of staphylococcal infections.[7,8] Equally important to the identification of S aureus as the cause of the infection is the susceptibility of the infecting isolate. Several available diagnostic tests are available for MRSA testing. Traditional culture-based methods using SBA can take up to 72 hours to detect MRSA. An oxacillin agar screening test is useful for detecting MRSA.[5] An oxacillin screen plate contains Mueller-Hinton agar supplemented with 4% NaCl and 6 μg/mL oxacillin.[169] Any growth is considered a positive test and interpreted as MRSA.[9] Selective chromogenic media-based culture can reduce the time to detection while improving recovery rates. This method incorporates a selective antibiotic and a chromogenic substrate that provides easy visual identification of selected colonies. Chromogenic agar has high sensitivity and specificity, and more than 85% of cases can be identified within 24 hours.[170–172] Several chromogenic media, including CHROMagar MRSA (Becton, Dickinson), CMRSA (Oxoid Limited), MRSA ID (bioMérieux), MRSASelect (Bio-Rad), and Spectra MRSA (Remel), are commercially available for surveillance cultures of MRSA in the clinical setting (Fig. 11).

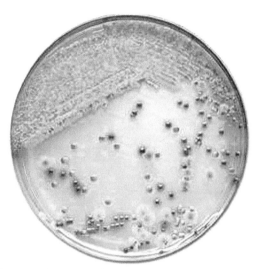

Fig. 11. Screening for MRSA by using a chromogenic medium. A CHROMagar MRSA (Becton, Dickinson, Sparks, Maryland) plate was inoculated with a nasal swab specimen and inoculated at 37°C for 24 hours. MRSA clones turned mauve while other bacterial colonies were inhibited, blue, or colorless.

Early diagnosis of severe infections caused by MRSA or CA-MRSA is crucial in guiding antimicrobial therapy. Blood culture using automated blood culture instruments with continuous monitoring remains the routine method for detecting staphylococcal bloodstream infections. Currently, definitive identification and antimicrobial susceptibility testing of staphylococci is time consuming, requiring 24 to 72 hours from the initial positive result for subculture, biochemical analysis, and antimicrobial susceptibility testing. This delay may lead to the unnecessary use of antimicrobial agents. Advanced laboratory techniques have been sought to rapidly identify staphylococcal isolates and determine antimicrobial susceptibility patterns. In particular, several molecular methods have been described to identify and differentiate staphylococcal isolates.[173,174] To take advantage of the rapid enrichment of automated blood culture instruments, several studies have reported that use of peptide or nucleic acid probes and conventional and real-time PCR can rapidly identify organisms from flagged blood cultures when staphylococci are detected.[173,175–178] The authors have reported two molecular systems, a StaphPlex system (Qiagen, Valencia, CA, USA)[8] (**Fig. 12**) and an IsoAmp Rapid Staph system (BioHelix, Beverly, MA, USA),[179] to rapidly detect and identify *S aureus* directly from staphylococci-presenting blood culture media. This may potentially better direct antibiotic usage when staphylococci are detected and thus lead to an overall reduction of use of vancomycin, which is often used empirically to treat patients until susceptibility results are available. The second version, IsoAmp Rapid Staph system, detects and characterizes *mecA* and *nuc* genes simultaneously in the same cassette (**Fig. 13**).

Traditional culture-based methods, especially those incorporating differential agar screening plates, are widely used for nasal MRSA screening. A rapid culture-based test measures adenylate kinase activity in an enriched selective broth culture, which produces results in 5 hours and has a negative predictive value of 90.4%.[180] Molecular

No.	Samples	epi	cons	haem	lug	homi	sim	nuc	mecA	ccrBI	ccrBII	ccrBIII	ccrBIV	pvl	aacA	ermA	ermC	tetM	tetK	iDS
01	S. epidermidis	1089	1870	20	33	26	28	10	2134	13	1833	3163	29	19	3093	2084	1894	4	9	16
02	S. haemolyticus	26	2959	2859	39	30	39	24	21	24	18	42	28	21	8	22	17	40	29	25
03	S. lugdunensis	45	3762	54	651	38	39	38	39	51	41	57	40	29	39	40	35	48	42	41
04	S. hominis	18	1772	27	27	756	14	20	2204	26	25	3812	31	24	2281	21	2268	3	35	25
05	S. simulans	13	1565	25	21	17	714	16	11	25	20	86	32	15	15	21	18	37	547	20
06	S. capitus	53	2519	52	54	41	34	55	78	32	36	54	57	50	40	56	33	47	25	48
07	S. warneri	17	3896	31	20	20	14	24	41	22	44	55	36	28	23	31	37	30	17	32
08	S. saprophyticus	31	2369	34	54	34	44	31	24	33	32	30	37	33	33	33	33	31	16	38
09	S. aureus (MSSA)	17	40	27	11	16	25	2229	53	23	41	40	29	24	34	26	17	35	19	20
10	HA-MRSA	20	44	41	40	25	20	2464	3557	17	3132	32	29	43	2900	3270	29	4461	38	26
11	HA-MRSA	25	51	40	24	7	34	990	3480	2845	25	27	28	27	17	18	14	4664	3499	25
12	HA-MRSA	1	43	22	20	12	19	924	3265	21	15	5357	35	20	658	2401	4120	4373	1132	20
13	CA-MRSA	14	30	15	15	28	9	1351	3563	36	39	22	4174	1874	22	14	29	30	17	44
14	Blank	10	21	8	2	9	11	4	13	14	7	17	22	11	3	8	12	18	8	10
15	CutOff	250	250	250	250	250	250	250	250	250	250	250	250	250	250	250	250	250	250	250

Fig. 12. Representative data from the StaphPlex system on selected prototype staphylococcal strains. Values are expressed as the median fluorescent intensity (MFI) value from the Luminex 200 (Austin, Texas). Each row represents a strain and each column represents one of 18 staphylococci-specific gene targets.

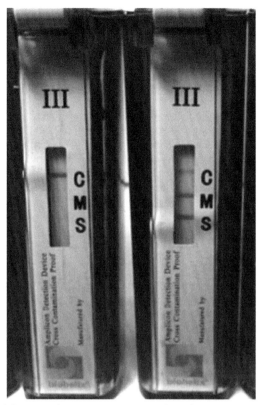

Fig. 13. Readout of the second version IsoAmp Rapid Staph BESt cassette (BioHelix, Beverly, Massachusetts). Positive reaction (*right*) and negative reaction (*left*) are shown. (*Photograph courtesy of* Huimin Kong, PhD, BioHelix Corp, Beverly, MA, USA.)

assays offer results that are available within hours, and they enable detection below the limit possible using conventional culture. Two molecular assays, including the BD GeneOhm MRSA (Becton, Dickinson) and the Cepheid Xpert MRSA (Cepheid) assays, are reported as sensitive and specific for detection and screening of MRSA nasal colonization.[29,181–184] The authors have developed an MVPlex assay to detect MRSA and vancomycin-resistant enterococci, two well-know causes of nosocomial infections, in one reaction tube.[185] A recent meta-analysis indicated that active screening for MRSA is more important than the type of test used. Because important and costly decisions, such as mandatory legislation for MRSA universal screening, are under consideration in many countries worldwide, policy makers should be aware of the limits and the heterogeneity of the available evidence.[186]

Adequate and precise typing of *S aureus* isolates that permits the monitoring of local outbreaks and wider-scale dissemination of specific dangerous clones is of great concern.[8,187,188] Differences in the various molecular methods used to define different genomic characteristics greatly affect their essential parameters, including discriminatory power and test turnaround time.[8,187,188] The most important methods currently used for MRSA typing are pulsed-field gel electrophoresis (PFGE),[17,189–191] multilocus sequence typing (MLST),[192,193] staphylococcal surface protein A (*spa*) typing,[187,190,194,195] multilocus variable tandem repeat analysis,[196,197] and repeat-element PCR (rep-PCR) typing.[191,198,199] These methods have been used to investigate the evolution of the MRSA clones that have emerged since the 1960s and to study their worldwide dissemination. **Table 1** contrasts commonly used molecular methods for S aureus typing.

Tremendous progress in molecular-typing methods has been made, with optimization and standardization of sequence-based technologies offering broad applicability and high throughput; however, no single S aureus typing method has yet provided rapid and reliable information that is sufficient to permit prompt action to control infections. Other bacterial genes (eg, coa) have been targeted for S aureus typing.[34] PCR coupled to electrospray ionization–mass spectrometry recently was reported for rapid molecular genotyping and clonal complex assignment of S aureus isolates.[200,201] Recently, a direct linear analysis was described to enable rapid, large-scale mapping of whole genomes by directly analyzing single linearized fragments of genomic DNA molecules of up to 250 kilobases in length from a simple restriction enzyme digest.[202] This approach was applied for molecular typing of S aureus. The process can be completed within 8 hours with a discriminatory power comparable to that of PFGE.[202,203]

TREATMENT AND PROGNOSIS

The treatment of S aureus infections generally consists of two aspects. When both aspects are properly addressed, the prognosis is excellent. The first aspect of treatment is appropriate antimicrobial therapy. This may involve topical agents, oral agents, or intravenous agents. The resistance traits exhibited by this pathogen continue to complicate the selection of appropriate antimicrobial therapy. Oral therapy is often a problem, particularly with CA-MRSA strains. Trimethoprim-sulfamethoxazole or clindamycin is usually used for S aureus skin and soft tissue infections in children when CA-MRSA is suspected.[204] The second aspect is drainage of staphylococcal abscesses. As S aureus infections often result in abscesses in whatever tissue is infected, drainage of these abscesses is essential. Bedside ultrasound is useful in determining the presence of occult abscess formation and prevents unnecessary invasive procedures.[205]

The treatment of severe staphylococcal skin and soft tissue infections can be much more problematic than the treatment of minor skin and soft tissue infection. Such treatment involves four fundamental management principles[125]: (1) early diagnosis and differentiation of necrotizing versus non-necrotizing fasciitis, (2) early initiation of appropriate intravenous antimicrobial therapy, (3) aggressive surgical intervention for drainage or débridement of necrotic tissue, and (4) timely identification of staphylococcal resistance traits and virulence factors. In addition, the treatment of severe S aureus infection should include admission to an intensive care unit[206,207] and consultation with an infectious diseases specialist.[208,209] Surgical consultation may also be required for drainage of staphylococcal abscesses or débridement of necrotic tissue.

The treatment of toxin-related staphylococcal infection raises some interesting possibilities. Commercial intravenous immunoglobulin (IVIG) neutralizes staphylococcal exotoxins, including the TSST-1.[210,211] Neutralization of S aureus PVL by IVIG may also prove useful because commercial IVIG preparations neutralize PVL.[212] This suggests that the use of IVIG for the treatment of severe staphylococcal infections in which such toxins are suspected is warranted.[213,214]

IMMUNITY

Immunity to staphylococcal infections is generally not seen; recurrent staphylococcal infections remain an important clinical problem.[215] S aureus infection produces

Table 1
Commonly used molecular methods for *S aureus* typing

Method	Data Output	Principle	Advantages	Disadvantages	Comments
PFGE	Image	Macrorestriction enzyme profile of entire bacterial genome	High discriminatory power to explore clonal diversity	Labor intensive and time consuming; hard to monitor long-term epidemic	Classic gold standard; limited and restricted database (PulseNet) is available
MLST	Nucleic acid sequences	Sequence variations of seven housekeeping genes	Universal database (http://www.mlst. net); objective and reproducible results	Costly and time consuming; hard to monitor rapid epidemic trends	eBURST is available to "blast" database containing more than 1000 sequence types
Spa sequencing	Nucleic acid sequences	Sequences and numbers of multiple repeats in the variable X region of the protein A gene	Fast and less labor intensive; amenable to high-throughput	Moderate discriminatory power; misclassification bias may happen	Spa databases are available via eGenomics and Ridom
Rep-PCR	Image	Random amplification of multicopy elements in entire bacterial genome	Rapid procedure; a high-throughput screening tool	Variable discriminatory power; poor reproducibility	A commercial kit along with a database is available from bioMérieux[199]

antigens that in recurrent staphylococcal infections result in increased titers of anti–*S aureus* antibody. For example, patients with an initial staphylococcal furuncle do not have elevated anti–*S aureus* antibody titers whereas those with repeated furuncles (ie, furunculosis) have high titers of anti–*S aureus* antibody.[216,217] These higher titers, however, do not seem to prevent or reduce recurrent staphylococcal furunculosis.[218] The possibility that antibodies against *S aureus* might prove useful, however, in preventing more invasive disease continues to spur vaccine studies.[219] *S aureus* capsular polysaccharides are important in the pathogenesis of infection[220] and are considered likely candidates for the development of vaccines.[221] Few, if any, of these vaccines have proved useful.[222] Finally, staphylococcal exotoxins also produce an immune response[215,223] and might be another vaccine avenue for future exploration.

REFERENCES

1. Kluytmans J, van Belkum A, Verbrugh H. Nasal carriage of *Staphylococcus aureus*: epidemiology, underlying mechanisms, and associated risks. Clin Microbiol Rev 1997;10(3):505–20.
2. Kwok AY, Chow AW. Phylogenetic study of Staphylococcus and Macrococcus species based on partial hsp60 gene sequences. Int J Syst Evol Microbiol 2003;53(Pt 1):87–92.
3. Hammond RK, White DC. Inhibition of carotenoid hydroxylation in *Staphylococcus aureus* by mixed-function oxidase inhibitors. J Bacteriol 1970;103(3):607–10.
4. Liu GY, Essex A, Buchanan JT, et al. *Staphylococcus aureus* golden pigment impairs neutrophil killing and promotes virulence through its antioxidant activity. J Exp Med 2005;202(2):209–15.
5. Lally RT, Ederer MN, Woolfrey BF. Evaluation of mannitol salt agar with oxacillin as a screening medium for methicillin-resistant *Staphylococcus aureus*. J Clin Microbiol 1985;22(4):501–4.
6. Ratner HB, Stratton CW. Thermonuclease test for same-day identification of *Staphylococcus aureus* in blood cultures. J Clin Microbiol 1985;21(6):995–6.
7. Miller MB, Tang YW. Basic concepts of microarrays and potential applications in clinical microbiology. Clin Microbiol Rev 2009;22(4):611–33.
8. Tang YW, Kilic A, Yang Q, et al. StaphPlex system for rapid and simultaneous identification of antibiotic resistance determinants and Panton-Valentine leukocidin detection of staphylococci from positive blood cultures. J Clin Microbiol 2007;45(6):1867–73.
9. Chambers HF. Methicillin resistance in staphylococci: molecular and biochemical basis and clinical implications. Clin Microbiol Rev 1997;10(4):781–91.
10. Katayama Y, Ito T, Hiramatsu K. A new class of genetic element, staphylococcus cassette chromosome mec, encodes methicillin resistance in *Staphylococcus aureus*. Antimicrob Agents Chemother 2000;44(6):1549–55.
11. Noto MJ, Kreiswirth BN, Monk AB, et al. Gene acquisition at the insertion site for SCCmec, the genomic island conferring methicillin resistance in *Staphylococcus aureus*. J Bacteriol 2008;190(4):1276–83.
12. Baba T, Takeuchi F, Kuroda M, et al. Genome and virulence determinants of high virulence community-acquired MRSA. Lancet 2002;359(9320):1819–27.
13. Okuma K, Iwakawa K, Turnidge JD, et al. Dissemination of new methicillin-resistant *Staphylococcus aureus* clones in the community. J Clin Microbiol 2002;40(11):4289–94.

14. Francis JS, Doherty MC, Lopatin U, et al. Severe community-onset pneumonia in healthy adults caused by methicillin-resistant *Staphylococcus aureus* carrying the Panton-Valentine leukocidin genes. Clin Infect Dis 2005;40(1):100–7.
15. Gonzalez BE, Hulten KG, Dishop MK, et al. Pulmonary manifestations in children with invasive community-acquired *Staphylococcus aureus* infection. Clin Infect Dis 2005;41(5):583–90.
16. Ito T, Ma XX, Takeuchi F, et al. Novel type V staphylococcal cassette chromosome mec driven by a novel cassette chromosome recombinase, ccrC. Antimicrob Agents Chemother 2004;48(7):2637–51.
17. Kilic A, Li H, Stratton CW, et al. Antimicrobial susceptibility patterns and staphylococcal cassette chromosome mec types of, as well as Panton-Valentine leukocidin occurrence among, methicillin-resistant *Staphylococcus aureus* isolates from children and adults in middle Tennessee. J Clin Microbiol 2006;44(12):4436–40.
18. Naimi TS, LeDell KH, Como-Sabetti K, et al. Comparison of community- and health care-associated methicillin-resistant *Staphylococcus aureus* infection. JAMA 2003;290(22):2976–84.
19. Berg AA. A case of acute osteomyelitis of the femur, with feneral systemic *Staphylococcus aureus* infection, teminating in recovery. Ann Surg 1900; 31(3):332–9.
20. Ogston A. Micrococcus poisoning. J Anat 1882;16(4):526–67.
21. Shinefield HR, Ruff NL. Staphylococcal infections: a historical perspective. Infect Dis Clin North Am 2009;23(1):1–15.
22. Vandenbergh MF, Verbrugh HA. Carriage of *Staphylococcus aureus*: epidemiology and clinical relevance. J Lab Clin Med 1999;133(6):525–34.
23. Popovich KJ. *Staphylococcus aureus*: not always right under your nose. Infect Control Hosp Epidemiol 2009;30(8):727–9.
24. Reighard A, Diekema D, Wibbenmeyer L, et al. *Staphylococcus aureus* nasal colonization and colonization or infection at other body sites in patients on a burn trauma unit. Infect Control Hosp Epidemiol 2009;30(8):721–6.
25. Vandenbergh MF, Yzerman EP, van Belkum A, et al. Follow-up of *Staphylococcus aureus* nasal carriage after 8 years: redefining the persistent carrier state. J Clin Microbiol 1999;37(10):3133–40.
26. Wertheim HF, Melles DC, Vos MC, et al. The role of nasal carriage in *Staphylococcus aureus* infections. Lancet Infect Dis 2005;5(12):751–62.
27. Bischoff WE, Wallis ML, Tucker KB, et al. *Staphylococcus aureus* nasal carriage in a student community: prevalence, clonal relationships, and risk factors. Infect Control Hosp Epidemiol 2004;25(6):485–91.
28. de Almeida Silva H, Steffen Abdallah VO, Carneiro CL, et al. Infection and colonization by *Staphylococcus aureus* in a high risk nursery of a Brazilian teaching hospital. Braz J Infect Dis 2003;7(6):381–6.
29. Farley JE, Stamper PD, Ross T, et al. Comparison of the BD GeneOhm methicillin-resistant *Staphylococcus aureus* (MRSA) PCR assay to culture by use of BBL CHROMagar MRSA for detection of MRSA in nasal surveillance cultures from an at-risk community population. J Clin Microbiol 2008;46(2):743–6.
30. Lowy FD. *Staphylococcus aureus* infections. N Engl J Med 1998;339(8):520–32.
31. Nulens E, Gould I, MacKenzie F, et al. *Staphylococcus aureus* carriage among participants at the 13th European Congress of Clinical Microbiology and Infectious Diseases. Eur J Clin Microbiol Infect Dis 2005;24(2):145–8.
32. Peacock SJ, Justice A, Griffiths D, et al. Determinants of acquisition and carriage of *Staphylococcus aureus* in infancy. J Clin Microbiol 2003;41(12): 5718–25.

33. Sdougkos G, Chini V, Papanastasiou DA, et al. Community-associated *Staphylococcus aureus* infections and nasal carriage among children: molecular microbial data and clinical characteristics. Clin Microbiol Infect 2008;14(11): 995–1001.
34. Shopsin B, Mathema B, Martinez J, et al. Prevalence of methicillin-resistant and methicillin-susceptible *Staphylococcus aureus* in the community. J Infect Dis 2000;182(1):359–62.
35. Ellis MW, Hospenthal DR, Dooley DP, et al. Natural history of community-acquired methicillin-resistant *Staphylococcus aureus* colonization and infection in soldiers. Clin Infect Dis 2004;39(7):971–9.
36. Kenner J, O'Connor T, Piantanida N, et al. Rates of carriage of methicillin-resistant and methicillin-susceptible *Staphylococcus aureus* in an outpatient population. Infect Control Hosp Epidemiol 2003;24(6):439–44.
37. Zhang W, Shen X, Zhang H, et al. Molecular epidemiological analysis of methicillin-resistant *Staphylococcus aureus* isolates from Chinese pediatric patients. Eur J Clin Microbiol Infect Dis 2009;28(7):861–4.
38. Qu F, Cui E, Guo T, et al. Nasal colonization and clonal transmission of methicillin-susceptible *Staphylococcus aureus* in Chinese military volunteers. J Clin Microbiol 2009;48(1):64–9.
39. Al-Rawahi GN, Schreader AG, Porter SD, et al. Methicillin-resistant *Staphylococcus aureus* nasal carriage among injection drug users: six years later. J Clin Microbiol 2008;46(2):477–9.
40. Graham PL 3rd, Lin SX, Larson EL. A U.S. population-based survey of *Staphylococcus aureus* colonization. Ann Intern Med 2006;144(5):318–25.
41. Reed AC, Stiles FE. Staphylococcus septicemia. Cal West Med 1927;26(4):492.
42. Skinner D, Keefer CS. Significance of bacteremia caused by *Staphylococcus aureus*. Arch Intern Med 1941;68:851–75.
43. Hoyt RE, Bissell FE. *Staphylococcus aureus* endocarditis: treatment with penicillin. Cal West Med 1941;63:226–7.
44. Beigelman PM, Rantz LA. The clinical importance of coagulase-positive, penicillin-resistant *Staphylococcus aureus*. N Engl J Med 1950;242(10):353–8.
45. Spink WW, Ferris V. Penicillin-resistant staphylococci: mechanisms involved in the development of resistance. J Clin Invest 1947;26(3):379–93.
46. Lacey RW. Genetic basis, epidemiology, and future significance of antibiotic resistance in *Staphylococcus aureus*: a review. J Clin Pathol 1973;26(12): 899–913.
47. Lacey RW. Antibiotic resistance plasmids of *Staphylococcus aureus* and their clinical importance. Bacteriol Rev 1975;39(1):1–32.
48. Chabbert YA, Roussel A. Taxonomy and epidemiology of R plasmids as molecular species. J Antimicrob Chemother 1977;3(Suppl C):25–33.
49. Lacey RW, Richmond MH. The genetic basis of antibiotic resistance in *S. aureus*: the importance of gene transfer in the evolution of this organism in the hospital environment. Ann N Y Acad Sci 1974;236(0):395–412.
50. Jevons MP. "Celbenin"-resistant staphylococci. Br Med J 1961;1:124–5.
51. Jevons MP, Parker MT. The evolution of new hospital strains of *Staphylococcus aureus*. J Clin Pathol 1964;17:243–50.
52. Boyce JM, White RL, Spruill EY. Impact of methicillin-resistant *Staphylococcus aureus* on the incidence of nosocomial staphylococcal infections. J Infect Dis 1983;148(4):763.
53. Boyce JM. Are the epidemiology and microbiology of methicillin-resistant *Staphylococcus aureus* changing? JAMA 1998;279(8):623–4.

54. Chambers HF. The changing epidemiology of *Staphylococcus aureus*? Emerg Infect Dis 2001;7(2):178–82.
55. Lubbe J. Secondary infections in patients with atopic dermatitis. Am J Clin Dermatol 2003;4(9):641–54.
56. Herold BC, Immergluck LC, Maranan MC, et al. Community-acquired methicillin-resistant *Staphylococcus aureus* in children with no identified predisposing risk. JAMA 1998;279(8):593–8.
57. Gardam MA. Is methicillin-resistant *Staphylococcus aureus* an emerging community pathogen? A review of the literature. Can J Infect Dis 2000;11(4):202–11.
58. Ho KM, Robinson JO. Risk factors and outcomes of methicillin-resistant *Staphylococcus aureus* bacteraemia in critically ill patients: a case control study. Anaesth Intensive Care 2009;37(3):457–63.
59. Benito N, Miro JM, de Lazzari E, et al. Health care-associated native valve endocarditis: importance of non-nosocomial acquisition. Ann Intern Med 2009; 150(9):586–94.
60. Moore CL, Hingwe A, Donabedian SM, et al. Comparative evaluation of epidemiology and outcomes of methicillin-resistant *Staphylococcus aureus* (MRSA) USA300 infections causing community- and healthcare-associated infections. Int J Antimicrob Agents 2009;34(2):148–55.
61. Tenover FC, Goering RV. Methicillin-resistant *Staphylococcus aureus* strain USA300: origin and epidemiology. J Antimicrob Chemother 2009;64(3):441–6.
62. Jarvis WR, Martone WJ. Predominant pathogens in hospital infections. J Antimicrob Chemother 1992;29(Suppl A):19–24.
63. Stone AM, Tucci VJ, Isenberg HD, et al. Wound infection: a prospective study of 7519 operations. Am Surg 1976;42(11):849–52.
64. Richards MJ, Edwards JR, Culver DH, et al. Nosocomial infections in combined medical-surgical intensive care units in the United States. Infect Control Hosp Epidemiol 2000;21(8):510–5.
65. Haley RW, Hightower AW, Khabbaz RF, et al. The emergence of methicillin-resistant *Staphylococcus aureus* infections in United States hospitals. Possible role of the house staff-patient transfer circuit. Ann Intern Med 1982;97(3):297–308.
66. Thompson RL, Cabezudo I, Wenzel RP. Epidemiology of nosocomial infections caused by methicillin-resistant *Staphylococcus aureus*. Ann Intern Med 1982; 97(3):309–17.
67. Albrich WC, Harbarth S. Health-care workers: source, vector, or victim of MRSA? Lancet Infect Dis 2008;8(5):289–301.
68. Temime L, Opatowski L, Pannet Y, et al. Peripatetic health-care workers as potential superspreaders. Proc Natl Acad Sci U S A 2009;106(43):18420–5.
69. Hsu CC, Macaluso CP, Special L, et al. High rate of methicillin resistance of *Staphylococcus aureus* isolated from hospitalized nursing home patients. Arch Intern Med 1988;148(3):569–70.
70. Bradley SF. Methicillin-resistant *Staphylococcus aureus* in nursing homes. Epidemiology, prevention and management. Drugs Aging 1997;10(3): 185–98.
71. Zetola N, Francis JS, Nuermberger EL, et al. Community-acquired meticillin-resistant *Staphylococcus aureus*: an emerging threat. Lancet Infect Dis 2005; 5(5):275–86.
72. King MD, Humphrey BJ, Wang YF, et al. Emergence of community-acquired methicillin-resistant *Staphylococcus aureus* USA 300 clone as the predominant cause of skin and soft-tissue infections. Ann Intern Med 2006;144(5):309–17.

73. Hidron AI, Low CE, Honig EG, et al. Emergence of community-acquired meticillin-resistant *Staphylococcus aureus* strain USA300 as a cause of necrotising community-onset pneumonia. Lancet Infect Dis 2009;9(6):384–92.

74. Gonzalez BE, Rueda AM, Shelburne SA 3rd, et al. Community-associated strains of methicillin-resistant *Staphylococcus aureus* as the cause of healthcare-associated infection. Infect Control Hosp Epidemiol 2006;27(10):1051–6.

75. Skov RL, Jensen KS. Community-associated meticillin-resistant *Staphylococcus aureus* as a cause of hospital-acquired infections. J Hosp Infect 2009;73(4): 364–70.

76. Iwatsuki K, Yamasaki O, Morizane S, et al. Staphylococcal cutaneous infections: invasion, evasion and aggression. J Dermatol Sci 2006;42(3):203–14.

77. Tristan A, Ferry T, Durand G, et al. Virulence determinants in community and hospital meticillin-resistant *Staphylococcus aureus*. J Hosp Infect 2007; 65(Suppl 2):105–9.

78. Carrillo-Marquez MA, Hulten KG, Hammerman W, et al. USA300 is the predominant genotype causing *Staphylococcus aureus* septic arthritis in children. Pediatr Infect Dis J 2009;28(12):1076–80.

79. Bocchini CE, Hulten KG, Mason EO Jr, et al. Panton-Valentine leukocidin genes are associated with enhanced inflammatory response and local disease in acute hematogenous *Staphylococcus aureus* osteomyelitis in children. Pediatrics 2006;117(2):433–40.

80. Kempker R, Difrancesco L, Martin-Gorgojo A, et al. Expanding spectrum of illness due to community-associated methicillin-resistant *Staphylococcus aureus*: a case report. Cases J 2009;2:7437.

81. Fraser JD, Proft T. The bacterial superantigen and superantigen-like proteins. Immunol Rev 2008;225:226–43.

82. Lappin E, Ferguson AJ. Gram-positive toxic shock syndromes. Lancet Infect Dis 2009;9(5):281–90.

83. Miller LG, Perdreau-Remington F, Rieg G, et al. Necrotizing fasciitis caused by community-associated methicillin-resistant *Staphylococcus aureus* in Los Angeles. N Engl J Med 2005;352(14):1445–53.

84. Genestier AL, Michallet MC, Prevost G, et al. *Staphylococcus aureus* Panton-Valentine leukocidin directly targets mitochondria and induces Bax-independent apoptosis of human neutrophils. J Clin Invest 2005;115(11): 3117–27.

85. Yamasaki O, Kaneko J, Morizane S, et al. The association between *Staphylococcus aureus* strains carrying panton-valentine leukocidin genes and the development of deep-seated follicular infection. Clin Infect Dis 2005;40(3): 381–5.

86. Gillet Y, Issartel B, Vanhems P, et al. Association between *Staphylococcus aureus* strains carrying gene for Panton-Valentine leukocidin and highly lethal necrotising pneumonia in young immunocompetent patients. Lancet 2002; 359(9308):753–9.

87. Labandeira-Rey M, Couzon F, Boisset S, et al. *Staphylococcus aureus* Panton-Valentine leukocidin causes necrotizing pneumonia. Science 2007;315(5815): 1130–3.

88. Corey GR. *Staphylococcus aureus* bloodstream infections: definitions and treatment. Clin Infect Dis 2009;48(Suppl 4):S254–9.

89. Hill PC, Birch M, Chambers S, et al. Prospective study of 424 cases of *Staphylococcus aureus* bacteraemia: determination of factors affecting incidence and mortality. Intern Med J 2001;31(2):97–103.

90. Mylotte JM, McDermott C, Spooner JA. Prospective study of 114 consecutive episodes of *Staphylococcus aureus* bacteremia. Rev Infect Dis 1987;9(5): 891–907.
91. Blot SI, Vandewoude KH, Hoste EA, et al. Outcome and attributable mortality in critically ill patients with bacteremia involving methicillin-susceptible and methicillin-resistant *Staphylococcus aureus*. Arch Intern Med 2002;162(19):2229–35.
92. Kaech C, Elzi L, Sendi P, et al. Course and outcome of *Staphylococcus aureus* bacteraemia: a retrospective analysis of 308 episodes in a Swiss tertiary-care centre. Clin Microbiol Infect 2006;12(4):345–52.
93. Swingle EL. Studies on small colony variants of *Staphylococcus aureus*. J Bacteriol 1935;29(5):467–89.
94. Looney WJ. Small-colony variants of *Staphylococcus aureus*. Br J Biomed Sci 2000;57(4):317–22.
95. McNamara PJ, Proctor RA. *Staphylococcus aureus* small colony variants, electron transport and persistent infections. Int J Antimicrob Agents 2000;14(2):117–22.
96. Agarwal H, Verrall R, Singh SP, et al. Small colony variant *Staphylococcus aureus* multiorgan infection. Pediatr Infect Dis J 2007;26(3):269–71.
97. Proctor RA, von Eiff C, Kahl BC, et al. Small colony variants: a pathogenic form of bacteria that facilitates persistent and recurrent infections. Nat Rev Microbiol 2006;4(4):295–305.
98. von Eiff C, Peters G, Becker K. The small colony variant (SCV) concept—the role of staphylococcal SCVs in persistent infections. Injury 2006;37(Suppl 2): S26–33.
99. Proctor RA, Kahl B, von Eiff C, et al. Staphylococcal small colony variants have novel mechanisms for antibiotic resistance. Clin Infect Dis 1998;27(Suppl 1): S68–74.
100. Kipp F, Becker K, Peters G, et al. Evaluation of different methods to detect methicillin resistance in small-colony variants of *Staphylococcus aureus*. J Clin Microbiol 2004;42(3):1277–9.
101. Besier S, Ludwig A, Ohlsen K, et al. Molecular analysis of the thymidine-auxotrophic small colony variant phenotype of *Staphylococcus aureus*. Int J Med Microbiol 2007;297(4):217–25.
102. Chatterjee I, Kriegeskorte A, Fischer A, et al. In vivo mutations of thymidylate synthase (encoded by thyA) are responsible for thymidine dependency in clinical small-colony variants of *Staphylococcus aureus*. J Bacteriol 2008;190(3): 834–42.
103. Spearman P, Lakey D, Jotte S, et al. Sternoclavicular joint septic arthritis with small-colony variant *Staphylococcus aureus*. Diagn Microbiol Infect Dis 1996; 26(1):13–5.
104. Sendi P, Rohrbach M, Graber P, et al. *Staphylococcus aureus* small colony variants in prosthetic joint infection. Clin Infect Dis 2006;43(8):961–7.
105. Neut D, van der Mei HC, Bulstra SK, et al. The role of small-colony variants in failure to diagnose and treat biofilm infections in orthopedics. Acta Orthop 2007;78(3):299–308.
106. Vaudaux P, Kelley WL, Lew DP. *Staphylococcus aureus* small colony variants: difficult to diagnose and difficult to treat. Clin Infect Dis 2006;43(8):968–70.
107. Spanu T, Romano L, D'Inzeo T, et al. Recurrent ventriculoperitoneal shunt infection caused by small-colony variants of *Staphylococcus aureus*. Clin Infect Dis 2005;41(5):e48–52.
108. Seifert H, Wisplinghoff H, Schnabel P, et al. Small colony variants of *Staphylococcus aureus* and pacemaker-related infection. Emerg Infect Dis 2003;9(10):1316–8.

109. Kahl B, Herrmann M, Everding AS, et al. Persistent infection with small colony variant strains of *Staphylococcus aureus* in patients with cystic fibrosis. J Infect Dis 1998;177(4):1023–9.
110. Agarwal A, Singh KP, Jain A. Medical significance and management of staphylococcal biofilm. FEMS Immunol Med Microbiol 2009;19:19.
111. Anderson KL, Roberts C, Disz T, et al. Characterization of the *Staphylococcus aureus* heat shock, cold shock, stringent, and SOS responses and their effects on log-phase mRNA turnover. J Bacteriol 2006;188(19):6739–56.
112. Costerton JW. Cystic fibrosis pathogenesis and the role of biofilms in persistent infection. Trends Microbiol 2001;9(2):50–2.
113. Sheagren JN. Staphylococcal infections of the skin and skin structures. Cutis 1985;36(5A):2–6.
114. Lemonick DM. Non-tropical pyomyositis caused by methicillin-resistant *Staphylococcus aureus*: an unusual cause of bilateral leg pain. J Emerg Med 2009. [Epub ahead of print].
115. Dryden MS. Skin and soft tissue infection: microbiology and epidemiology. Int J Antimicrob Agents 2009;34(Suppl 1):S2–7.
116. Lopez FA, Lartchenko S. Skin and soft tissue infections. Infect Dis Clin North Am 2006;20(4):759–72, v–vi.
117. Haridas M, Malangoni MA. Predictive factors for surgical site infection in general surgery. Surgery 2008;144(4):496–501 [discussion: 501–3].
118. Pessaux P, Atallah D, Lermite E, et al. Risk factors for prediction of surgical site infections in "clean surgery". Am J Infect Control 2005;33(5):292–8.
119. Suchard JR. "Spider bite" lesions are usually diagnosed as skin and soft-tissue infections. J Emerg Med 2009. [Epub ahead of print].
120. Smolin G, Hall JM, Okumoto M, et al. Effect of systemic corticosteroids on antibody-forming cells in the eye and draining lymph nodes. Ann Ophthalmol 1977; 9(11):1417–21.
121. Zimmerman RK. *Staphylococcus aureus* hordeolum as a cause of bacteremia and secondary foci. J Fam Pract 1989;29(4):433–5.
122. Nalmas S, Bishburg E, Shah M, et al. Skin and soft tissue abscess: 1 year's experience. J Cutan Med Surg 2009;13(5):257–61.
123. Schrock JW, Laskey S, Cydulka RK. Predicting observation unit treatment failures in patients with skin and soft tissue infections. Int J Emerg Med 2008; 1(2):85–90.
124. Stulberg DL, Penrod MA, Blatny RA. Common bacterial skin infections. Am Fam Physician 2002;66(1):119–24.
125. Napolitano LM. Severe soft tissue infections. Infect Dis Clin North Am 2009; 23(3):571–91.
126. Teng CS, Lo WT, Wang SR, et al. The role of antimicrobial therapy for treatment of uncomplicated skin and soft tissue infections from community-acquired methicillin-resistant *Staphylococcus aureus* in children. J Microbiol Immunol Infect 2009;42(4):324–8.
127. Todd JK. Staphylococcal toxin syndromes. Annu Rev Med 1985;36:337–47.
128. Krasagakis K, Samonis G, Maniatakis P, et al. Bullous erysipelas: clinical presentation, staphylococcal involvement and methicillin resistance. Dermatology 2006;212(1):31–5.
129. Gemmell CG. Staphylococcal scalded skin syndrome. J Med Microbiol 1995; 43(5):318–27.

130. Amagai M, Matsuyoshi N, Wang ZH, et al. Toxin in bullous impetigo and staphylococcal scalded-skin syndrome targets desmoglein 1. Nat Med 2000;6(11): 1275–7.
131. Nishifuji K, Sugai M, Amagai M. Staphylococcal exfoliative toxins: "molecular scissors" of bacteria that attack the cutaneous defense barrier in mammals. J Dermatol Sci 2008;49(1):21–31.
132. Balaban N, Rasooly A. Staphylococcal enterotoxins. Int J Food Microbiol 2000; 61(1):1–10.
133. Le Loir Y, Baron F, Gautier M. *Staphylococcus aureus* and food poisoning. Genet Mol Res 2003;2(1):63–76.
134. Thomas D, Chou S, Dauwalder O, et al. Diversity in *Staphylococcus aureus* enterotoxins. Chem Immunol Allergy 2007;93:24–41.
135. Corpening A, Foxhall EP. Outbreak of food poisoning, probably due to *Staphylococcus aureus*. Am J Public Health Nations Health 1935;25(8): 938–40.
136. Gilbert RJ, Wieneke AA, Lanser J, et al. Serological detection of enterotoxin in foods implicated in staphylococcal food poisoning. J Hyg (Lond) 1972;70(4): 755–62.
137. Edmondson HT, Rhode CM, Seago RW. Necrotizing fasciitis caused by hemolytic *Staphylococcus aureus*. Am Surg 1972;38(9):523–6.
138. Todd J, Fishaut M, Kapral F, et al. Toxic-shock syndrome associated with phage-group-I staphylococci. Lancet 1978;2(8100):1116–8.
139. Green J, Lynn WA. Presentation and clinical features of severe sepsis. J R Coll Physicians Lond 2000;34(5):418–23.
140. McCormick JK, Yarwood JM, Schlievert PM. Toxic shock syndrome and bacterial superantigens: an update. Annu Rev Microbiol 2001;55:77–104.
141. Bradley SF. *Staphylococcus aureus* pneumonia: emergence of MRSA in the community. Semin Respir Crit Care Med 2005;26(6):643–9.
142. Fernandez Guerrero ML, Gonzalez Lopez JJ, Goyenechea A, et al. Endocarditis caused by *Staphylococcus aureus*: a reappraisal of the epidemiologic, clinical, and pathologic manifestations with analysis of factors determining outcome. Medicine (Baltimore) 2009;88(1):1–22.
143. Karadimas EJ, Bunger C, Lindblad BE, et al. Spondylodiscitis. A retrospective study of 163 patients. Acta Orthop 2008;79(5):650–9.
144. Gonzalez-Lopez JJ, Gorgolas M, Muniz J, et al. Spontaneous epidural abscess: analysis of 15 cases with emphasis on diagnostic and prognostic factors. Eur J Intern Med 2009;20(5):514–7.
145. Mylona E, Samarkos M, Kakalou E, et al. Pyogenic vertebral osteomyelitis: a systematic review of clinical characteristics. Semin Arthritis Rheum 2009; 39(1):10–7.
146. Shirtliff ME, Mader JT. Acute septic arthritis. Clin Microbiol Rev 2002;15(4):527–44.
147. Pintado V, Meseguer MA, Fortun J, et al. Clinical study of 44 cases of *Staphylococcus aureus* meningitis. Eur J Clin Microbiol Infect Dis 2002;21(12):864–8.
148. Arias CA, Murray BE. Antibiotic-resistant bugs in the 21st century—a clinical super-challenge. N Engl J Med 2009;360(5):439–43.
149. Deresinski S. Methicillin-resistant *Staphylococcus aureus*: an evolutionary, epidemiologic, and therapeutic odyssey. Clin Infect Dis 2005;40(4):562–73.
150. Menzies BE. The role of fibronectin binding proteins in the pathogenesis of *Staphylococcus aureus* infections. Curr Opin Infect Dis 2003;16(3):225–9.

151. Vercellotti GM, Lussenhop D, Peterson PK, et al. Bacterial adherence to fibronectin and endothelial cells: a possible mechanism for bacterial tissue tropism. J Lab Clin Med 1984;103(1):34–43.

152. Shuter J, Hatcher VB, Lowy FD. *Staphylococcus aureus* binding to human nasal mucin. Infect Immun 1996;64(1):310–8.

153. Trivier D, Houdret N, Courcol RJ, et al. The binding of surface proteins from *Staphylococcus aureus* to human bronchial mucins. Eur Respir J 1997;10(4): 804–10.

154. Hoefnagels-Schuermans A, Peetermans WE, Jorissen M, et al. *Staphylococcus aureus* adherence to nasal epithelial cells in a physiological in vitro model. In Vitro Cell Dev Biol Anim 1999;35(8):472–80.

155. Holland DB, Bojar RA, Farrar MD, et al. Differential innate immune responses of a living skin equivalent model colonized by *Staphylococcus epidermidis* or *Staphylococcus aureus*. FEMS Microbiol Lett 2009;290(2):149–55.

156. DeLeo FR, Diep BA, Otto M. Host defense and pathogenesis in *Staphylococcus aureus* infections. Infect Dis Clin North Am 2009;23(1):17–34.

157. Foster TJ. Immune evasion by staphylococci. Nat Rev Microbiol 2005;3(12): 948–58.

158. Larkin EA, Carman RJ, Krakauer T, et al. *Staphylococcus aureus*: the toxic presence of a pathogen extraordinaire. Curr Med Chem 2009;16(30):4003–19.

159. Fowler T, Wann ER, Joh D, et al. Cellular invasion by *Staphylococcus aureus* involves a fibronectin bridge between the bacterial fibronectin-binding MSCRAMMs and host cell beta1 integrins. Eur J Cell Biol 2000;79(10):672–9.

160. Sinha B, Fraunholz M. *Staphylococcus aureus* host cell invasion and post-invasion events. Int J Med Microbiol 2009;300(2–3):170–5.

161. Kubica M, Guzik K, Koziel J, et al. A potential new pathway for *Staphylococcus aureus* dissemination: the silent survival of *S. aureus* phagocytosed by human monocyte-derived macrophages. PLoS One 2008;3(1):e1409.

162. Anwar S, Prince LR, Foster SJ, et al. The rise and rise of *Staphylococcus aureus*: laughing in the face of granulocytes. Clin Exp Immunol 2009;157(2):216–24.

163. Kerr A Jr, Tan JS. Biopsies of the Janeway lesion of infective endocarditis. J Cutan Pathol 1979;6(2):124–9.

164. Narita S, Kaneko J, Chiba J, et al. Phage conversion of Panton-Valentine leukocidin in *Staphylococcus aureus*: molecular analysis of a PVL-converting phage, phiSLT. Gene 2001;268(1–2):195–206.

165. Deurenberg RH, Vink C, Kalenic S, et al. The molecular evolution of methicillin-resistant *Staphylococcus aureus*. Clin Microbiol Infect 2007;13(3):222–35.

166. Ben Zakour NL, Guinane CM, Fitzgerald JR. Pathogenomics of the staphylococci: insights into niche adaptation and the emergence of new virulent strains. FEMS Microbiol Lett 2008;289(1):1–12.

167. Lindsay JA. Genomic variation and evolution of *Staphylococcus aureus*. Int J Med Microbiol 2009;300(2–3):98–103.

168. Novick RP. Mobile genetic elements and bacterial toxinoses: the superantigen-encoding pathogenicity islands of *Staphylococcus aureus*. Plasmid 2003;49(2): 93–105.

169. CLSI. Performance standards for antimicrobial susceptibility testing. 10th Informational Supplement, M100-S18. Wayne (PA): Clinical and Laboratory Standards Institute; 2009.

170. Peterson JF, Riebe KM, Hall GS, et al. SpectraTM MRSA, a new chromogenic agar medium to screen for methicillin-resistant *Staphylococcus aureus*. J Clin Microbiol 2009;48(1):215–9.

171. Diederen B, van Duijn I, van Belkum A, et al. Performance of CHROMagar MRSA medium for detection of methicillin-resistant *Staphylococcus aureus*. J Clin Microbiol 2005;43(4):1925–7.
172. Flayhart D, Hindler JF, Bruckner DA, et al. Multicenter evaluation of BBL CHROMagar MRSA medium for direct detection of methicillin-resistant *Staphylococcus aureus* from surveillance cultures of the anterior nares. J Clin Microbiol 2005;43(11):5536–40.
173. Fujita S, Senda Y, Iwagami T, et al. Rapid identification of staphylococcal strains from positive-testing blood culture bottles by internal transcribed spacer PCR followed by microchip gel electrophoresis. J Clin Microbiol 2005;43(3):1149–57.
174. Martineau F, Picard FJ, Ke D, et al. Development of a PCR assay for identification of staphylococci at genus and species levels. J Clin Microbiol 2001;39(7):2541–7.
175. Carroll KC, Leonard RB, Newcomb-Gayman PL, et al. Rapid detection of the staphylococcal *mecA* gene from BACTEC blood culture bottles by the polymerase chain reaction. Am J Clin Pathol 1996;106(5):600–5.
176. Chapin K, Musgnug M. Evaluation of three rapid methods for the direct identification of *Staphylococcus aureus* from positive blood cultures. J Clin Microbiol 2003;41(9):4324–7.
177. Oliveira K, Procop GW, Wilson D, et al. Rapid identification of *Staphylococcus aureus* directly from blood cultures by fluorescence in situ hybridization with peptide nucleic acid probes. J Clin Microbiol 2002;40(1):247–51.
178. Paule SM, Pasquariello AC, Thomson RB Jr, et al. Real-time PCR can rapidly detect methicillin-susceptible and methicillin-resistant *Staphylococcus aureus* directly from positive blood culture bottles. Am J Clin Pathol 2005;124(3):404–7.
179. Goldmeyer J, Li H, McCormac M, et al. Identification of *Staphylococcus aureus* and determination of methicillin resistance directly from positive blood cultures by isothermal amplification and a disposable detection device. J Clin Microbiol 2008;46(4):1534–6.
180. Johnson G, Millar MR, Matthews S, et al. Evaluation of BacLite Rapid MRSA, a rapid culture based screening test for the detection of ciprofloxacin and methicillin resistant *S. aureus* (MRSA) from screening swabs. BMC Microbiol 2006;6:83.
181. Boyce JM, Havill NL. Comparison of BD GeneOhm methicillin-resistant *Staphylococcus aureus* (MRSA) PCR versus the CHROMagar MRSA assay for screening patients for the presence of MRSA strains. J Clin Microbiol 2008;46(1):350–1.
182. Paule SM, Hacek DM, Kufner B, et al. Performance of the BD GeneOhm methicillin-resistant *Staphylococcus aureus* test before and during high-volume clinical use. J Clin Microbiol 2007;45(9):2993–8.
183. Rossney AS, Herra CM, Brennan GI, et al. Evaluation of the Xpert methicillin-resistant *Staphylococcus aureus* (MRSA) assay using the GeneXpert real-time PCR platform for rapid detection of MRSA from screening specimens. J Clin Microbiol 2008;46(10):3285–90.
184. Wolk DM, Picton E, Johnson D, et al. Multicenter evaluation of the Cepheid Xpert methicillin-resistant *Staphylococcus aureus* (MRSA) test as a rapid screening method for detection of MRSA in nares. J Clin Microbiol 2009;47(3):758–64.
185. Podzorski RP, Li H, Han J, et al. MVPlex assay for direct detection of methicillin-resistant *Staphylococcus aureus* in naris and other swab specimens. J Clin Microbiol 2008;46(9):3107–9.

186. Tacconelli E, De Angelis G, de Waure C, et al. Rapid screening tests for meticillin-resistant *Staphylococcus aureus* at hospital admission: systematic review and meta-analysis. Lancet Infect Dis 2009;9(9):546–54.
187. Shopsin B, Kreiswirth BN. Molecular epidemiology of methicillin-resistant *Staphylococcus aureus*. Emerg Infect Dis 2001;7(2):323–6.
188. Struelens MJ, Hawkey PM, French GL, et al. Laboratory tools and strategies for methicillin-resistant *Staphylococcus aureus* screening, surveillance and typing: state of the art and unmet needs. Clin Microbiol Infect 2009;15(2):112–9.
189. Prevost G, Pottecher B, Dahlet M, et al. Pulsed field gel electrophoresis as a new epidemiological tool for monitoring methicillin-resistant *Staphylococcus aureus* in an intensive care unit. J Hosp Infect 1991;17(4):255–69.
190. Tang YW, Waddington MG, Smith DH, et al. Comparison of protein A gene sequencing with pulsed-field gel electrophoresis and epidemiologic data for molecular typing of methicillin-resistant *Staphylococcus aureus*. J Clin Microbiol 2000;38(4):1347–51.
191. Tenover FC, Gay EA, Frye S, et al. Comparison of typing results obtained for methicillin-resistant *Staphylococcus aureus* isolates with the DiversiLab system and pulsed-field gel electrophoresis. J Clin Microbiol 2009;47(8):2452–7.
192. Enright MC, Day NP, Davies CE, et al. Multilocus sequence typing for characterization of methicillin-resistant and methicillin-susceptible clones of *Staphylococcus aureus*. J Clin Microbiol 2000;38(3):1008–15.
193. Maiden MC, Bygraves JA, Feil E, et al. Multilocus sequence typing: a portable approach to the identification of clones within populations of pathogenic microorganisms. Proc Natl Acad Sci U S A 1998;95(6):3140–5.
194. Frenay HM, Bunschoten AE, Schouls LM, et al. Molecular typing of methicillin-resistant *Staphylococcus aureus* on the basis of protein A gene polymorphism. Eur J Clin Microbiol Infect Dis 1996;15(1):60–4.
195. Stephens AJ, Inman-Bamber J, Giffard PM, et al. High-resolution melting analysis of the spa repeat region of *Staphylococcus aureus*. Clin Chem 2008;54(2):432–6.
196. Moser SA, Box MJ, Patel M, et al. Multiple-locus variable-number tandem-repeat analysis of meticillin-resistant *Staphylococcus aureus* discriminates within USA pulsed-field gel electrophoresis types. J Hosp Infect 2009;71(4):333–9.
197. Sabat A, Krzyszton-Russjan J, Strzalka W, et al. New method for typing *Staphylococcus aureus* strains: multiple-locus variable-number tandem repeat analysis of polymorphism and genetic relationships of clinical isolates. J Clin Microbiol 2003;41(4):1801–4.
198. Deplano A, Schuermans A, Van Eldere J, et al. Multicenter evaluation of epidemiological typing of methicillin-resistant *Staphylococcus aureus* strains by repetitive-element PCR analysis. J Clin Microbiol 2000;38(10):3527–33.
199. Ross TL, Merz WG, Farkosh M, et al. Comparison of an automated repetitive sequence-based PCR microbial typing system to pulsed-field gel electrophoresis for analysis of outbreaks of methicillin-resistant *Staphylococcus aureus*. J Clin Microbiol 2005;43(11):5642–7.
200. Hall TA, Sampath R, Blyn LB, et al. Rapid molecular genotyping and clonal complex assignment of *Staphylococcus aureus* isolates by PCR coupled to electrospray ionization-mass spectrometry. J Clin Microbiol 2009;47(6):1733–41.
201. Wolk DM, Blyn LB, Hall TA, et al. Pathogen profiling: rapid molecular characterization of *Staphylococcus aureus* by PCR/electrospray ionization-mass

spectrometry and correlation with phenotype. J Clin Microbiol 2009;47(10): 3129–37.

202. White EJ, Fridrikh SV, Chennagiri N, et al. *Staphylococcus aureus* strain typing by single-molecule DNA mapping in fluidic microships with fluorescent tags. Clin Chem 2009;55(12):2121–9.

203. Tang YW. Progress toward rapid and accurate *Staphylococcus aureus* strain typing. Clin Chem 2009;55(12):2074–6.

204. Hyun DY, Mason EO, Forbes A, et al. Trimethoprim-sulfamethoxazole or clindamycin for treatment of community-acquired methicillin-resistant *Staphylococcus aureus* skin and soft tissue infections. Pediatr Infect Dis J 2009;28(1):57–9.

205. Ramirez-Schrempp D, Dorfman DH, Baker WE, et al. Ultrasound soft-tissue applications in the pediatric emergency department: to drain or not to drain? Pediatr Emerg Care 2009;25(1):44–8.

206. Miles F, Voss L, Segedin E, et al. Review of *Staphylococcus aureus* infections requiring admission to a paediatric intensive care unit. Arch Dis Child 2005; 90(12):1274–8.

207. Verhagen DW, van der Meer JT, Hamming T, et al. Management of patients with *Staphylococcus aureus* bacteraemia in a university hospital: a retrospective study. Scand J Infect Dis 2003;35(8):459–63.

208. Jenkins TC, Price CS, Sabel AL, et al. Impact of routine infectious diseases service consultation on the evaluation, management, and outcomes of *Staphylococcus aureus* bacteremia. Clin Infect Dis 2008;46(7):1000–8.

209. Lahey T, Shah R, Gittzus J, et al. Infectious diseases consultation lowers mortality from *Staphylococcus aureus* bacteremia. Medicine (Baltimore) 2009; 88(5):263–7.

210. Takei S, Arora YK, Walker SM. Intravenous immunoglobulin contains specific antibodies inhibitory to activation of T cells by staphylococcal toxin superantigens [comment]. J Clin Invest 1993;91(2):602–7.

211. Yanagisawa C, Hanaki H, Natae T, et al. Neutralization of staphylococcal exotoxins in vitro by human-origin intravenous immunoglobulin. J Infect Chemother 2007;13(6):368–72.

212. Gauduchon V, Cozon G, Vandenesch F, et al. Neutralization of *Staphylococcus aureus* Panton Valentine leukocidin by intravenous immunoglobulin in vitro. J Infect Dis 2004;189(2):346–53.

213. Powell JP, Wenzel RP. Antibiotic options for treating community-acquired MRSA. Expert Rev Anti Infect Ther 2008;6(3):299–307.

214. Schlievert PM. Use of intravenous immunoglobulin in the treatment of staphylococcal and streptococcal toxic shock syndromes and related illnesses. J Allergy Clin Immunol 2001;108(Suppl 4):S107–10.

215. Schaffer AC, Lee JC. Staphylococcal vaccines and immunotherapies. Infect Dis Clin North Am 2009;23(1):153–71.

216. Espersen F, Hedstrom SA. Recurrent staphylococcal furunculosis: antibody response against *Staphylococcus aureus*. Scand J Infect Dis 1984;16(4):413–4.

217. Tsuda S. Immunological aspects of staphylococcal skin infection. J Dermatol 1977;4(4):123–8.

218. El-Gilany AH, Fathy H. Risk factors of recurrent furunculosis. Dermatol Online J 2009;15(1):16.

219. Shinefield HR. Use of a conjugate polysaccharide vaccine in the prevention of invasive staphylococcal disease: is an additional vaccine needed or possible? Vaccine 2006;24(Suppl 2):S2-65–9.

220. O'Riordan K, Lee JC. *Staphylococcus aureus* capsular polysaccharides. Clin Microbiol Rev 2004;17(1):218–34.
221. Foster TJ. Potential for vaccination against infections caused by *Staphylococcus aureus*. Vaccine 1991;9(4):221–7.
222. Middleton JR. *Staphylococcus aureus* antigens and challenges in vaccine development. Expert Rev Vaccines 2008;7(6):805–15.
223. Krakauer T. Immune response to staphylococcal superantigens. Immunol Res 1999;20(2):163–73.

Chikungunya

Ann M. Powers, PhD

KEYWORDS

• Chikungunya virus • Alphavirus • Mosquito-borne arbovirus

OVERVIEW

Chikungunya virus is a zoonotic, vector-borne pathogen that has been responsible for numerous outbreaks of febrile arthralgia since its discovery in the early 1950s. In the past decade, the virus has re-emerged more frequently, causing massive epidemics that have moved from Africa throughout the Indian Ocean to India and Southeast Asia. A discussion of the virus, its epidemiology, diagnostic criteria, and immunity are presented in this article.

MICROBIOLOGY

Chikungunya virus (CHIKV) is one of 29 recognized species within the genus *Alphavirus* in the family *Togaviridae* (**Table 1**).[1] Like all alphaviruses, the virus contains a positive-sense, single-stranded, nonsegmented RNA genome of approximately 11.8 kilobase in length. The genome encodes 4 nonstructural proteins that are responsible for the cytoplasmic replication of the viral genome and 5 structural proteins that are encoded in the 3' one-third of the genome and translated from a subgenomic messenger RNA.[2] The resulting virions, which are generated by budding through the plasma membrane, are approximately 70 nm in diameter (**Fig. 1**).

EPIDEMIOLOGY

The first documented outbreak of Chikungunya fever occurred in 1952 to 53 on the Makonde plateau of Tanganyika. During this period, a high proportion of residents of all ages were affected by a distinctive disease with "very sharp onset of crippling joint pains, severe fever, and eventually, the conspicuous rash." The elders of the Makonde tribes could not recall any previous, similar epidemics, suggesting that this was indeed a new illness.[3–5] After that, only minor outbreaks occurred periodically in Africa, but some major epidemics were reported in the 1960s and 70s in India and Southeast Asia.[6,7] These Asian outbreaks were the first documented urban epidemics and led to the realization that 2 distinct transmission cycles existed. In Asia, the virus was found to circulate between mosquitoes and naïve human hosts in a cycle similar to that of dengue viruses. This cycle was in stark contrast to the sylvatic cycle described in

Centers for Disease Control and Prevention, Division of Vector-Borne Infectious Diseases, 3150 Rampart Road, Fort Collins, CO 80521, USA
E-mail address: apowers@cdc.gov

Clin Lab Med 30 (2010) 209–219
doi:10.1016/j.cll.2009.10.003
0272-2712/10/$ – see front matter. Published by Elsevier Inc.

labmed.theclinics.com

Table 1				
The 29 distinct alphaviruses by disease association in their vertebrate hosts				
Affecting Humans— Causing Encephalitis	Affecting Humans— Causing Febrile Arthralgia	Affecting Humans— Causing Febrile or Other Illness	Affecting Animals— Causing Disease of Any Nature	No Known Disease
Eastern equine encephalitis virus	Barmah Forest virus	Everglades virus	Eastern equine encephalitis virus	Aura virus
Tonate virus	Chikungunya virus	Mucambo virus	Getah virus	Bebaru virus
Venezuelan equine encephalitis virus	Mayaro virus	Rio Negro virus	Highlands J virus	Cabassou virus
Western equine encephalitis virus	O'nyong nyong virus	Semliki Forest virus	Middelburg virus	Fort Morgan virus
	Ross River virus	Tonate virus	Mucambo virus	Mosso das Pedras virus
	Sindbis virus		Ross River virus	Ndumu virus
	Una virus		Salmon pancreas disease virus	Pixuna virus
			Venezuelan equine encephalitis virus	Southern elephant seal virus
			Western equine encephalitis virus	Trocara virus
				Whataroa virus

Africa, where the virus was maintained in a zoonotic cycle involving nonhuman primates and forest-dwelling *Aedes* species mosquitoes (**Fig. 2**).[8,9] However, large outbreaks in Africa were thought to be vectored by *Aedes aegypti*, the same mosquito identified as an urban vector in Asia. After a 1973 outbreak in India ended, only sporadic activity occurred over the next 30 years, with no major outbreaks until 2004 when a large epidemic started on the coast of Kenya. This outbreak initiated a spreading epidemic that reached numerous islands of the Indian Ocean, India, and parts of Southeast Asia (**Fig. 3**) and reached at least 18 countries throughout Asia, Europe, and North America via imported cases.[10–13] Over the course of 5 years, an estimate of more than 2 million cases occurred, with outbreaks in several countries where the virus had never before been documented. Because the populations of these areas were completely naïve, attack rates were as high as 70%,[14] producing tremendous drains on both public health and economic resources.[15,16] During the course of this massive outbreak, molecular epidemiology of the virus was monitored, allowing assessment of changes that could modulate transmission, virulence, and further spread of the virus.

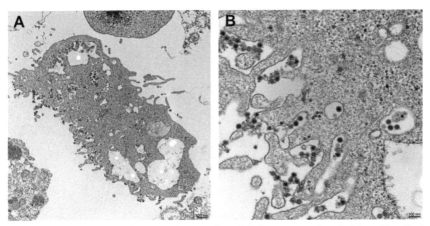

Fig. 1. (*A, B*) Thin section electron micrographs of Chikungunya virus in Vero E6 cells. In-fected cells showed an abundance of viral particles that tended to associate with the plasma membrane. (*Courtesy of* Cynthia Goldsmith, MS and James A. Comer, PhD.)

   Molecular genetic studies of the virus indicated that the origin of the 2004 outbreak was coastal Kenya. Two communities were affected in 2004 with tens of thousands of cases identified. In early 2005, the virus was found to have moved to the island nation of Comoros, where an attack rate of 63% suggested that approximately 215,000 cases occurred in a matter of months.[10,17] Movement of the virus continued to other islands of the Indian Ocean, including La Reunion, where it was estimated that 40,000 cases per week occurred during the peak of the epidemic. The virus continued to spread, reaching India where more than 1.3 million cases were suspected in the first year alone.[18] From India, an infected individual transported the virus to Italy where autochthonous transmission was reported in 2007.[19] Genetics of the virus in all these areas revealed that the virus was a member of the Central/East African genotype and was undergoing microevolution throughout the course of the epidemic.[20–22]

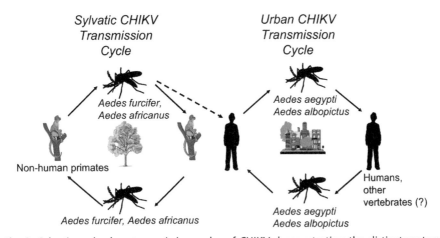

Fig. 2. Sylvatic and urban transmission cycles of CHIKV demonstrating the distinct vectors and vertebrate hosts used.

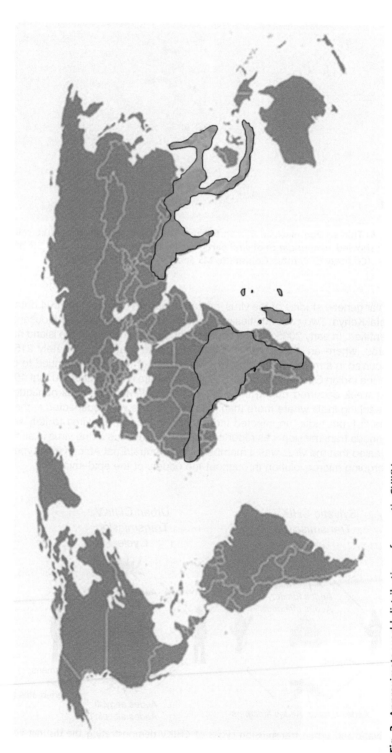

Fig. 3. Approximate world distribution of enzootic CHIKV.

CLINICAL PRESENTATION

The classical presentation of chikungunya fever includes the rapid onset of high fever (>102°F), severe and incapacitating joint pain, and rash.[23] These 3 symptoms have been documented from the earliest outbreaks and remain the most prevalent disease pattern to this day. Furthermore, the vast majority of infected individuals show clinical illness, with as few as 3% of cases remaining asymptomatic.[24,25] Symptoms can appear within 2 days postinfection with the acute phase typically lasting from a few days to weeks. Fever is usually the first symptom, with an abrupt onset occurring as early as 2 days postinfection and persisting for days. Shortly after fever onset, virtually all cases develop severe and incapacitating joint pain. The debilitating polyarthralgias are most common in the peripheral small joints and can persist for months. Rash is the least reliable symptom, presenting in as few as 19% of patients. When rash is present, it is typically maculopapular in nature, but recent studies have also noted vesiculobullous lesions with desquamation, aphthouslike ulcers, and vasculitic lesions.[13,26–28]

Additional symptoms that have been reported in CHIKV-infected patients include headache, fatigue, nausea, vomiting, and conjunctivitis, all occurring with varying frequency and severity. Furthermore, neurologic manifestations, which had been infrequently reported from the earliest epidemics, have been increasingly documented during the most recent outbreak. These neuroinvasive complications include meningoencephalitis, myeloneuropathy, Guillan-Barré syndrome, acute flaccid paralysis, and palsies.[29–32] In one recent study, as many as 16% of the patients demonstrated neurologic involvement associated with CHIKV infection.[32] Mortality has also been reported recently in association with CHIKV infection, but a causal relationship has yet to be established. When mortality does occur, underlying conditions appear to represent a common risk factor.[33,34]

PATHOGENESIS

Because CHIKV has historically been understudied, little is known regarding the specific mechanisms of viral pathogenesis. However, a closely related alphavirus manifesting with similar clinical presentation, Ross River virus (RRV), has been more fully evaluated for disease development. During RRV infection, the T-cell–mediated immune response is postulated to play a role in persistence of symptoms. Patients who quickly recover from RRV have a predominance of CD8+ T cells in contrast to patients with chronic disease where CD4+ cells are more prevalent in the synovial fluid.[35] Furthermore, treatment of in vitro infected macrophages with CD8+ T cells generated by vaccination of mice with RRV capsid protein results in complete clearance of the infection.[36]

Another possible mechanism of pathogenesis due to RRV infection involves the activity of the signaling receptor, complement receptor 3 (CR3). CR3 deficiency in recombinant mice diminished the expression of certain proinflammatory and cytotoxic effectors within infected tissues, resulting in decreased tissue destruction.[37]

Finally, viral antigen in the synovial fluid of RRV patients with chronic joint pain attracted inflammatory infiltrates to the affected joints. It is hypothesized that persistently infected macrophages directly cause pathogenesis via tissue destruction, because clearance of macrophage from infected tissue has been associated with a decrease in symptoms.[38] Because RRV infects macrophages, it is likely that chemokines secreted by these infected cells attract additional macrophages that are subsequently infected, thus propagating the cycle.[39,40] Although no virus could be cultured from synovial fluid in a small cohort of CHIKV patients with prolonged joint pain,[41] the presence of high-titered specific antibodies suggests persistent antigen presence, and the similarities to RRV infection warrant further investigation of possible shared pathogenic mechanisms.

DIAGNOSIS

Depending on the availability, timing of collection, and sample volume, CHIKV infection can be diagnosed and confirmed by direct virus detection, viral RNA detection, or presence of CHIKV-specific antibodies. An acute serum sample collected within 7 days of illness onset is likely to have high levels of viremia (up to $10^{6.8}$ pfu/mL)[12,42] making the best options for diagnosis either nucleic acid detection or virus isolation. Both approaches are extremely sensitive and specific and can be completed within a few hours (nucleic acid detection) or in less than 2 days (virus isolation). Nucleic acid detection has the advantage of being quicker and not requiring biosafety level 3 facilities; however, obtaining an isolate using culture techniques provides additional options for downstream studies not possible using limited nucleic acid techniques.

Serologic testing to detect anti-CHIKV IgM or IgG antibodies from acute or convalescent samples can also be diagnostic. Most commonly, the detection platform is ELISA (enzyme-linked immunosorbent assay)-based with confirmation including neutralization assays. IgM antibodies are frequently present within 7 days postinfection and can persist for several months, making this a good indicator of recent infection.[12,42] In the absence of IgM antibody, virus, or nucleic acid from the acute sample, a 4-fold change in antibody titers between the acute and convalescent samples can also be diagnostic.

DIFFERENTIAL DIAGNOSIS

Laboratory confirmation of CHIKV infection using CHIKV-specific tests is critical for accurate diagnosis, because the clinical presentation can be similar to numerous other sympatric pathogens. Malaria and dengue viruses cause a clinical syndrome mimicking that of CHIKV infection. In fact, the 2004 epidemic in Lamu, Kenya was originally thought to be malarial, and in 2005 in Comoros, the outbreak was first reported as a denguelike epidemic.[14,17] Other arboviruses that must also be considered are West Nile virus, O'nyong nyong virus (ONNV), RRV, and Sindbis virus. Laboratory confirmation is particularly important to distinguish between CHIKV and ONNV; ONNV is genetically the closest relative to CHIKV, and there is some degree of serologic cross-reactivity between these viruses.[43] Antibodies raised against CHIKV can inhibit ONNV replication in neutralization assays but ONNV-specific antibodies do not inhibit CHIKV.[44–47] Clinically, cervical lymphadenopathy is more common in ONNV infection but can also be present in CHIKV cases, making this an unreliable diagnostic parameter, particularly in Central Africa where the viruses coexist.[48,49]

As further support for CHIKV-specific laboratory confirmation being essential for accurate diagnosis, many clinical laboratory parameters for CHIKV infections can be variable and are not present consistently enough to aid in diagnosis. For example, results may include thrombocytopenia, leukocytosis, or hypocalcemia.[50–53] However, these are highly variable and are often more prominent in alternative causes (eg, thrombocytopenia is far more common in dengue virus infections).[54–56] Another parameter, the erythrocyte sedimentation rate, may be slightly elevated in CHIKV infections but is also suggestive of rheumatoid arthritis (RA).[52,57] Diagnosis is facilitated during large epidemics with hundreds of cases, whereas small outbreaks or isolated cases must also be distinguished from more severe diseases, such as rheumatic fever, brucellosis, rubella, or hepatitis.[52]

TREATMENT, PROGNOSIS, AND LONG-TERM OUTCOMES

Because there is no specific treatment available, supportive treatment of symptoms, including rest, fluids, antipyretics and analgesics, is the only option. Several antiviral drugs have been tested for their efficacy against chikungunya fever. These include ribavirin, sulfated polysaccharides, interferon, corticosteroids, and chloroquine.[58–60] Although there has been some evidence that these options may provide some relief, side effects exist and the long-term benefits and cost-effectiveness are unclear. However, preliminary results are encouraging and suggest that additional testing including multidrug regimes should be undertaken.

Although most patients recover completely from the illness within a matter of weeks with no residual sequelae, persistence of symptoms is noted in some patients. Prolonged symptoms that can last several months include fatigue, incapacitating joint pain, and tenosynovitis or edematous polyarthritis. In a small percentage of cases, symptoms have even been reported to last for years; up to 64% of patients with chikungunya fever reported joint stiffness and/or pain more than a year after the initial infection, with 12% reporting symptoms 3 to 5 years later.[41,61,62] Additionally, one recent study suggested that CHIKV infection may contribute to the initiation of RA. Twenty-one patients were diagnosed with RA 4 to 18 months after confirmation of CHIKV illness.[57] Finally, it has recently been suggested that there is a genetic association with long-term pathology,[63,64] but additional studies are necessary to clarify this relationship.

IMMUNITY AND REINFECTION

Infection with CHIKV, like all arboviruses, is presumed to result in lifelong immunity. CHIKV-specific neutralizing antibodies have been detected as early as 2 weeks postinfection, and IgG antibodies have been documented to persist for years suggesting that immunologic memory would provide protection on rechallenge.

Although no commercial vaccine is available for CHIKV, a live-attenuated strain has been developed and extensively characterized for its vaccine potential. This strain, designated 181/25, was shown to induce neutralizing antibodies in 98% of subjects receiving the CHIKV vaccine in a phase 2 clinical trial. Furthermore, more than 85% were still seropositive at 1 year.[65] Interest in further evaluating this vaccine along with new candidates has resurged as the 2004 to 2009 CHIKV epidemic continues. Because the 181/25 vaccine was developed against a CHIKV strain from the Asian genotype, the suitability of this vaccine to protect against recent outbreak strains that have emerged from the Central/East African genotype was questioned. The antisera from patients infected with a Central/East African strain were shown to neutralize

Table 2
Results of cross-neutralization assays using serum collected during a CHIKV outbreak in Comoros in 2005 and homologous virus (isolated from a human case) or the vaccine strain 181/25. Results are the average neutralization titers of 40 samples

Human Serum Samples	Homologous Titer	Heterologous Titer (181/25)
Negative	<10	<10
IgM+/IgG−	90	850
IgM+/IgG+	122	495
IgM−/IgG+	127	891

Asian genotype vaccine more efficiently than homologous virus (**Table 2**), indicating that any CHIKV vaccine would probably protect against strains from all genotypes. Further development of vaccine and therapeutic options for CHIKV infection are needed as the virus continues its global expansion.

REFERENCES

1. Weaver SC, Frey TK, Huang HV, et al. *Togaviridae*. In: Fauquet CM, Mayo MA, Maniloff J, et al, editors. Virus taxonomy: eighth report of the international committee on taxonomy of viruses. Amsterdam: Elsevier Academic Press; 2005. p. 999–1008.
2. Strauss EG, Strauss JH. Structure and replication of the alphavirus genome. In: Schlesinger S, Schlesinger M, editors. The Togaviruses and Flaviviruses. New York: Plenum Press; 1986. p. 35–90.
3. Robinson MC. An epidemic of virus disease in Southern province, tanganyika territory, in 1952–53. I. clinical features. Trans R Soc Trop Med Hyg 1955;49(1): 28–32.
4. Ross RW. The Newala epidemic.III. The virus: isolation, pathogenic properties and relationship to the epidemic. J Hyg 1956;54:177–91.
5. Lumsden WH, Robinson MC. Investigations on an epidemic of dengue-like disease at Newala, Tanganyika Territory Part I - clinical picture, epidemiology, and entomology. Entebbe: Virus Research Institute; 1953.
6. Nimmannitya S, Halstead SB, Cohen SN, et al. Dengue and chikungunya virus infection in man in Thailand, 1962–1964. I. Observations on hospitalized patients with hemorrhagic fever. Am J Trop Med Hyg 1969;18(6):954–71.
7. Padbidri VS, Gnaneswar TT. Epidemiological investigations of chikungunya epidemic at Barsi, Maharashtra state, India. J Hyg Epidemiol Microbiol Immunol 1979;23(4):445–51.
8. Jupp PG, McIntosh BM. Chikungunya virus disease. In: Monath TP, editor, The arbovirus: epidemiology and ecology, vol. II. Boca Raton, Florida: CRC Press; 1988. p. 137–57.
9. Powers AM, Logue CH. Changing patterns of Chikungunya virus: re-emergence of a zoonotic arbovirus. J Gen Virol 2007;88(Pt 9):2363–77.
10. Kariuki Njenga M, Nderitu L, Ledermann JP, et al. Tracking epidemic Chikungunya virus into the Indian Ocean from East Africa. J Gen Virol 2008;89(Pt 11): 2754–60.
11. Ravi V. Re-emergence of Chikungunya virus in India. Indian J Med Microbiol 2006;24(2):83–4.
12. Lanciotti RS, Kosoy OL, Laven JJ, et al. Chikungunya virus in US travelers returning from India, 2006. Emerg Infect Dis 2007;13(5):764–7.
13. Borgherini G, Poubeau P, Staikowsky F, et al. Outbreak of chikungunya on Reunion Island: early clinical and laboratory features in 157 adult patients. Clin Infect Dis 2007;44(11):1401–7.
14. Sergon K, Njuguna C, Kalani R, et al. Seroprevalence of Chikungunya virus (CHIKV) infection on Lamu Island, Kenya, October 2004. Am J Trop Med Hyg 2008;78(2):333–7.
15. Gopalan SS, Das A. Household economic impact of an emerging disease in terms of catastrophic out-of-pocket health care expenditure and loss of productivity: investigation of an outbreak of Chikungunya in Orissa, India. J Vector Borne Dis 2009;46(1):57–64.

16. Seyler T, Hutin Y, Ramanchandran V, et al. Estimating the burden of disease and the economic cost attributable to Chikungunya, Andhra Pradesh, India, 2005–2006. Trans R Soc Trop Med Hyg 2010;104(2):133–8.
17. Sergon K, Yahaya AA, Brown J, et al. Seroprevalence of Chikungunya Virus Infection on Grande Comore Island, Union of the Comoros, 2005. Am J Trop Med Hyg 2007;76(6):1189–93.
18. Staples JE, Breiman RF, Powers AM. Chikungunya Fever: an epidemiological review of a re-emerging infectious disease. Clin Infect Dis 2009;49(6): 942–8.
19. Angelini R, Finarelli AC, Angelini P, et al. An outbreak of Chikungunya fever in the province of Ravenna, Italy. Euro Surveill 2007;12(9):E070906 070901.
20. Schuffenecker I, Iteman I, Michault A, et al. Genome microevolution of Chikungunya viruses causing the Indian Ocean outbreak. PLoS Med 2006;3(7): e263.
21. Cherian SS, Walimbe AM, Jadhav SM, et al. Evolutionary rates and timescale comparison of Chikungunya viruses inferred from the whole genome/E1 gene with special reference to the 2005–07 outbreak in the Indian subcontinent. Infect Genet Evol 2009;9(1):16–23.
22. Powers AM, Brault AC, Tesh RB, et al. Re-emergence of Chikungunya and O'nyong-nyong viruses: evidence for distinct geographical lineages and distant evolutionary relationships. J Gen Virol 2000;81(Pt 2):471–9.
23. Robinson MC. An epidemic of a dengue-like fever in the southern province of Tanganyika. Cent Afr J Med 1956;2(11):394–6.
24. Queyriaux B, Simon F, Grandadam M, et al. Clinical burden of Chikungunya virus infection. Lancet Infect Dis 2008;8(1):2–3.
25. Sissoko D, Moendandze A, Malvy D, et al. Seroprevalence and risk factors of chikungunya virus infection in Mayotte, Indian Ocean, 2005–2006: a population-based survey. PLoS One 2008;3(8):e3066.
26. Inamadar AC, Palit A, Sampagavi VV, et al. Cutaneous manifestations of Chikungunya fever: observations made during a recent outbreak in south India. Int J Dermatol 2008;47(2):154–9.
27. Bandyopadhyay D, Ghosh SK. Mucocutaneous features of Chikungunya fever: a study from an outbreak in West Bengal, India. Int J Dermatol 2008;47(11): 1148–52.
28. Robin S, Ramful D, Zettor J, et al. Severe bullous skin lesions associated with Chikungunya virus infection in small infants. Eur J Pediatr 2009;169:67–72.
29. Wielanek AC, Monredon JD, Amrani ME, et al. Guillan-Barré syndrome complicating a Chikungunya virus infection. Neurology 2007;69(22):2105–7.
30. Rampal SM, Meena H. Neurological complications in Chikungunya fever. J Assoc Physicians India 2007;55:765–9.
31. Singh SS, Manimunda SP, Sugunan AP, et al. Four cases of acute flaccid paralysis associated with Chikungunya virus infection. Epidemiol Infect 2008;136(9): 1277–80.
32. Chandak NH, Kashyap RS, Kabra D, et al. Neurological complications of Chikungunya virus infection. Neurol India 2009;57(2):177–80.
33. Tandale BV, Sathe PS, Arankalle VA, et al. Systemic involvements and fatalities during Chikungunya epidemic in India, 2006. J Clin Virol 2009;46(2):145–9.
34. Economopoulou A, Dominguez M, Helynck B, et al. Atypical Chikungunya virus infections: clinical manifestations, mortality and risk factors for severe disease during the 2005–2006 outbreak on Reunion. Epidemiol Infect 2009;137(4): 534–41.

35. Fraser JR, Becker GJ. Mononuclear cell types in chronic synovial effusions of Ross River virus disease. Aust N Z J Med 1984;14(4):505–6.
36. Linn ML, Mateo L, Gardner J, et al. Alphavirus-specific cytotoxic T lymphocytes recognize a cross-reactive epitope from the capsid protein and can eliminate virus from persistently infected macrophages. J Virol 1998;72(6):5146–53.
37. Morrison TE, Simmons JD, Heise MT. Complement receptor 3 promotes severe ross river virus-induced disease. J Virol 2008;82(22):11263–72.
38. Lidbury BA, Simeonovic C, Maxwell GE, et al. Macrophage-induced muscle pathology results in morbidity and mortality for Ross River virus-infected mice. J Infect Dis 2000;181(1):27–34.
39. Mahalingam S, Friedland JS, Heise MT, et al. Chemokines and viruses: friends or foes? Trends Microbiol 2003;11(8):383–91.
40. Mateo L, La Linn M, McColl SR, et al. An arthrogenic alphavirus induces mono- cyte chemoattractant protein-1 and interleukin-8. Intervirology 2000;43(1): 55–60.
41. Brighton SW, Prozesky OW, de la Harpe AL. Chikungunya virus infection. A retro- spective study of 107 cases. S Afr Med J 1983;63(9):313–5.
42. Panning M, Grywna K, van Esbroeck M, et al. Chikungunya fever in travelers re- turning to Europe from the Indian Ocean region, 2006. Emerg Infect Dis 2008; 14(3):416–22.
43. Blackburn NK, Besselaar TG, Gibson G. Antigenic relationship between Chikun- gunya virus strains and o'nyong nyong virus using monoclonal antibodies. Res Virol 1995;146(1):69–73.
44. Chanas AC, Johnson BK, Simpson DI. Antigenic relationships of alphaviruses by a simple micro-culture cross-neutralization method. J Gen Virol 1976;32(2): 295–300.
45. Chanas AC, Johnson BK, Simpson DI. Characterization of two Chikungunya virus variants. Acta Virol 1979;23(2):128–36.
46. Karabatsos N. Antigenic relationships of group A arboviruses by plaque reduc- tion neutralization testing. Am J Trop Med Hyg 1975;24(3):527–32.
47. Williams MC, Woodall JP. O'nyong-nyong fever: an epidemic virus disease in East Africa. II. Isolation and some properties of the virus. Trans R Soc Trop Med Hyg 1961;55:135–41.
48. Colin de Verdiere N, Molina JM. Rheumatic manifestations caused by tropical viruses. Joint Bone Spine 2007;74(5):410–3.
49. Kiwanuka N, Sanders EJ, Rwaguma EB, et al. O'nyong-nyong fever in south- central Uganda, 1996–1997: clinical features and validation of a clinical case definition for surveillance purposes. Clin Infect Dis 1999;29(5):1243–50.
50. Deller JJ Jr, Russell PK. Chikungunya disease. Am J Trop Med Hyg 1968;17(1): 107–11.
51. Jadhav M, Namboodripad M, Carman RH, et al. Chikungunya disease in infants and children in Vellore: a report of clinical and haematological features of virolog- ically proved cases. Indian J Med Res 1965;53(8):764–76.
52. Tesh RB. Arthritides caused by mosquito-borne viruses. Annu Rev Med 1982;33: 31–40.
53. Shore H. O'nyong-nyong fever: an epidemic virus disease in East Africa. III. Some clinical and epidemiological observations in the Northern Province of Uganda. Trans R Soc Trop Med Hyg 1961;55:361.
54. Carey DE, Myers RM, DeRanitz CM, et al. The 1964 Chikungunya epidemic at Vellore, South India, including observations on concurrent dengue. Trans R Soc Trop Med Hyg 1969;63(4):434–45.

55. Halstead SB, Nimmannitya S, Margiotta MR. Dengue and Chikungunya virus infection in man in Thailand, 1962–1964. II. Observations on disease in outpatients. Am J Trop Med Hyg 1969;18(6):972–83.
56. Kularatne SA, Gihan MC, Weerasinghe SC, et al. Concurrent outbreaks of Chikungunya and Dengue fever in Kandy, Sri Lanka, 2006–07: a comparative analysis of clinical and laboratory features. Postgrad Med J 2009;85(1005):342–6.
57. Bouquillard E, Combe B. Rheumatoid arthritis after Chikungunya fever: a prospective follow-up study of 21 cases. Ann Rheum Dis 2009;68(9):1505–6.
58. Brighton SW. Chloroquine phosphate treatment of chronic Chikungunya arthritis. An open pilot study. S Afr Med J 1984;66(6):217–8.
59. Briolant S, Garin D, Scaramozzino N, et al. In vitro inhibition of Chikungunya and Semliki Forest viruses replication by antiviral compounds: synergistic effect of interferon-alpha and ribavirin combination. Antiviral Res 2004;61(2):111–7.
60. de Lamballerie X, Ninove L, Charrel RN. Antiviral treatment of Chikungunya virus infection. Infect Disord Drug Targets 2009;9(2):101–4.
61. Borgherini G, Poubeau P, Jossaume A, et al. Persistent arthralgia associated with Chikungunya virus: a study of 88 adult patients on reunion island. Clin Infect Dis 2008;47(4):469–75.
62. Sissoko D, Malvy D, Ezzedine K, et al. Post-epidemic Chikungunya disease on Reunion Island: course of rheumatic manifestations and associated factors over a 15-month period. PLoS Negl Trop Dis 2009;3(3):e389.
63. Sudarsanareddy L, Sarojamma V, Ramakrishna V. Genetic predisposition to Chikungunya–a blood group study in Chikungunya affected families. J Virol 2009;6:77.
64. Fulsundar SR, Roy S, Manimunda SP, et al. Investigations on possible role of MIF gene polymorphism in progression of Chikungunya infection into cases of acute flaccid paralysis and chronic arthropathy. J Genet 2009;88(1):123–5.
65. Edelman R, Tacket CO, Wasserman SS, et al. Phase II safety and immunogenicity study of live Chikungunya virus vaccine TSI-GSD-218. Am J Trop Med Hyg 2000; 62(6):681–5.

Tick-Borne Flaviviruses

P. Rocco LaSala, MD[a],*, Michael Holbrook, PhD[b,c]

KEYWORDS

• Flavivirus • Vector • Host • Tick-borne • Encephalitis

Many of the human and zoonotic diseases caused by arthropod-borne flaviviruses have long been recognized—some were known centuries before the introduction of germ theory (eg, louping ill), while others helped to solidify its establishment (eg, yellow fever). As such, their inclusion in an edition of emerging infections might seem suspect without further considering the remarkable increases in tick-borne flaviviral disease incidence throughout the past 2 decades. Hence, a compelling case is made for their status as "re"-emerging entities. By contrast, other agents (eg, Alkhurma hemorrhagic fever virus, deer tick virus) have been characterized only very recently and do represent emerging pathogens in the truest sense of the word. While enhanced clinical awareness and improvements in laboratory diagnostic methods have contributed to this rising incidence, one must not fail to recognize that the transmission of tick-borne viruses, like other vector-borne agents, is impacted by a very broad set of factors, both natural (eg, climate and ecology) and man-made (eg, human mobility and agricultural patterns). As our encroachment into areas of virus endemicity intensifies, and as changes in global economic and environmental conditions continue to promote the expansion of tick populations, we will undoubtedly continue to observe attendant increases in rates of disease attributable to these vector-borne pathogens.

This article focuses on a few of the major tick-borne flaviviral diseases. Specifically, diseases caused by tick-borne encephalitis virus (TBEV), louping ill virus (LIV), Powassan virus (POWV), Kyasanur Forest disease virus (KFDV) and Omsk hemorrhagic fever virus (OHFV), as well as their subtypes, are discussed.

MICROBIOLOGY

The family *Flaviviridae* consists of 3 genera: (1) Pestivirus, which contains several virus species causing zoonotic infections, (2) Hepacivirus, consisting solely of human

[a] Clinical Microbiology Laboratory, Department of Pathology, West Virginia University, 2190 Health Sciences North, PO Box 9203, Morgantown, WV 26506-9203, USA
[b] Department of Pathology, Robert Shope BSL-4 Laboratory, Emerging and High Risk Pathogens, University of Texas Medical Branch, 1.116 Keiller Building, 301 University Boulevard, Galveston, TX 77555-0609, USA
[c] NIAID Integrated Research Facility, Frederick, MD 21702, USA
* Corresponding author.
E-mail address: plasala@hsc.wvu.edu

Clin Lab Med 30 (2010) 221–235
doi:10.1016/j.cll.2010.01.002
0272-2712/10/$ – see front matter © 2010 Elsevier Inc. All rights reserved.

hepatitis C virus and [tentatively] GB virus, and (3) Flavivirus. The latter genus is comprised of over 70 species, nearly all of which are arthropod-borne (ie, are arboviruses) and produce a variety of disease manifestations in humans. Members of the Flavivirus genus are divided into those that are mosquito-borne, those that are tick-borne, and those for which no arthropod vector is required or has been identified. Phylogenetic analyses based on various gene/peptide sequences as well as antigenic studies using neutralizing sera generally support this biologic subgrouping scheme.[1,2] Similarly, species of flaviviruses transmitted predominately by ticks can be classified as those hosted by mammals and those hosted by seabirds. This delineation is also supported by phylogenetic data (**Fig. 1**).

Congruencies between phylogeny and biogeographic properties, such as principal tick vector, principal vertebrate host, global distribution, and so forth, lend clues to the evolutionary history of these agents.[3] In contrast to their mosquito-borne counterparts, the tick-borne flaviviruses (TBF) associated with human disease show considerably less overall diversity. TBF appear to have evolved more slowly and in a continuous, clinal fashion across the Eurasian land mass.[4] Put differently, beginning in Far Eastern Asia with POWV representing the ancestral (hard-tick associated) phylogenetic node,

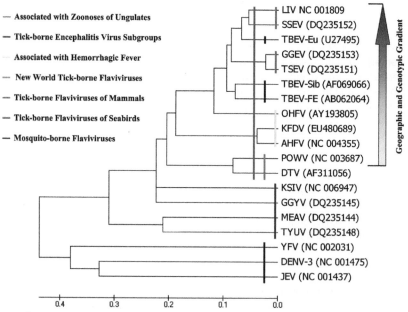

Fig. 1. Phylodendrogram showing evolutionary history of 19 Flavivirus species (GenBank Accession) inferred from 9929 base pair positions using the Minimum Evolution method and MEGA4 software. Evolutionary distances were computed using the Maximum Composite Likelihood method. Phylogenetic groups sharing biologic similarities are indicated. The geographic/genotypic gradient is drawn from earliest to latest node branches, representing TBF species distributed from East Asia through Western Europe. AHFV, Alkhurma hemorrhagic fever virus; DEN-3, dengue virus, serotype 3; DTV, deer tick virus; GGEV, Greek goat encephalitis virus; GGYV, Gadgets Gully virus; JEV, Japanese encephalitis virus; KFDV, Kyasanur forest disease virus; KSIV, Karshi virus; LIV, louping ill virus; MEAV, Meaban virus; OHFV, Omsk hemorrhagic fever virus; POWV, Powassan virus; SSEV, Spanish sheep encephalitis virus; TBEV-Eu, tick-borne encephalitis virus, European subtype; TBEV-FE, tick-borne encephalitis virus, Far Eastern subtype; TBEV-Sib, tick-borne encephalitis virus, Siberian subtype; TSEV, Turkish sheep encephalitis virus; TYUV, Tyuleniy virus; YFV, yellow fever virus.

one generally observes incrementally greater genotypic relatedness among geographically proximate TBF species when moving toward Western Europe, where LIV and its subgroups circulate, representing the most recently diverged clades (see **Fig. 1**). This observation is substantiated by recent analysis revealing higher genetic identity between LIV and the European subtype of TBEV (TBEV-Eu) than among TBEV subtypes.[2] However, the identification of new viral species and appreciation of wider distributions for known species could contradict this.

Like all Flaviviruses, the tick-borne agents have a spherical virion appearance by electron microscopy, measure 40 to 50 nm in diameter, and are enclosed by a host-derived lipid envelope (**Fig. 2**). The flavivirus genome consists of one, single-stranded, positive-sense RNA molecule, approximately 11 kb in length, which encodes 3 structural and 7 nonstructural proteins in a single open reading frame (ORF) (**Fig. 3**). Variable-length 3'- and 5'-untranslated regions flank either side of the ORF and assist in translation, cellular localization, and virion packaging.[5] The infectious genome directly serves as template for cellular transcription, and the resulting polyprotein is co- and posttranslationally cleaved by host-derived and viral-derived enzymes into functional components.

EPIDEMIOLOGY

The TBF are maintained in nature via complex cycles of invertebrate-vertebrate-invertebrate transmission. Successful viral maintenance and potential for human exposure are dependent on many factors, including: (1) population density and distribution of tick vectors and intermediate vertebrate hosts, (2) feeding predilections of particular tick species and/or instar forms, (3) local environmental conditions that influence questing, (4) infection rates within local tick populations, and (5) frequency/duration of human traffic within tick habitats. The TBF of mammals are transmitted primarily

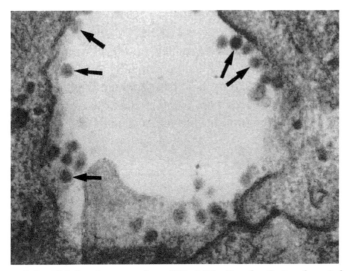

Fig. 2. Transmission EM showing egression of West Nile (Sarafend) virus from infected Vero cells at 16 h post infection. Numerous virus particles are seen budding from the plasma membrane (*arrows*). (*From* Nf ML, Yeong FM, Tan SH. Cryosubstitution technique reveals new morphology of flavivirus-induced structures. J Virol Methods 1994;49:305–14; with permission.)

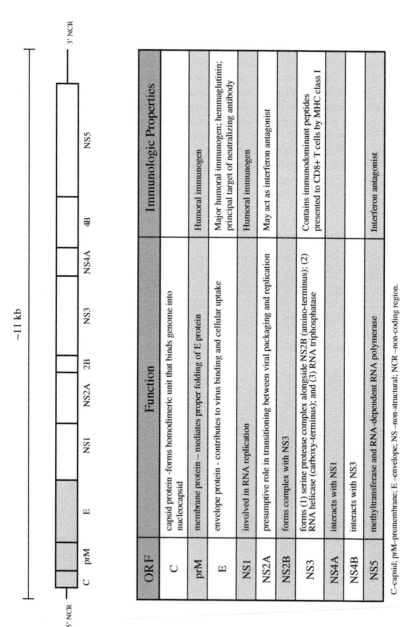

Fig. 3. Flavivirus RNA genome arrangement depicting both structural (*shaded*) and nonstructural gene products within the single ORF. General properties of each are outlined below.

C–capsid; prM–premembrane; E –envelope; NS –non-structural; NCR –non-coding region.

ORF	Function	Immunologic Properties
C	capsid protein –forms homodimeric unit that binds genome into nucleocapsid	
prM	membrane protein – mediates proper folding of E protein	Humoral immunogen
E	envelope protein - contributes to virus binding and cellular uptake	Major humoral immunogen; hemmaglutinin; principal target of neutralizing antibody
NS1	involved in RNA replication	Humoral immunogen
NS2A	presumptive role in transitioning between viral packaging and replication	May act as interferon antagonist
NS2B	forms complex with NS3	
NS3	forms (1) serine protease complex alongside NS2B (amino-terminus); (2) RNA helicase (carboxy-terminus); and (3) RNA triphosphatase	Contains immunodominant peptides presented to CD8+ T cells by MHC class I
NS4A	interacts with NS1	
NS4B	interacts with NS3	
NS5	methyltransferase and RNA-dependent RNA polymerase	Interferon antagonist

by hard ticks of the genera *Ixodes, Dermacentor*, and *Haemaphysalis*, and many are pathogenic to humans (**Table 1**). By contrast, TBF of seabirds are vectored chiefly by soft, argasid ticks and are not typically associated with human disease.

Transovarial passage of virus from adult to egg (and hence larva) occurs, ensuring long-term survival of viral species, but this phenomenon seems less important to natural maintenance than does transstadial passage, which provides a pool for horizontal transmission and viral amplification. One of the major factors in virus acquisition by uninfected ticks is the predilection of vector species to cofeed simultaneously alongside numerous other ticks on a single, multiply-infested host. Horizontal transmission during such a scenario is efficient even in the absence of detectable host viremia, a phenomenon called nonviremic trans-mission.[6] The degree to which tick-derived factors, particularly of salivary origin, contribute to such transmission appears considerable and has been the subject of investigation.[7] Intermediate hosts for the TBF include species of rodents, ungu-lates, lagomorphs, and birds; and the overall frequency, severity and outcome of their respective infections is variable. Unlike the reservoirs of the mosquito-borne flaviviruses, these vertebrates indirectly contribute to long-term virus survival not by maintaining subclinical viremia for long durations, but rather by providing short-term opportunity for horizontal tick transmission.[8]

Humans serve as incidental hosts and do not contribute to viral life cycle. Clinically apparent disease is generally more common among young to middle-aged adult males; and temporal seasonality is typical. Both of these observations likely reflect an increased probability for tick exposure. Although some variation in seasonal disease peak(s) exists between climatic regions, late spring to summer is common and correlates with the height of questing by local tick populations. Among nonimmu-nized persons in endemic areas, seroprevalence rates as high as 70% to 95% suggest that subclinical infection is common for some TBF.[9]

Throughout the twentieth century, diseases caused by TBEV were referred to as "Russian spring summer encephalitis," "Central European encephalitis," "Far Eastern encephalitis," "forest spring encephalitis," and "Früh-Sommer-meningoencephalitis" (among others) due to its broad distribution and variable clinical manifestations. Another designation, "biphasic milk disease," is derived from the distinct manner of virus acquisition via ingestion of raw sheep's or goat's milk and the near-invariable biphasic clinical syndrome. Genotypically, 3 subtypes of TBEV are recognized: Sibe-rian (TBEV-Sib) and Far Eastern (TBEV-FE) types are transmitted primarily by *Ixodes persulcatus*, whereas the European (TBEV-Eu) subtype is vectored by *Ixodes ricinus* (see **Table 1**). Infection by these strains represents the most prevalent of all tick-borne flaviviral diseases of humans, with annual rates totaling approximately 12,000 cases worldwide. Disease is exclusive to the Old World, with foci of endemicity extending from Siberia to Scandinavia and southward through regions of central Europe (**Fig. 4**). The incidence of disease varies tremendously between regions, however, with less than 0.82 cases per 100,000 population in Austria where vaccination rates are high, to more than 80 cases per 100,000 population in parts of Western Siberia.[10] As of 2007, TBE was a reportable disease in 16 European countries. Over the past 2 decades the overall incidence of TBEV infection has increased substantially, and new endemic foci have developed. However, year-to-year reductions in disease burden have also been noted sporadically in certain endemic foci, the reasons for which are unknown.[10]

The TBF with hemorrhagic manifestations (OHFV, KFDV and its subtype Alkhurma hemorrhagic fever virus [ALKV]) produce disease much less commonly and within more confined geographic areas than does TBEV (see **Fig. 4**). The distribution of

Table 1
Major tick-borne flaviviruses of medical significance including principal tick vector and vertebrate host(s)

Virus (Abbreviation)	Subtypes	Principal Vector	Intermediate Host(s)	Case Fatality Rate[b]
Tick-borne encephalitis virus (TBEV)	European subtype	*Ixodes ricinus*	Field mice, other rodents	0.5%–2%
	Far Eastern subtype	*I persulcatus* (also *Haemaphysalis concinna*)		5%–20%
	Siberian subtype	*I persulcatus* (also *H. concinna*)		1%–3%
Omsk hemorrhagic fever virus (OHFV)		*Dermacentor reticulatus*	Voles, muskrats	0.5%–3%
Kyasanur Forest disease virus (KFDV)		*H spinigera*	Rodents, shrews, birds, monkeys	2%–10%
	Alkhurma hemorrhagic fever virus (AHFV)	Unknown	Unknown (suspect goats, sheep and/or camels)	25%
Powassan virus (POWV)		*I cookei* (North America), *H longicornis* (East Asia)	Groundhogs, woodchucks, foxes, squirrels, skunks	20%
	Deer tick virus (DTV)	*I scapularis*	White-footed mice	Unknown
Louping ill virus (LIV)[a]	Greek goat encephalitis virus (GGEV) Turkish sheep encephalitis virus (TSEV) Spanish sheep encephalitis virus (SSEV)	*I ricinus*	Mountain hares, sheep, goats, grouse	Very rare

[a] Based on phylogenetic analysis of complete amino acid sequences, Grard and colleagues[2] have demonstrated that LIV and SSEV form a closely related sister group to the European subtype of TBEV, whereas TSEV and GGEV form a monophyletic lineage distinct from both TBEV and LIV. Although their work suggests a different taxonomic schema, this virus grouping was chosen based on biologic as well as phylogenetic data.

[b] Mortality figures are approximate and likely represent overestimates based on unknown numbers of subclinical infections and/or overall low case numbers.

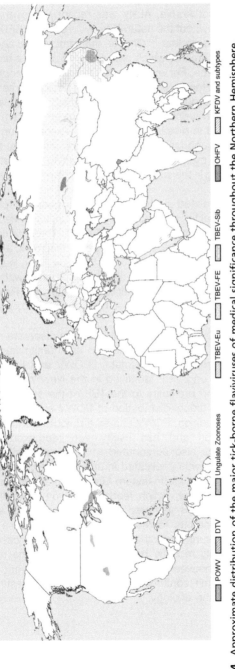

Fig. 4. Approximate distribution of the major tick-borne flaviviruses of medical significance throughout the Northern Hemisphere.

KFDV was thought to be limited to Karnataka State in the southwestern Indian subcontinent, where it is transmitted by *Haemaphysalis spinigera* to monkeys and humans. More recent data from the Middle East and China indicate that the distribution of viral subtypes (ALKV and Nanjianyin virus, respectively) is more widespread (see **Fig. 4**).[11,12] In Saudi Arabia, ALKV was recently recovered from the argasid tick, *Ornithodoros savignyi*, but the natural life cycle of these KFDV subtypes in China and Saudi Arabia remains unclear.[13] Of note, the hemorrhagic agents have a propensity to produce local outbreaks, which may occur at different times of year than the other TBF-related illnesses. For example, KFDV causes epizootics from December to May, corresponding to local *H spinigera* questing peak, whereas ALKV hemorrhagic fever has been diagnosed during the Muslim Hajj, perhaps in relation to high rates of animal importation and slaughter.[14,15] OHFV, vectored by *Dermacentor reticulatus*, was originally implicated in disease outbreaks in Siberia during the late 1940s and 1950s (see **Fig. 4**), although incidence has declined since that time. Direct contact with muskrat carcasses by hunters has been linked to disease more recently, with seasonal peaks occurring in the autumn-winter, later than might be expected for transmission by ticks.[8]

Louping ill virus and related subtypes (eg, Greek goat encephalitis virus [GGEV], Spanish sheep encephalitis virus [SSEV], and Turkish sheep encephalitis virus [TSEV]) are found in Western Europe (see **Fig. 4**). These viruses primarily cause encephalitic infections of domestic sheep and goats, leading to a characteristic neurologic symptom described centuries ago as "louping" (for leaping) by the Scots. Human disease is noted almost exclusively among persons with occupational exposure (eg, veterinarians, shepherds, abattoir workers, farmers). Rates of natural, human acquisition are low, however, and may even be outnumbered by accidental infections occurring in the laboratory setting.[16]

Similar to TBF of seabirds, POWV is distributed in disparate regions of the globe (see **Fig. 4**), from Asia, where it is maintained and transmitted by *Haemaphysalis longicornis* ticks, to North America. Notably, POWV and the closely related deer tick virus (DTV) are the only TBF identified in the New World. Given its ancestral phylogenetic position and proximity to the TBF of the seabirds clade (see **Fig. 1**), one may speculate that global distribution of POWV somehow relates to dispersal by migratory birds. In addition, POWV shares a unique amino acid residue with the mosquito-borne flavivirus and has itself been recovered from mosquitoes,[9] a feature that may have also contributed to its dissemination. During the latter twentieth century, POWV was implicated in approximately 30 cases of encephalitis in Ontario, Canada, and the Northeastern United States. In this region the virus is transmitted by *Ixodes cookei*, which feeds chiefly on groundhogs and rarely on humans. By contrast, DTV is vectored by *Ixodes scapularis*, whose proclivity for human blood meals accounts for many of the other diseases discussed in this issue. It is somewhat surprising, therefore, that the first case of human illness caused by DTV has only recently been documented.[17] The high degree of antigenic cross-reactivity between DTV and POWV, however, indicate that prior reports of POWV infection confirmed solely by serologic testing could potentially have mischaracterized the etiology.

CLINICAL PRESENTATION

As seen with the mosquito-borne flaviviruses, disease manifestations of TBF are broad-ranging. Many of the agents produce subclinical infection detected only incidentally by sero-surveillance studies. When apparent, clinical disease typically begins approximately 5 to 14 days following virus acquisition and manifests acutely as a plethora of mild to debilitating, nonspecific symptoms that include fever, headache, sore throat, malaise, nausea, and vomiting. A minority of patients recover from this stage with no additional untoward effects. In time, however, most will begin to exhibit various degrees of neurologic manifestations, often following a short period of apparent convalescence (the biphasic disease course). Meningitis, meningoencephalitis, meningoencephalomyelitis, and mono-/polyradiculitis have each been reported, leading to a range of signs and symptoms such as headache, photophobia, altered consciousness, seizures, paresis, paralysis, cranial nerve abnormalities, cognitive deficits, sensory disturbances, dysphagia, ataxia, or tremors. Complete neurologic recovery may require several weeks to several years, and a small proportion of patients will experience permanent sequelae of ataxic, dyskinetic, paralytic, or neuro-psychiatric disorders.

Some studies suggest that disease course is somewhat milder among children and adolescents than adults (**Fig. 5**).[18] Yet morbidity is also clearly dependent on the relative virulence of infecting viral species or subtype.[9,19] Clinical characteristics may overlap among patients within the same outbreak or who are infected by similar viruses (eg, KFDV and ALKV causing hemorrhagic diatheses; TBEV-Eu and LIV causing biphasic illness). Overall mortality rates vary by virus type, ranging from less than 1% for TBE-Eu and LIV to as high as around 25% for some of the hemorrhagic flaviviruses (see **Table 1**).

A fascinating aspect of TBF is the reported ability to produce chronic, indolent disease either via long-term, low-level viral persistence or, possibly, through a mechanism of viral latency and recrudescence.[9] This phenomenon has been described extensively in the Russian literature, and is noted most commonly in association with the Siberian subtype of TBEV.[20] Syndromes are characterized by slowly progressive neurologic dysfunction that may begin years after initial exposure to virus. Causality has been inferred based on observations that virus can be recovered in culture for long durations from patients with long-standing disease and from affected regions of the central nervous system (CNS) in postmortem samples.[9]

Among the hemorrhagic TBF, KFDV and its subtypes may be associated with encephalitis, whereas OHFV more commonly produces a biphasic illness devoid of symptomatic neurologic manifestations. For OHFV, signs and symptoms may include

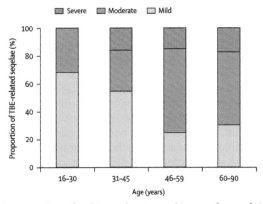

Fig. 5. Age-related proportion of mild, moderate, and severe form of tick-borne encephalitis in a prospective study from Lithuania. (*From* Lindquist L, Vapalahti O. Tick-borne encephalitis. Lancet 2008;371:1861; with permission.)

papulovesicular or petechial cutaneous rash, lymphadenopathy, ocular suffusion, and capillary perturbations, leading to oral and nasal mucosal bleeding as well as scattered visceral hemorrhage.[8,9] Infection by KFDV and ALKV may present as epistaxis, hematemesis, cutaneous bleeding (eg, purpura, ecchymoses, or petechiae), melena, or oozing from venipuncture sites as well as neurologic symptoms similar to other TBF.[14,15] Of note, bleeding diathesis does not appear to portend a worse prognosis.

PATHOGENESIS AND IMMUNITY

The specific mechanisms of viral pathogenicity for TBF are largely unknown. As with all arthropod-borne viruses, TBF are thought to replicate locally or be taken up by dendritic cells (Langerhans cells) or macrophages following deposition into the skin.

The virus would then be transported to draining lymph nodes where it replicates further, stimulating the innate immune response with subsequent development of adaptive immunity. In the case of strains associated with encephalitis, the virus ultimately penetrates the blood-brain barrier (BBB) and enters the CNS where a significant amount of pathology is induced, largely as a result of the host inflammatory response. The process by which TBF, and encephalitic flaviviruses in general, cross the BBB is currently a topic of significant discussion as the precise mechanism is unclear. In mice, TBEV is able to penetrate the BBB in 4 to 6 days depending on the strain and age of mouse (M. Holbrook, unpublished results, 2006–2009).[21] There is little apparent pathology outside the CNS in either small animal models or cases of human disease, indicating a high tropism for neural tissue. Recent studies of TBEV-Eu infections using magnetic resonance imaging have shown significant pathology in the anterior horns of both thoracic and cervical vertebrae, lumbar nerve roots, basal ganglia, and the thalamus.[22–24] Further histologic studies suggest that TBEV-Eu targets neurons within the anterior pons, medulla oblongata, dentate nucleus, and Purkinje cells.[25] Similar studies are not available for infections with the other subtypes of TBEV, but it is likely that the pathology is similar. The chronic form of TBEV infection is curious. Several studies have investigated aspects of the disease process in nonhuman primates and hamsters, but it is still unclear why some virus subtypes cause a persistent disease.[9]

On presentation, TBE patients often have elevated IgM and IgG levels in their cerebrospinal fluid (CSF), with some patients demonstrating intrathecal production of IgM and IgG.[26] However, the presence of IgM or IgG in the CSF is not a prognostic indicator for the outcome of disease.[26,27] Patients with low serum IgG or CSF IgM early in the disease process are more inclined to develop more severe disease as there is a decreased ability to clear the virus, leading to an increased viremia. Individuals with TBE develop high neutralizing titers of IgG that peak toward the end of the illness. IgG titers wane somewhat, but residual titers are sufficient to protect patients against reinfection.[28] Unlike the case for sequential dengue virus infections, antibody-dependent enhancement has not been observed in the tick-borne flaviviral illnesses.

As the principal disease pathology for the TBEV is development of encephalitis or meningoencephalitis, efforts have been made to understand the development of inflammation and adaptive immunity in the brain. Recent studies have found that, along with having a necessary protective role in the infected brain, CD8+ T cells can also have a deleterious effect by inducing cell death or actively killing infected neurons.[29]

In the case of OHFV, the limited amount of information is based on the recently identified mouse model.[30] In this system, it has been shown that OHFV causes a primarily viscerotropic disease with infection of the spleen and liver, yet also has a neurologic component because the virus is able to get into the brain.[21] The specific mechanisms of viral pathogenicity are not well understood, although preliminary work points toward regulation of the T-cell response as an important component of the disease process (M. Holbrook, unpublished results, 2006–2009).

DIAGNOSIS

Aside from local, ongoing outbreaks for which practitioners may reach a presumptive diagnosis based on clinicoepidemiologic factors alone, TBF disease symptoms are nonspecific and the differential diagnosis is broad (**Table 2**). As a result, laboratory testing is essential for securing a diagnosis. Several testing approaches are available, and the optimal method depends in large part on the stage and manifestations of the disease process itself.

TBF can be readily cultivated in vitro on a variety of cells (eg, Vero, BHK, tick-derived lines) and is best achieved using serum, plasma, whole blood, or CSF specimens drawn during the viremic period within the first few days of disease onset. For diagnostic purposes, this approach is problematic given the facts that (1) most patients do not seek medical care until late in disease course when neurologic symptoms develop, at which point systemic virus has usually been cleared, and (2) propagation of TBF agents requires specialized laboratory facilities with BSL-3 or BSL-4 capabilities.

A second testing option is amplification of viral genomic RNA by reverse transcriptase-polymerase chain reaction (RT-PCR). This assay may use primers having broad-range, flavivirus specificity or ones specifically targeting TBF. In either case, samples testing positive require further analysis (eg, by sequencing or probe hybridization) of amplicon products for definitive identification of the infecting agent. Unfortunately, with the possible exception of KFDV,[14] this approach too is limited by the short duration of viremia, and detection of target RNA from peripheral blood and CSF is often unsuccessful during later disease stages.[15,31] Given its high sensitivity during the

Table 2	
Differential diagnoses of tick-borne flaviviral diseases	
Other viruses	Enterovirus
	Herpes simplex virus
	Varicella zoster virus
	Hepatitis C virus
Systemic/central nervous system bacterial infections	*Neisseria meningitides*
	Streptococcus pneumoniae
	Listeria monocytogenes
Other zoonotic/vector-borne agents Viral	Mosquito-borne flaviviruses
	Alphaviruses
	Rift Valley fever virus
	Crimean-Congo hemorrhagic fever virus
	Filoviruses
Bacterial	Granulocytic anaplasmosis
	Rickettsial disease
	Lyme borreliosis
Noninfectious	Multiple sclerosis
	Guillian-Barré syndrome
	Thrombotic thrombocytopenic purpura

acute phase, however, RT-PCR may be a reasonable testing alternative before sero-conversion in the appropriate epidemiologic setting.[32]

The most commonly relied upon test modality for the TBF agents is some form of serologic analysis. Historically, complement fixation (CF) and hemagglutination inhibition (HI) assays were used, although these methods were somewhat laborious and did not routinely delineate species-specific antibody. As a result, they did not provide diagnostic specificity. Rather, neutralization assays (NA) were and continue to be required for effectively defining antiflavivirus antibody specificity. By measuring a reduction in plaque formation, fluorescent foci, or enzymatic reaction on cell mono-layers as an end point, these assays establish the ability of patient sera to block culti-vation of various flaviviruses. Because NA also requires considerable expertise and adequate biocontainment facilities, its routine performance is generally reserved for specialized reference or research laboratories.

The enzyme-linked immunosorbent assay (ELISA) is employed by many clinical labo-ratories, as this format allows for high throughput and automation while also providing objective end points. Various formulations have been developed that use either purified viral lysate or recombinant viral protein(s) as antigen sources. Testing may be per-formed on serum and CSF alike. As with CF and HI assays, ELISA is also prone to cross-reactivity by heterologous flavivirus antibody. Yet it does afford the capability of easily detecting and delineating IgG and IgM. Furthermore, the IgM capture method used by some kits enhances test specificity by decreasing potential interference due to autoimmune and anti-isotype antibodies (eg, rheumatoid factor). Some laboratories have successfully adapted ELISA for quantitative results reporting.[33]

As with infectious agents, detection of IgM in acute phase serum or CSF or a fourfold increase in IgG titer between acute and convalescent periods usually defines a positive result. Important caveats to consider are: (1) an early IgG response, such that acute phase testing may already reveal high antibody titers (**Fig. 6**); (2) IgM persistence for weeks to months, such that recent past infections may be mistaken as current (see **Fig. 6**); (3) cross-reactivity with other flaviviruses, such that follow-up NA testing for definitive serotyping may be indicated; and (4) prior vaccination, which may impact assay interpretation as well as the ability of some persons to produce antibody following "breakthrough" infection.[34]

Ancillary laboratory data may also indirectly support a diagnosis of TBF infection. Parameters such as absolute leukopenia, thrombocytopenia, elevated hepatic trans-aminases, and lactate dehydrogenase are frequently reported, as are prolonged prothrombin time and activated partial thromboplastin time for the hemorrhagic TBF. For neuroinvasive infections, CSF abnormalities consist of neutrophilic pleocyto-sis that subsequently becomes lymphocyte predominant, and elevated protein levels. Laboratory indices reflecting renal, pulmonary, and cardiac functions are generally within normal ranges.

TREATMENT AND PREVENTION

One of the primary means for prevention of any tick-borne disease is to minimize phys-ical contact with the vector itself through (1) reduction in exposure to tick habitats, (2) use of environmental, personal, or pet acarisides, and (3) frequent "tick checks" to remove embedded ticks promptly. Given that flavivirus transmission is believed to occur very soon after feeding commences, however, the latter approach may not be as effective against TBF as for other tick-borne agents.[35]

Active immunization is another means for primary prevention of TBF disease. Several vaccines have been developed in different countries through the years,

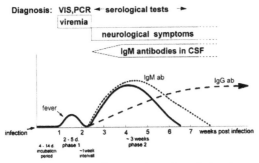

Fig. 6. Biphasic course of a TBE virus infection: detection of the virus or viral nucleic acids and development of specific antibodies (ab) in serum and cerebrospinal fluid (CSF). VIS, virus isolation; PCR, polymerase chain reaction. (*From* Heinz FX, Holzmann H. Tick-borne encephalitis. In: Service MW, editor. The encyclopedia of arthropod-transmitted infections. Wallingford (UK): CABI Publishing; 2001. p. 507–12; with permission.)

many of which have proven extremely effective in disease prevention. At present, those that are commercially available in Germany and Austria use purified, formalin-inactivated TBEV produced in chick embryo cells. Dosing schedule consists of 2 inoculations delivered 2 weeks to 3 months apart followed by a third inoculation given 9 to 12 months later. Seroconversion rates following the third dose exceed 98%, and available clinicoepidemiologic evidence suggests the vaccines are both safe and highly effective.[36] In Austria, where aggressive immunization campaigns have led to 85% to 90% of the population being vaccinated, the impact on disease has been remarkable. Yearly rates of disease reached as high as 700 cases in the prevaccination era compared with a current annual average of around 70 cases.[36]

Vaccines have also been developed in Russia and India using different virus species or strains, with formalin inactivation being the most commonly employed method of production. Alternative strategies, including live attenuated virus preparations, genetically engineered chimeric viruses, protein subunit, and RNA vaccines continue to be explored.

Therapy for the TBF-induced disease is largely supportive. No specific antiviral agents have demonstrable efficacy against TBF agents. Hyperimmune serum is available and in use for secondary immunoprophylaxis for those persons exposed to TBF.

REFERENCES

1. Calisher CH, Karabatsos N, Dalrymple JM, et al. Antigenic relationships between flaviviruses as determined by cross-neutralization tests with polyclonal antisera. J Gen Virol 1989;70:37–43.
2. Grard G, Moureau G, Charrel RN, et al. Genetic characterization of tick-borne flaviviruses: new insights into evolution, pathogenetic determinants and taxonomy. Virology 2007;361(1):80–92.
3. Gould EA, de Lamballerie X, Zanotto PM, et al. Evolution, epidemiology, and dispersal of flaviviruses revealed by molecular phylogenies. Adv Virus Res 2001;57:71–103.
4. Zanotto PM, Gao GF, Gritsun T, et al. An arbovirus cline across the northern hemisphere. Virology 1995;210(1):152–9.

5. Lindenbach BD, Thiel HJ, Rice CM. Flaviviridae: the viruses and their replication. In: Knipe DM, Howley PM, editors. Fields virology. 5th edition. Philadelphia: Lippincott-Williams; 2007.

6. Jones LD, Gaunt M, Hails RS, et al. Transmission of louping ill virus between infected and uninfected ticks co-feeding on mountain hares. Med Vet Entomol 1997;11:172–6.

7. Nuttall PA, Labuda M. Tick-host interactions: saliva-activated transmission. Parasitology 2004;129(Suppl):S177–89.

8. Charrel RN, Attoui H, Butenko AM, et al. Tick-borne virus diseases of human interest in Europe. Clin Microbiol Infect 2004;10:1040–55.

9. Gritsun TS, Nuttall PA, Gould EA. Tick-borne encephalitis. Adv Virol Res 2003;61: 317–71.

10. Süss J. Tick-borne encephalitis in Europe and beyond—the epidemiological situation as of 2007. Euro Surveill 2008;13:1–8.

11. Charrel RN, Zaki AM, Attoui H, et al. Complete coding sequence of the Alkhurma virus, a tick-borne flavivirus causing severe hemorrhagic fever in humans in Saudi Arabia. Biochem Biophys Res Commun 2001;287:455–61.

12. Wang J, Zhang H, Fu S, et al. Isolation of Kyasanur forest disease virus from febrile patient, Yunnan, China. Emerg Infect Dis 2009;15:326–8.

13. Charrel RN, Fagbo S, Moureau G, et al. Alkhurma hemorrhagic fever virus in Ornithodoros savignyi ticks. Emerg Infect Dis 2007;13:153–5.

14. Pattnaik P. Kyasanur forest disease: an epidemiological view in India. Rev Med Virol 2006;16:151–65.

15. Madani TA. Alkhumra virus infection, a new viral hemorrhagic fever in Saudi Arabia. J Infect 2005;51:91–7.

16. Davidson MM, Williams H, Macleod JA. Louping ill in man: a forgotten disease. J Infect 1991;23(3):241–9.

17. Tavakoli NP, Wang H, Dupuis M, et al. Fatal case of deer tick virus encephalitis. N Engl J Med 2009;360:2099–107.

18. Lesnicar G, Poljak M, Seme K, et al. Pediatric tick-borne encephalitis in 371 cases from an endemic region in Slovenia, 1959 to 2000. Pediatr Infect Dis J 2003;22:612–7.

19. Lindquist L, Vapalahti O. Tick-borne encephalitis. Lancet 2008;371:1861–71.

20. Gritsun TS, Frolova TV, Zhankov AI, et al. Characterization of a siberian virus isolated from a patient with progressive chronic tick-borne encephalitis. J Virol 2003; 77:25–36.

21. Tigabu B, Juelich T, Bertrand J, et al. Clinical evaluation of highly pathogenic tick-borne flavivirus infection in the mouse model. J Med Virol 2009;81:1261–9.

22. Alkadhi H, Kollias SS. MRI in tick-borne encephalitis. Neuroradiology 2000;42: 753–5.

23. Bender A, Schulte-Altedorneburg G, Walther EU, et al. Severe tick borne encephalitis with simultaneous brain stem, bithalamic, and spinal cord involvement documented by MRI. J Neurol Neurosurg Psychiatry 2005;76:135–7.

24. Pfefferkorn T, Feddersen B, Schulte-Altedorneburg G, et al. Tick-borne encephalitis with polyradiculitis documented by MRI. Neurology 2007;68:1232–3.

25. Gelpi E, Preusser M, Garzuly F, et al. Visualization of Central European tick-borne encephalitis infection in fatal human cases. J Neuropathol Exp Neurol 2005;64: 506–12.

26. Kaiser R, Holzmann H. Laboratory findings in tick-borne encephalitis—correlation with clinical outcome. Infection 2000;28:78–84.

27. Günther G, Haglund M, Lindquist L, et al. Intrathecal IgM, IgA and IgG antibody response in tick-borne encephalitis. Long-term follow-up related to clinical course and outcome. Clin Diagn Virol 1997;8:17–29.
28. Klockmann U, Bock HL, Kwasny H, et al. Humoral immunity against tick-borne encephalitis virus following manifest disease and active immunization. Vaccine 1991;9:42–6.
29. Růžek D, Salát J, Palus M, et al. CD8 + T-cells mediate immunopathology in tick-borne encephalitis. Virology 2009;384:1–6.
30. Holbrook MR, Aronson JF, Campbell GA, et al. An animal model for the tickborne flavivirus—Omsk hemorrhagic fever virus. J Infect Dis 2005;191:100–8.
31. Puchhammer-Stöckl E, Kunz C, Mandl CW, et al. Identification of tick-borne encephalitis virus ribonucleic acid in tick suspensions and in clinical specimens by a reverse transcription-nested polymerase chain reaction assay. Clin Diagn Virol 1995;4:321–6.
32. Saksida A, Duh D, Lotric-Furlan S, et al. The importance of tick-borne encephalitis virus RNA detection for early differential diagnosis of tick-borne encephalitis. J Clin Virol 2005;33:331–5.
33. Holzmann H, Kundi M, Stiasny K, et al. Correlation between ELISA, hemagglutination inhibition, and neutralization tests after vaccination against tick-borne encephalitis. J Med Virol 1996;48:102–7.
34. Holzmann H. Diagnosis of tick-borne encephalitis. Vaccine 2003;21(Suppl 1): S36–40.
35. Ebel GD, Kramer LD. Short report: duration of tick attachment required for transmission of Powassan virus by deer ticks. Am J Trop Med Hyg 2004;71:268–71.
36. Kunz C. TBE vaccination and the Austrian experience. Vaccine 2003;21(Suppl 1): S50–5.

Yellow Fever: A Reemerging Threat

Christina L. Gardner, PhD, Kate D. Ryman, PhD*

KEYWORDS

• Yellow fever virus • Mosquito-borne
• Transmission • Vaccine • Emerging disease

Yellow fever (YF) is a viral disease, endemic to tropical regions of Africa and the Americas. YF principally affects humans and nonhuman primates, and is transmitted via the bite of infected mosquitoes. The agent of YF, yellow fever virus (YFV), can cause devastating epidemics of potentially fatal, hemorrhagic disease. We rely on mass vaccination campaigns to prevent and control these outbreaks. However, the risk of major YF epidemics, especially in densely populated, poor urban settings, both in Africa and South America, has greatly increased due to: (1) reinvasion of urban settings by the mosquito vector of YF, *Aedes aegypti*; (2) rapid urbanization, particularly in parts of Africa, with populations shifting from rural to predominantly urban; and (3) waning immunization coverage. Consequently, YF is considered an emerging, or reemerging disease of considerable importance.

A BRIEF HISTORY OF YELLOW FEVER RESEARCH

YF originated in Africa, and was imported into Europe and the Americas as a consequence of the slave trade between these continents.[1] In the Western Hemisphere, the first recorded epidemic of disease believed to have been YF occurred in the Yucatan in 1648.[2] Throughout the eighteenth and nineteenth centuries explosive YF outbreaks ravaged tropical South and Central America, as well as port cities on the eastern seaboard of North America and in Europe.[3] Although it was realized early on that the disease was not contagious, the source was wrongly attributed to environmental miasmas. It was Carlos Finlay, a Cuban scientist, who first determined in the late 1800s that mosquitoes were responsible for disseminating the disease. Dispatched to Cuba by the United States government to investigate the cause of YF, Walter Reed and colleagues confirmed that the primary mode of YF transmission to humans was the *Aedes aegypti* mosquito (**Fig. 1**) and, in ground-breaking virologic studies, demonstrated that the disease was caused by an agent that could be filtered from the blood of infected individuals.[4] Campaigns to eradicate *Ae aegypti*, the so-called

Center for Vaccine Research, Department of Microbiology and Molecular Genetics, University of Pittsburgh, 3501 Fifth Avenue, Pittsburgh, PA 15261, USA
* Corresponding author.
E-mail address: ryman@pitt.edu

Clin Lab Med 30 (2010) 237–260
doi:10.1016/j.cll.2010.01.001
0272-2712/10/$ – see front matter © 2010 Elsevier Inc. All rights reserved.

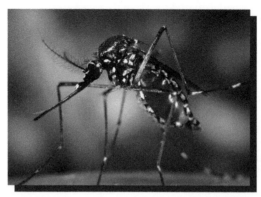

Fig. 1. The yellow fever mosquito. The *Aedes aegypti* mosquito is the primary vector responsible for the transmission of yellow fever virus (YFV) between humans. Known as the YF mosquito, this vector is responsible for explosive outbreaks of urban yellow fever (YF) in African, South American, and Central American cities. Image from the Public Health Image Library, Centers for Disease Control. Photo, James Gathany; contributor Frank Collins. (*Courtesy of* the Centers for Disease Control and Prevention; with permission.)

yellow fever mosquito, from Cuba and Panama were highly successful in eliminating urban YF cases. Unfortunately, the goal of YF eradication was thwarted by YF being a zoonotic disease, maintained by sylvatic mosquito species and nonhuman primates in the Amazon jungle. This aspect is discussed further in the Epidemiology section.

The causative agent of YF disease, YFV, was first isolated in 1927 from a Ghanaian patient named Asibi,[4] and the Asibi YFV strain is still widely used by scientists today. In the 1930s, Max Theiler and colleagues[5–7] produced a live-attenuated vaccine strain, designated 17D, which was attenuated for viscerotropic disease in monkeys and humans, but remained immunogenic. The YF vaccine used today derives from the original 17D strain, and Theiler was awarded the Nobel Prize for his life-saving research in 1951. Almost concurrently a second live-attenuated vaccine was developed from a YFV strain isolated in Senegal, in 1927. This vaccine was widely used from the 1940s to the 1960s in French-speaking African countries, virtually eradicating the disease, until its use was discontinued in 1980.

MICROBIOLOGY OF YELLOW FEVER VIRUS

YFV is the prototypic member of the genus *Flavivirus*, family Flaviviridae; *flavus* being Latin for yellow. The 3 genera in this family contain a large number of major human and veterinary pathogens,[8] including dengue (DENV), Japanese encephalitis (JEV) and West Nile (WNV) viruses in the *Flavivirus* genus, bovine viral diarrhea (BVDV) and classic swine fever (CSFV) viruses in the *Pestivirus* genus, and hepatitis C virus (HCV) in the *Hepacivirus* genus. Here, descriptions of YFV structure and replication are extrapolated from studies with this and other *Flavivirus* genus members.

Virion Structure

Mature YFV virions are icosahedral and comprise a nucleocapsid, composed of capsid (C) protein subunits, surrounded by a lipid bilayer derived from host membranes. The viral envelope is studded with dimers of envelope (E) glycoprotein and membrane (M) protein (**Fig. 2**). The diameter of the virion is approximately 40 nm, with surface projections of 5 to 10 nm. The E glycoprotein is the major component of the virion surface[9] and possesses most of the biologic activity, including

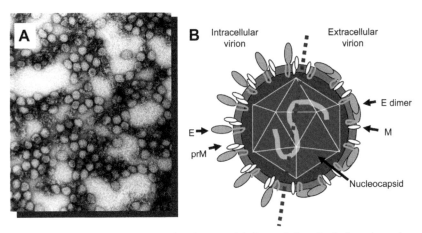

Fig. 2. The yellow fever virus virion. The virus particle is small, icosahedral, and enveloped. (A) Photomicrograph showing multiple YFV virions (original magnification ×234,000). Image from the Public Health Image Library, Centers for Disease Control. (B) The immature (intracellular) and mature (extracellular) infectious virion. The single-stranded, infectious RNA genome is packaged in an icosahedral nucleoside with a lipid envelope and viral spike proteins, prM/M and E. The prM protein is processed to M by furin-mediated cleavage immediately before egress. (*Courtesy of* the Centers for Disease Control and Prevention; with permission.)

cell-surface receptor binding, virion assembly and fusion activity at low pH, and immunogenicity.[10]

The genome packaged inside the YFV virion is a single-stranded, positive-polarity, infectious RNA molecule, approximately 11 kb in length[11] (**Fig. 3**). Similar to host messenger RNAs (mRNAs), the genome possesses a cap structure at the 5′ terminus but, unlike most host mRNAs, it lacks 3′ terminal polyadenylation.[11] Instead, the 3′-terminal nucleotides form a very stable, highly conserved stem-loop structure, serving to stabilize the genome and provide signals for initiation of translation and RNA synthesis,[12] discussed further below. All of the viral proteins are encoded in a single open reading frame (ORF), produced as a polyprotein and processed by proteolytic cleavage.[9,11] The structural proteins (C, M, and E) that form the virion are encoded in the 5′-quarter of the genome, while the nonstructural (NS) proteins (NS1, NS2A, NS2B, NS3, NS4A, NS4B, and NS5) that form the viral replicase are encoded in the remaining three-quarters.[9,11]

Virus Replication

At the molecular level, YFV and other flaviviruses appear simple, producing only 10 proteins in the infected cell (see **Fig. 3**). However, it is increasingly evident that the interaction between virus and cell is extremely complex, as the virus has adapted to exploit the host's machinery for macromolecular synthesis for its own propagation and to antagonize or circumvent antiviral responses.[13] These pathogens modulate pattern recognition receptors, stress granules, and membranous structures to promote crucial steps in their life cycle.[13] By elucidating these processes at the molecular level, scientists hope to identify points of vulnerability in the virus amplification cycle that can be targeted with antiviral drugs or used in the design of vaccine candidates.

Extracellular flavivirus particles bind to target cells by interaction with cell-surface receptors which have yet to be identified, and are internalized by receptor-mediated

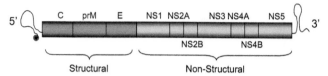

Fig. 3. The yellow fever virus genome. The genome is a single-stranded RNA molecule of positive polarity (ie, can be translated), with highly structured 5′ and 3′ nontranslated regions, a 5′ terminal cap, and a single open reading frame encoding the 10 viral proteins, 3 structural and 7 nonstructural.

endocytosis. A conformational rearrangement of the E glycoprotein occurs in the lower pH environment of the endosome, which facilitates fusion of the viral lipid envelope with the endosomal membrane and release of the nucleocapsid into the cell's cytoplasm.[14,15] After the nucleocapsid disassembles, replication proceeds with the immediate translation of the genome. Two short, conserved repeats (CS1 and CS2) are found 5′ to the 3′ putative secondary structure sequence. It has been postulated that base-pairing of these terminal sequences circularizes the genome to facilitate genome translation, replication, or packaging.[16]

Cap-dependent translation of the long ORF initiates at an AUG codon near the 5′ end of the genome,[9] for which the virus presumably borrows host eukaryotic translation initiation factors (eIFs) such as components of the eIF4F complex, membrane-bound ribosomes, and various other proteins (**Fig. 4**, step 1). Of note, flaviviruses may also use a novel, cap-independent translation mechanism under certain circumstances,[17] perhaps to better compete with the translation of host mRNAs. Co- and posttranslational processing of the polyprotein into individual mature proteins involves tightly regulated, sequential cleavages mediated by proteases of both host and viral origin (see **Fig. 4**, step 2).[9,13,18]

The NS proteins include the large, highly conserved proteins NS1, NS3, NS5, and the 4 small, hydrophobic proteins NS2A, NS2B, NS4A, and NS4B.[11] Current knowledge of NS protein functions is summarized here.

- The NS1 glycoprotein is an unusual protein that seems to be integral to virulence and pathogenesis. This protein can be cell associated,[19] on the cell surface,[19,20] and extracellular,[21–23] and plays a role in pathogenesis by inhibiting complement cascade activity.[24] On the other hand, NS1-specific antibodies provide protective immunity[20,25,26] via Fc receptor-dependent and independent mechanisms.[27,28]
- NS3 is an enzyme with central importance in the flavivirus life cycle. The N-terminal serine protease functions with its essential cofactor NS2B in the processing of the polyprotein, while the C-terminal NTPase/helicase performs ATP-dependent RNA strand separation during replication.[29–37]
- The NS5 protein has 2 distinct enzymatic activities, separated by an interdomain region: the S-adenosyl methyltransferase is located in the N-terminus and responsible for capping the nascent RNA,[38–40] while the RNA-dependent RNA polymerase (RdRp) responsible for replicating the viral RNA genome is found in the C-terminus.[41–43]
- The NS2A, NS2B, NS4A, and NS4B polypeptides consist mainly of multiple hydrophobic, potential membrane-spanning domains. These membrane-associated proteins are believed to participate in the assembly of viral replication complexes by localization of NS3 and NS5 to membranes via protein-protein interactions.[18]

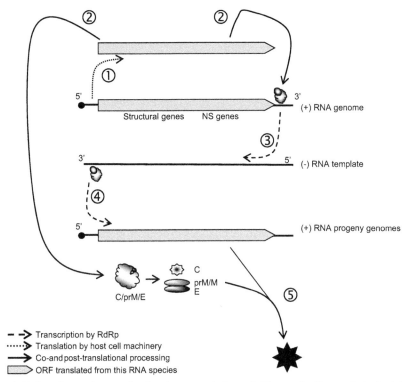

Fig. 4. Yellow fever virus replication in a permissive cell. The replication cycle is depicted as a series of temporally regulated steps: (1) Translation of the polyprotein; (2) co- and post-translational processing to produce the structural proteins (C, prM, and E) and the nonstructural proteins (NS1, NS2A, NS2B, NS3, NS4A, NS4B and NS5); (3) synthesis of complementary, negative-sense RNA by the RNA-dependent RNA polymerase NS5 and other viral replicase components; (4) synthesis of progeny genomes by transcription of the negative strand; (5) progeny genomes are packaged into nucleocapsids and bud intracellularly to acquire envelope.

The newly translated and processed viral NS proteins associate to form the replicase. The replicase recognizes secondary structure in the 3′ terminus of the genomic RNA and the NS5 RdRp initiates the synthesis of full-length negative-sense RNA copies from the genome template (see **Fig. 4**, step 3). These negative-sense RNAs are rapidly transcribed to produce progeny positive-sense RNA genomes (see **Fig. 4**, step 4). RNA replication is asymmetric with positive-strand synthesis considerably more efficient than negative-strand synthesis, probably because the different stem-loop structures present at the 3′-terminal ends of the positive and negative strands may affect the efficiency of initiation of a replication complex.[16]

Flavivirus replication occurs associated with host cell membranes.[44] Infection causes dramatic proliferation of spherical invaginations known as vesicle packets (VP) in the perinuclear region of the endoplasmic reticulum (ER),[45–48] at least in part through activity of the NS4A protein.[44,49] The localization of several viral NS proteins and dsRNA replicative intermediates in VPs[48,50] suggests they are the site of viral replication. Sequestration of the viral factory within these membranous structures may serve to concentrate viral and host components and improve the efficiency of replication, to anchor the viral replication complex, and to conceal the viral RNA repli-cative intermediates from host cell surveillance mechanisms.[51] The potential impor-tance of this immune evasion strategy to flavivirus pathogenesis remains to be elucidated.

Depending on the virus strain and cell type, the synthesis of YFV RNA is detectable within 3 to 6 hours after infection, and progeny virions are released by about 12 hours. Immature, noninfectious virions assemble within the ER, where viral RNA complexes with the C protein and is packaged into an ER-derived lipid bilayer containing hetero-dimers of the prM and E proteins,[52,53] indicating that budding through the host cell membrane occurs intracellularly. Subcellular transport of immature flavivirus particles to the cell surface is thought to occur by the translocation of immature virion-contain-ing vesicles from membranous components of the cell to the plasma membrane. Fusion of these vesicles with the plasma membrane then releases the vesicle contents including virions into the extracellular environment.[54] During assembly and transport of immature virions, the precursor to the M protein (prM) protects E proteins from undergoing irreversible conformational changes in acidic compartments of the secre-tory pathway.[55] Virion maturation occurs in the trans-Golgi network by a delayed furin-mediated cleavage of the prM to M[56,57] triggering rearrangements in the E protein that promote infectivity.[9] Infectious, mature virus particles are released by exocytosis into the extracellular medium (see **Fig. 4**, step 5).

EPIDEMIOLOGY OF YELLOW FEVER

Central to the epidemiology of YFV is the requirement for mosquito-borne transmis-sion to primate hosts. The majority of flaviviruses are transmitted to man (and other vertebrates) by the bite of an arthropod vector, primarily mosquitoes and ticks. Despite the presence of virus in the blood and bodily secretions during acute infection, flavivirus infections are not contagious (ie, transmitted directly from human to human). Consequently, available reservoirs of infectious virus and high levels of vector popu-lations are prerequisites for epidemic outbreaks. In addition, vertical or transovarial transmission of virus in mosquitoes is important in the maintenance of YFV.[58,59]

Transmission Cycles of Yellow Fever Virus

YFV infects humans and nonhuman primates in tropical areas of Africa and the Amer-icas, transmitted between primate hosts in the saliva of infected mosquitoes. The natural epidemiology of YF on both continents is a cycling of the virus between forest mosquitoes and wild primates. Secondary transmission to humans occurs in 3 cycles: sylvatic, intermediate, and urban (**Fig. 5**).[60] The *sylvatic (jungle) YF transmission cycle* occurs in the tropical rainforests of Africa and South America, where the virus is endemically transmitted between several monkey species and mosquitoes inhabiting the forest canopy. Occasionally, the virus is "accidentally" transmitted to humans who enter these areas, causing sporadic cases, usually in male forestry workers. The *inter-mediate YF transmission cycle* results in small-scale epidemics in rural villages of the African savannah when infected mosquitoes of semidomestic species indiscriminately feed on both monkey and human hosts. This type of outbreak has been the most common in Africa in recent decades.

The major cause for concern comes from the *urban YF transmission cycle*, initiated when virus is introduced into areas with high human population density and mosqui-toes transmit YFV from human to human, resulting in explosive, large-scale epidemics. In the urban cycle, humans are the primary host and the urban mosquito species, *Ae aegypti*, is the vector. Urban YF occurs indiscriminately among naïve

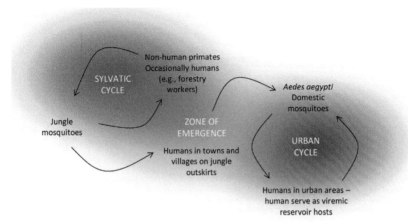

Fig. 5. Yellow fever transmission cycles. The yellow fever virus is transmitted between human and nonhuman primate hosts by mosquitoes in 3 cycles: the sylvatic (jungle) cycle in which mosquitoes of the forest canopy transmit virus to monkeys and secondarily to humans entering the jungle; the intermediate cycle (or zone of emergence) in which virus enters rural towns and villages bordering jungle areas; and the urban cycle in which humans serve as the viremic host and virus is transmitted from human to human by the domesticated *Aedes aegypti* mosquito.

humans, spread either by the movement of viremic human hosts or by the accidental transportation of infected mosquitoes (eg, in used tires). Any outbreak in which *Ae aegypti* is the vector is classified as urban YF by the World Health Organization (WHO), regardless of the area, while outbreaks involving other mosquito species are classified as jungle YF.[61] On the edge of the jungle the cycles intermingle, and infected workers returning from jungle areas often form the focus of an urban outbreak.

Epidemiology of Yellow Fever Today

Historically, devastating urban YF epidemics have occurred in Europe, Africa, and South, Central, and North America.[62] In the absence of a sylvatic cycle, improved sanitation and mosquito abatement programs eliminated epidemic urban YF from North American and European cities, with the last outbreak occurring in New Orleans in 1905.[3] However, it is estimated that YF continues to affect over 200,000 persons annually in tropical regions of Africa, South America, and Central America, with at least 30,000 fatalities.[63] Forty-four countries in Africa (**Fig. 6**A) and South and Central America (see **Fig. 6**B) are within the modern YF endemic zone, with almost 900 million people at risk of infection.[64] This total includes an estimated 508 million people in 32 African countries, and the remainder in 12 South and Central American countries (**Table 1**).[65] Most YF cases occur in sub-Saharan Africa, including periodic, unpredictable outbreaks of urban YF. An alarming resurgence of virus circulation and expansion of the endemic zones have been detected in Africa[66,67] and South America[68] in recent years, setting the scene for an explosion of urban epidemics.[69] The current situation in Africa, the Americas, and worldwide is described in more detail in this section.

Yellow fever in Africa

In Africa, YFV is endemic in many nonhuman primate species, causing a subclinical infection and a balanced relationship between the host and the virus. In the African

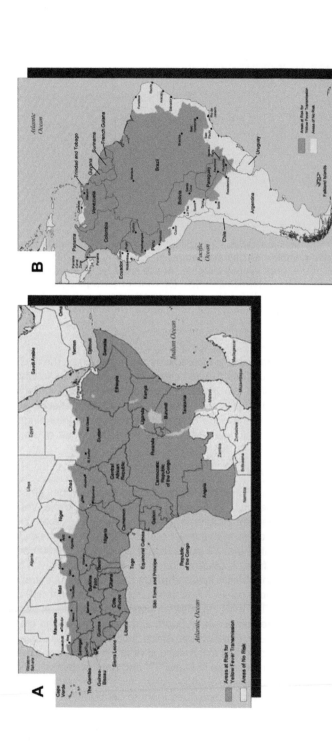

Fig. 6. The yellow fever endemic zone. The maps depict the areas in (*A*) Africa and (*B*) the Americas that are at risk for yellow fever virus transmission in 2009. (*From* Brunette GW, Kozarsky PE, Magill AJ, et al. CDC Health Information for International Travel 2010. Elsevier; 2009.)

Table 1
Countries in Africa and the Americas at risk of yellow fever

Africa	
West Africa	Benin, Burkina Faso, Cape Verde, Côte d'Ivoire, Equatorial Guinea, Gambia, Ghana, Guinea, Guinea-Bissau, Liberia, Mali, Mauritania, Niger, Nigeria, Sao Tome and Principe, Senegal, Sierra Leone, Togo
Central Africa	Angola, Burundi, Cameroon, Central African Republic, Chad, Democratic Republic of the Congo, Gabon, Rwanda
East Africa	Ethiopia, Kenya, Somalia, Sudan, Tanzania, Uganda
The Americas	
Central America	Panama
South America	Argentina, Bolivia, Brazil, Colombia, Ecuador, Guyana, French Guyana, Paraguay, Peru, Suriname, Trinidad and Tobago, Venezuela

sylvatic cycle, the virus is most frequently vectored by the *Aedes africanus* mosquito. Because *Ae africanus* is a night feeder, preferentially takes blood meals from monkeys, and rarely bites man, cases of true jungle YF in humans are uncommon in Africa. Infection of man with the forest virus typically occurs through the semidomesticated mosquito species *Aedes simpsonii*, known as a "bridging vector" because it feeds indiscriminately on nonhuman primates and humans. Although this appears to be a minor distinction, it has important epidemiologic implications. Exposure to infection results from the proximity of man's habitation to the forest and consequently all members of the household are equally exposed.

Due to mass vaccination campaigns in the 1940s and efforts to remove *Ae aegypti* breeding sites, urban YF was dramatically controlled in Africa, particularly in French-speaking West African countries where vaccination with the French neurotropic vaccine (FNV) was made compulsory.[70] By the 1960s, however, in areas where vaccine coverage had waned or was absent, thousands of YF cases occurred in West Africa and in Ethiopia, where the disease had not previously been reported. A further expansion in the late 1980s produced approximately 120,000 cases with 20% fatality in Nigeria alone.[71] These expansions were rooted in an amplification of the enzootic transmission cycle, exacerbated by poor or nonexistent vaccine coverage.

With each passing year, the risk of explosive urban YF epidemics in African cities becomes greater. The use of FNV was discontinued in the 1980s due to the risk of postvaccinal encephalitis, and current vaccination coverage with the 17D vaccine is inadequate. Another major contributing factor is the extremely rapid urbanization occurring in Africa, with cities becoming larger and more numerous and urban populations increasing by 4% annually. The effect of this rural to urban population shift is to crowd naïve populations into areas with poor housing, inadequate sanitation, and little access to running water. Drinking water is often stored near dwellings in large open containers; the preferred breeding sites of *Ae aegypti* mosquitoes.

The last decade has seen an increase in the number of African countries reporting YF activity to the WHO, particularly in West Africa; this reveals a disconcerting increase in the circulation of the virus in nonimmune human populations and reemergence in geographic areas that have long been free of YF. As a result, several large cities have already experienced YF outbreaks in the past few years: Abidjan, Côte d'Ivoire (2001); Dakar, Senegal (2002); Touba, Senegal (2002); Conakry, Guinea (2002); and Bobo Dioulasso, Burkina Faso (2004). The outbreaks were rapidly controlled by emergency reactive vaccination campaigns involving the administration of millions of vaccine doses to at-risk populations, and the number of YF cases has remained low. For example, in the 2001 outbreak in Abidjan, 2.61 million people were vaccinated in a 12-day period. However, multiple outbreaks occurring simultaneously in different locations tremendously stress the response capacity of affected countries, as well as the support capabilities of the international community, and significantly deplete vaccine stockpiles.

Yellow fever in the Americas
Historically, urban YF was a major endemic and epidemic disease terrorizing cities in South and Central America and the southeastern United States. Similar to the situation in Africa, by the 1940s mosquito abatement programs to control and eradicate the domestic vector, *Ae aegypti*, and mass vaccination campaigns resulted in the disappearance of urban YF. However, it was clearly impossible to eradicate the jungle *Haemagogus* spp mosquito vectors or the nonhuman primate reservoir hosts and thus jungle YF continues to occur, primarily afflicting young male forestry and agricultural workers in the Orinoco and Amazon river basins. Probably reflecting the more recent introduction of YFV into the Americas, several nonhuman primates that are effective viremic hosts succumb to fatal disease. Large die-offs of these animals in the forests signal local YF activity and are helpful to surveillance efforts.[72]

In the last few years, the Pan-American Health Organization (PAHO) reports intensely increased circulation of jungle YF in the Americas, affecting Argentina, Paraguay, and Brazil in the southern part of the continent, Colombia and Venezuela in the Andean region, and Trinidad and Tobago in the Caribbean. It is disturbing that *Ae aegypti* mosquitoes have reinfested most major urban centers in Central and South America, including cities that were historically centers of urban YF and are now inhabited by large nonimmune populations. Immunization coverage has dropped, placing these areas at greater risk of urban epidemics today than at any time in the past 50 years. The last documented urban YF epidemic in the Americas occurred in 1928 in Rio de Janeiro, Brazil.[68] Although there have been reports of sporadic cases in residents of urban areas in Brazil (1942), Trinidad (1954), and Bolivia (1999), verification of a true urban YF cycle in which humans serve as the primary host and virus is transmitted by *Ae aegypti* is controversial.[72] Most recently, after a 34-year absence, YF returned to Paraguay in 2008, causing a cluster of possible urban YF cases in Asunción.[65] Two million vaccine doses were urgently requested from the global stockpile (already sorely depleted by African outbreaks in the same year) and the outbreak was successfully contained by mass vaccination amidst public panic.

Yellow fever in travelers
YF poses a significant threat to unvaccinated travelers in the YF endemic zone.[73] The traveler's risk of YFV infection is dependent on immunization status, travel destination, season, length of visit, and activities. The ease of international travel also makes the introduction and spread of YF into new areas infested with competent *Ae aegypti* vectors possible, theoretically placing parts of Asia, Australia, Europe, and North America at risk. During recent decades there have been several documented cases of the human importation of YFV to nonendemic areas. Since 1964, a total of 9 YF cases have been documented in European and North American tourists after returning home from visits to West Africa and South America,[66] but secondary transmission has not yet occurred. It is not certain why YFV has not spread to new regions infested with *Ae aegypti*, in particular Asia, but clearly the traditional geographic barriers to YF are breaking down. Although YF outbreaks in developed countries will probably be

identified and controlled quickly, the impact on public emotion and the medical system would be significant.

Coping with the threat of future urban yellow fever epidemics
The strategies for YF control are routine infant immunization for children aged 6 months or older, mass vaccination campaigns to prevent epidemics, outbreak detection and rapid response, and control of *Ae aegypti* in urban centers. In 1988, the WHO recommended that vaccination against YF be included in routine infant immunization programs. As of 2009, 22 African countries and 14 South American countries have done so.

The Yellow Fever Initiative was launched in 2006 to procure the resources to confront the challenge presented by YF worldwide which, if not addressed, might result in large-scale urban epidemics, affecting millions of people. The Initiative assesses risk of YF outbreaks at the district level based on location in an ecological risk area, notification of suspected or confirmed cases since 1960 in this or an adjacent district, the number of these cases and the number of years since 1960 in which they have been reported, and the susceptibility of the population (ie, the proportion not covered by vaccination). During the first stage of the initiative in 2007, 12 African countries with large nonimmune populations are considered to be at high risk, and immunization efforts are being intensified. Vaccine coverage rates are high in South America and a few African countries, and are increasing in many others.

CLINICAL PRESENTATION OF YELLOW FEVER INFECTION

Described as "the original viral hemorrhagic fever (VHF)," severe YF is a pansystemic viral sepsis with viremia, fever, prostration, hepatic, renal, and myocardial injury, hemorrhage, shock, and 20% to 50% lethality.[74] However, human YF varies from an almost inapparent, abortive infection in which symptoms abate rapidly after the first phase to an invariably fatal, fulminating disease with symptoms following a biphasic course.[10] YF shares clinical features with other VHFs such as Dengue hemorrhagic fever, Lassa fever, and Crimean-Congo hemorrhagic fever.

YFV is introduced subcutaneously into the primate host by injection of the saliva of an infected mosquito (**Fig. 7**). A 3- to 6-day incubation period is followed by the abrupt onset of symptoms. In mild, abortive YF cases, symptoms of infection are typically nonspecific, manifested as fever, headache and constitutional problems. In such cases, patients recover in a few days with no lasting sequelae. In more severe cases, patients experience fever, chills, malaise, headache, lower back pain, generalized myalgia, nausea, and dizziness, often manifesting Faget's sign (increasing temperature with decreasing pulse rate). During this so-called period of infection, which lasts several days, viremic titers are sufficiently high for transmission to biting mosquitoes. This stage is often followed by a "period of remission," with rapid abatement of fever and other symptoms lasting up to 24 hours, and clearance of virus from the circulation. At this point, many YF infections resolve without further symptoms.

In approximately 20% of patients, illness reappears in a more severe form, the "period of intoxication," with high fever, vomiting, epigastric pain, prostration, and dehydration. Hepatic-induced coagulopathy produces severe hemorrhagic manifestations including petechiae, ecchymoses, epistaxis (bleeding of the gums), and the characteristic "black vomit" (hematemesis; gastrointestinal hemorrhage). YF is distinguished from other VHFs by the characteristic severity of liver damage and appearance of jaundice (hence *flavus*; Latin for yellow). Moreover, damage to the kidneys frequently leads to extreme albuminuria and acute renal failure. Antibodies can be detected at this stage, while viremia is usually absent. Late central nervous system

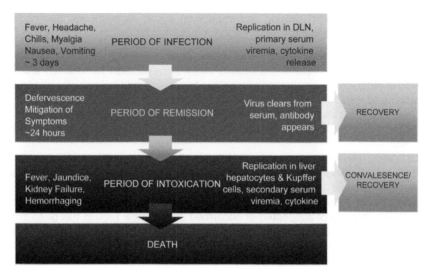

Fig. 7. The phases of yellow fever, indicating the clinical symptoms in the periods of infection, remission, and intoxication, alongside the pathogenesis of infection.

(CNS) manifestations, such as confusion, seizure, and coma, presage death, which typically follows within 7 to 10 days of onset.

Pathology of Human Yellow Fever Virus Infection

Gross pathology of fatal human YF reveals that the kidneys are generally grossly enlarged, congested, and edematous. The heart is also often enlarged. The liver, the characteristic organ of YF infection, is normal or slightly enlarged in size and icteric, with lobular markings obliterated.[75] Microscopic pathologic changes in the liver include swelling and necrosis of hepatocytes in the midzone of the liver lobule, with sparing of cells in the portal area and surrounding the central veins. The presence of Councilman bodies, coincident with disarray of the midzonal hepatocyte plate and microvesicular lipid accumulation, are considered to be hallmarks of fatal human YF infection.[10,76] Viral antigen and RNA are demonstrable by immunocytochemistry and nucleic acid hybridization in cells undergoing these pathologic changes, and cytopathology appears to be mediated by direct viral injury[10,76] via apoptosis.[77] Inflammatory changes, remarkably, are absent or minimal, and patients with hepatitis who recover do not develop residual scarring or cirrhosis.

The kidneys show acute tubular necrosis, probably the result of reduced perfusion of blood rather than direct viral injury. Focal degeneration of muscle cells may be present in the heart.[76] Spleen and lymph nodes show necrosis of B-cell areas.[75] The brain shows edema and petechial hemorrhages, but viral invasion and encephalitis are very rare events. Hemorrhage results principally from decreased synthesis of clotting factors by the liver and consequent disseminated intravascular coagulation (DIC). During acute YF, hemorrhagic symptoms and fatal outcome are strongly correlated with highly elevated pro- and anti-inflammatory cytokines,[78] suggesting a contribution to disease. Although the source of the cytokines is not known, hepatocytes,[77] endothelial cells,[79] or activated macrophages[80] may contribute. Furthermore, immune clearance attempts may exacerbate viral pathogenesis.

DIAGNOSIS OF YELLOW FEVER VIRUS INFECTION

YF surveillance is critical for the monitoring of the incidence of disease and to allow the prediction and early detection of outbreaks, and the monitoring of control measures and case reporting is required by International Health Regulations. The prompt detection of YF and rapid response through emergency vaccination campaigns are essential for the control of outbreaks. However, underreporting is a tremendous concern and the true number of cases is estimated to be up to 250 times what is now being reported. One confirmed case of YF in an unvaccinated population should be considered an outbreak, and a confirmed case in any context must be fully investigated, particularly in any area where most of the population has been vaccinated. Investigation teams must assess and respond to the outbreak with both emergency measures and longer-term immunization plans. The WHO recommends that every at-risk country have at least one national laboratory where basic YF blood tests can be performed.

Clinical Diagnosis of Yellow Fever

YF should be suspected in patients in endemic areas (or with recent travel to endemic areas) who present with a sudden fever, relative bradycardia, and signs of jaundice (**Table 2**). Complete blood count, urinalysis, liver function tests, coagulation tests, viral blood culture, and serologic tests should be obtained. Leukopenia with a relative neutropenia, thrombocytopenia, prolonged clotting, and increased prothrombin time are common. Bilirubin and aminotransferase levels may be elevated acutely and for several months. Albuminuria occurs in 90% of patients and aids in differentiating YF from other forms of hepatitis.

Clinical diagnosis of YF in the field, particularly diagnosis of isolated cases, remains difficult for several reasons. Case-by-case differences in severity, and in the clusters of symptoms observed, make this a difficult disease to recognize and mild disease often escapes diagnosis. Although classic cases should be easily recognized, jaundice is more often absent than present, and YF may not be included in the differential diagnosis of patients presenting symptoms of headache, nausea, backache, and fever, especially during the early stages of the infection. YF is easily confused with Dengue fever, Lassa fever, Ebola fever, malaria, typhoid, hepatitis, and other diseases, as well as poisoning (**Table 3**).

Laboratory Diagnosis of Yellow Fever

Laboratory confirmation of YF is pivotal to diagnosis, but unfortunately requires highly trained laboratory staff with access to specialized equipment and materials (**Table 4**). Laboratory criteria for diagnosis are any one of the following: (1) the presence of YFV-specific IgM or a fourfold or greater increase in IgG levels between acute and convalescent sera in the absence of recent vaccination; (2) isolation of YFV; (3) positive postmortem liver histopathology; (4) detection of YFV antigen in tissues by immunohistochemistry; or (5) detection of YFV genomic sequences in blood or organs by polymerase chain reaction. Frequently YF is not diagnosed until the patient has either recovered or succumbed, if a diagnosis is ever made. Case definitions state that a suspected case is characterized by acute onset of fever followed by jaundice within 2 weeks of the onset of the first symptoms, while a confirmed YF case additionally requires laboratory confirmation or an epidemiologic link to a laboratory-confirmed case or outbreak.

TREATMENT OF YELLOW FEVER VIRUS INFECTION

There is no specific treatment for YF infection and consequently supportive care is critical. Of course, most patients with YF are unable to benefit from state-of-the-art

Table 2
Laboratory workup for suspected yellow fever

CBC count	• Leukopenia with relative neutropenia • Thrombocytopenia (associated with consumptive coagulopathy) • Early hemoconcentration with increased hemoglobin and hematocrit levels • Subsequent hemorrhage and hemodilution with decreasing complete blood cell counts
Coagulation analyses	• Reduced fibrinogen and clotting factors II, V, VII, VIII, IX, and X • Presence of fibrin split products (indicate disseminated intravascular coagulation) • Decreased clotting factor synthesis • Elevated prothrombin time • Prolonged clotting time
Blood chemistry	• Elevated serum creatinine level • Hypoglycemia secondary to hepatic dysfunction • Metabolic acidosis
Urinalysis	• Elevated urinary protein levels • Elevated urobilinogen levels
Liver function tests	• Transaminitis precedes the appearance of jaundice, and the degree of liver dysfunction in the acute phase may be predictive of the clinical course • Serum aspartate transferase levels exceed alanine transferase levels • Elevated direct bilirubin levels
Other	• Hypoalbuminemia-albuminuria, decreased synthesis, and extravasation of albumin through damaged capillary endothelium • Chest radiography may show pulmonary edema or secondary bacterial pulmonary infections • Brain computed tomography scan may show intracranial hemorrhage late in the illness • Electrocardiogram and cardiac monitoring for arrhythmias

medical care.[81] Ideally a severely ill patient is admitted to the intensive care unit (ICU) and provided with vasoactive medications, fluid resuscitation, and ventilator support. Symptoms including DIC, hemorrhage, renal and hepatic dysfunction, and possible secondary infection are treated. The use of salicylates is contraindicated in YF cases because of the increased risk of bleeding. Although YFV cannot be transmitted person to person, viremic patients should be isolated with mosquito netting in areas with potential vector transmission and until differential diagnoses are eliminated.

Although no specific antiviral drug is available, several compounds with in vitro antiviral activity have been described, including ribavirin and interferon-α. However, trials with ribavirin in experimentally infected monkeys have yielded conflicting results.[82] Interferon-γ treatment of monkeys resulted in delayed onset of viremia and illness, but had no effect on survival.[83]

YELLOW FEVER VIRUS VACCINATION

Two YF vaccines were developed almost concurrently in the 1930s, but attenuation was achieved by distinctly different methods. Both FNV and 17D strains had lost

Table 3 Differential diagnoses for yellow fever	
Viral hemorrhagic fevers	eg, Dengue hemorrhagic fever, Rift Valley, Venezuelan, Bolivian, Argentine, Lassa, Crimean-Congo, Marburg, and Ebola fevers
Viral hepatitis	eg, Hepatitis A, hepatitis B, hepatitis C, hepatitis E
Viral febrile syndromes	eg, Influenza, Chikungunya fever, Dengue fever, and many other viral infections
Other	Louse-borne relapsing fever Toxic hepatitis Malaria Relapsing fever Typhoid Typhus Acanthamoeba Toxin-mediated hepatitis Liver failure from other causes

the ability to cause visceral YF in primates, but retained their immunogenicity. Furthermore, neither vaccine strain is mosquito competent; an important consideration for a live-attenuated vaccine to prevent reversion to virulence and vector transmission.

Development of Live-attenuated Yellow Fever Vaccines

The FNV vaccine strain was derived by performing 128 serial passages in mouse brain of the wild-type French viscerotropic virus (FVV), isolated in Senegal in 1927.[4] In the 1940s and early 1950s, nearly 40 million doses of FNV were administered (mostly by scarification of the skin along with the smallpox vaccine) in French-speaking countries of West Africa[4] in a mandatory vaccination campaign. YF cases declined dramatically in these countries, but unfortunately administration of FNV was associated with a high incidence of encephalitis in children. In 1961, FNV vaccination in children under the age of 10 was abandoned and manufacture was discontinued in the 1980s.

The 17D vaccine was developed by Theiler and Smith in 1937.[7] The original Asibi YFV isolate was empirically attenuated by 176 serial passages in murine and chick embryo tissue cultures, resulting in loss of viscerotropism and mosquito

Table 4 Laboratory diagnostic tests	
Serologic/immunologic	• IgM antibody-capture enzyme-linked immunosorbent assay to detect YFV-specific IgM; a single positive serum titer is diagnostic in the absence of recent vaccination • 4-fold increase in YFV-specific IgG antibody titer in a patient with no history of recent vaccination • Important to rule out cross-reactivity with other flaviviruses, often by likelihood of exposure • Lesions compatible with those of YF or detection of virus in tissue using immunohistochemical staining. Often post-mortem as liver biopsy is contraindicated due to high risk of hemorrhage
Molecular	• Detection of YFV antigen by in serum specimens • Detection of viral genomic RNA in tissue, blood or other body fluid using reverse transcriptase-polymerase chain reaction

competence.[7] Initial problems with over- or underattenuation were resolved by establishing of a virus seed lot system in 1945; WHO requirements are that no vaccine shall be manufactured that is more than one passage level from a seed lot that has passed all safety tests. The 17D vaccine strain is generally regarded as one of the safest and most effective live-attenuated viral vaccines ever developed.[84,85]

Two substrains of 17D (17D-204 and 17DD) are used as vaccines today, and more than 500 million doses have been administered. At present there are 4 sites of vaccine manufacture worldwide (Institut Pasteur in Dakar, Senegal; Bio-Manguinhos, Fio Cruz, Rio de Janeiro, Brazil; and Sanofi Pasteur in the USA and France), which produce a total of 20 to 25 million doses annually. As described previously, for protection in areas at high risk of YF transmission, the WHO's dual strategy for prevention of YF epidemics relies on preventative mass immunization campaigns followed by infant routine immunization. One vaccine dose, containing approximately 10^5 plaque-forming units (pfu) of virus, provides protective immunity for at least 10 years, after which the WHO recommends revaccination. Approximately 90% of vaccinees seroconvert by 10 days and 99% of vaccinees seroconvert by 30 days post immunization.[85–87] YFV-specific neutralizing antibodies are detectable for more than 35 years.[88,89]

Immune Response to Vaccination

During the first few days after immunization with the live-attenuated 17D vaccine, low levels of circulating viral RNA and infectious virus are detectable (<100 pfu/mL) in blood.[87] The live-attenuated 17D vaccine strain infects human DCs very poorly in vitro,[90] but stimulates their activation and maturation via multiple Toll-like receptors.[91,92] In vaccinees, proinflammatory cytokines interleukin-1β[93] and tumor necrosis factor -α[87,94] are released, and markers of the type I interferon (interferon-α/β) response are expressed by peripheral blood cells.[95,96] Humoral immunity, involving CD4$^+$ T-cell and B-cell activation, and rapid elicitation of YFV-specific IgM and neutralizing antibodies is believed to play a major role in host defense against YFV infection.[83,95] Neutralizing antibodies are used as the correlate of protection by the WHO. However, the potential importance of cell-mediated immunity, especially class I–restricted CD8$^+$ T cells, in controlling primary YFV infections should not be underestimated.[87,97,98]

Molecular Determinants of 17D Vaccine Attenuation

Over the last 20 years, nucleotide sequence analyses of the genomes of wild-type YFV isolates and their attenuated derivatives have provided clues as to the molecular basis of virulence/attenuation,[99–101] but the large number of mutations and their distribution across the entire genome have complicated interpretation of these comparative data. Comparison of the complete genomic sequences of 17D-204 and 2 other 17D substrains, 17DD and 17D-213 (the original 17D virus is not available),[11,102,103] with those of wild-type YFV isolates including the parental Asibi strain[99] has identified 48 nucleotide and 20 amino acid differences common to all 17D substrains, scattered throughout the genome.[102] As these mutations arose before divergence of the 17D-204 and 17DD substrains from the common attenuated lineage at passage 176, these changes are considered to be the primary candidates that contribute to the molecular basis of attenuation. Five mutations clustered in the E protein occur at sites conserved in natural YFV isolates from Africa and South America, and consequently are likely to be implicated in the attenuation process. The location of these mutations relative to functional domains in the E protein lends credence to this hypothesis. Two of the mutated amino acids (E-52 and E-200) lie in the fusion domain.[56] Moreover, mutations at E-173 and E-305 are integral components of neutralizing epitopes mapped by monoclonal antibody escape mutants.[104,105] The loss of a 17D-204 substrain-specific epitope from the 17D virus, selected for neutralization escape, resulted in dramatic changes in neurovirulence ranging from avirulence to increased virulence.[104] Although less well studied, mutations in other locations, particularly in the nonstructural proteins, are also being considered as determinants of YFV virulence.[101,106,107]

Vaccine-Associated Adverse Events

The 17D vaccine is often cited as one of the most successful vaccines ever developed, with only mild side effects reported by approximately 25% of vaccines, including injection site pain or redness, headache, malaise, and myalgia. However, in recent years several issues have arisen that must be addressed. Vaccine production technology has not changed since 1945 when the seed-lot system was introduced, contributing to limited production potential. The 17D virus is propagated in embryonated eggs, with each egg yielding around 400 vaccine doses. The eggs must be free of adventitious agents such as avian retrovirus. The inability to rapidly replace vaccine stockpiles has critical implications for availability.

In the last 10 years 2 categories of severe adverse events associated with vaccination have been recognized: (1) vaccine-associated neurotropic disease (YEL-AND)[108–110] and (2) vaccine-associated viscerotropic disease (YEL-AVD).[111–117] YEL-AND was first described in the 1940s as "post-vaccinal encephalitis," most often in young children. Consequently, in 1945 vaccination was contraindicated for infants younger than 6 months and only recommended for those older than 9 months, which complicates inclusion in routine infant immunization programs. Moreover, a monkey neurovirulence test for vaccine seeds was introduced. Together, these measures resulted in a reduction in YEL-AND, but the development of the vaccine adverse event reporting system (VAERS) in the United States revealed that YEL-AND was not so a rare a phenomenon, occurring at a frequency of 4 to 5 per million doses and with case fatality rates of less than 5%. The second category of adverse event, YEL-AVD, was first described in 1999 in Brazil, resembling wild-type YF with pansystemic disease and high virus titers in many organs, especially the liver.[111,113,117,118] VAERS demonstrated that YEL-AVD occurred with a frequency of 3 to 4 per million doses administered but, significantly, the case fatality rate is 60%. The host genes and host immune response have been proposed to be at least in part responsible for YEL-AVD.[119] However, there has been no one apparent causal factor that explains all cases. A recent cluster of 4 deaths and 1 nonfatal case of YEL-AVD in Ica, Peru, in October 2007[65] following administration of 42,742 doses from one vaccine lot (ie, 1 in 10,000 vaccinees died following administration of this vaccine lot) has caused this hypothesis to be reassessed.

At present, the US Advisory Committee on Immunization Practices and the WHO Global Advisory Committee on Vaccine Safety are reviewing the vaccine and contraindications for the vaccine,[120] and the WHO Expert Committee on Biological Standardization met in late 2008 to discuss the manufacturing and quality control processes for the vaccine. This committee last reviewed the vaccine in 1998.[121] Given the above, there are discussions on the need to improve the current 17D vaccine. Is there a need for a new vaccine? The process from discovery to licensure for a new vaccine is at least 15 years. Furthermore, risk-benefit evaluations of the current 17D vaccine indicate that it is highly efficacious and that its withdrawal would leave a huge number of unprotected people in disease endemic areas. Finally, there has been a considerable investment in using the current 17D vaccine virus as a backbone for chimeric vaccines that have the structural protein genes of a particular flavivirus in a 17D backbone. This so-called ChimeriVax platform is being used by Sanofi Pasteur and Acambis to develop candidate DENV, WNV, and JEV vaccines.[122]

FUTURE PERSPECTIVES

There are many unanswered questions remaining about YF disease and its agent, YFV, while the threat of urban outbreaks and endemic zone expansion continues to increase. A major gap in our knowledge of YF and YFV is in management and treatment of patients with this disease or with serious vaccine-associated adverse events. Treatment of YF by supportive care is virtually ineffective, and even admission to the ICU does not seem to improve the prognosis or change the mortality rate. There is a desperate need for the development of specific antiviral drugs and improved rapid diagnostic tests for this and other flaviviral diseases. Finally, the 17D vaccine, on which disease control entirely rests, has been associated recently with fatal adverse events. Consequently, improvements to the vaccine's safety will be required. To address these issues, a greatly improved understanding of complex interactions between the virus and host cell factors that control replication, as well as innate and adaptive immune responses, will be required.

REFERENCES

1. Barrett AD, Monath TP. Epidemiology and ecology of yellow fever virus. Adv Virus Res 2003;61:291–315.
2. Carter HR. Yellow fever: an epidemiological and historical study of its place of origin. Baltimore (MD): Williams & Wilkins; 1931.
3. Tomlinson W, Hodgson RS. Centennial year of yellow fever eradication in New Orleans and the United States, 1905–2005. La State Med Soc 2005;157(2): 216–7.
4. Staples JE, Monath TP. Yellow fever: 100 years of discovery. JAMA 2008;300(8): 960–2.
5. Smith HH, Theiler M. The adaptation of unmodified strains of yellow fever virus to cultivation in vitro. J Exp Med 1937;65(6):801–8.
6. Theiler M, Smith HH. The effect of prolonged cultivation in vitro upon the pathogenicity of yellow fever virus. J Exp Med 1937;65(6):767–86.
7. Theiler M, Smith HH. The use of yellow fever virus modified by in vitro cultivation for human immunization. J Exp Med 1937;65(6):787–800.
8. Gould EA, Solomon T. Pathogenic flaviviruses. Lancet 2008;371(9611):500–9.
9. Chambers TJ, McCourt DW, Rice CM. Production of yellow fever virus proteins in infected cells: identification of discrete polyprotein species and analysis of cleavage kinetics using region-specific polyclonal antisera. Virology 1990; 177(1):159–74.
10. Burke DS, Monath TP. Flaviviruses. In: Knipe DM, Howley PM, editors. Fields virology. Philadelphia: Lippincott, Williams & Wilkins; 2001. p. 1043–125.
11. Rice CM, Lenches EM, Eddy SR, et al. Nucleotide sequence of yellow fever virus: implications for flavivirus gene expression and evolution. Science 1985; 229(4715):726–33.
12. Brinton MA, Fernandez AV, Dispoto JH. The 3'-nucleotides of flavivirus genomic RNA form a conserved secondary structure. Virology 1986;153(1):113–21.
13. Fernandez-Garcia MD, Mazzon M, Jacobs M, et al. Pathogenesis of flavivirus infections: using and abusing the host cell. Cell Host Microbe 2009;5(4):318–28.
14. Bressanelli S, Stiasny K, Allison SL, et al. Structure of a flavivirus envelope glycoprotein in its low-pH-induced membrane fusion conformation. EMBO J 2004;23(4):728–38.
15. Modis Y, Ogata S, Clements D, et al. Structure of the dengue virus envelope protein after membrane fusion. Nature 2004;427(6972):313–9.

16. Brinton MA, Dispoto JH. Sequence and secondary structure analysis of the 5'-terminal region of flavivirus genome RNA. Virology 1988;162(2):290–9.
17. Edgil D, Polacek C, Harris E. Dengue virus utilizes a novel strategy for translation initiation when cap-dependent translation is inhibited. J Virol 2006;80(6):2976–86.
18. Lindenbach BD, Rice CM. Molecular biology of flaviviruses. Adv Virus Res 2003; 59:23–61.
19. Westaway EG. Flavivirus replication strategy. Adv Virus Res 1987;33:45–90.
20. Schlesinger JJ, Brandriss MW, Putnak JR, et al. Cell surface expression of yellow fever virus non-structural glycoprotein NS1: consequences of interaction with antibody. J Gen Virol 1990;71:593–9.
21. Lee JM, Crooks AJ, Stephenson JR. The synthesis and maturation of a non-structural extracellular antigen from tick-borne encephalitis virus and its relationship to the intracellular NS1 protein. J Gen Virol 1989;70(Pt 2):335–43.
22. Mason PW. Maturation of Japanese encephalitis virus glycoproteins produced by infected mammalian and mosquito cells. Virology 1989;169:354–64.
23. Winkler G, Randolph VB, Cleaves GR, et al. Evidence that the mature form of the flavivirus nonstructural protein NS1 is a dimer. Virology 1988;162(1):187–96.
24. Chung KM, Liszewski MK, Nybakken G, et al. West Nile virus nonstructural protein NS1 inhibits complement activation by binding the regulatory protein factor H. Proc Natl Acad Sci U S A 2006;103(50):19111–6.
25. Bray M, Zhao BT, Markoff L, et al. Mice immunized with recombinant vaccinia virus expressing dengue 4 virus structural proteins with or without nonstructural protein NS1 are protected against fatal dengue virus encephalitis. J Virol 1989; 63(6):2853–6.
26. Zhang YM, Hayes EP, McCarty TC, et al. Immunization of mice with dengue structural proteins and nonstructural protein NS1 expressed by baculovirus recombinant induces resistance to dengue virus encephalitis. J Virol 1988;62(8): 3027–31.
27. Chung KM, Nybakken GE, Thompson BS, et al. Antibodies against West Nile Virus nonstructural protein NS1 prevent lethal infection through Fc gamma receptor-dependent and -independent mechanisms. J Virol 2006;80(3):1340–51.
28. Chung KM, Thompson BS, Fremont DH, et al. Antibody recognition of cell surface-associated NS1 triggers Fc-gamma receptor-mediated phagocytosis and clearance of West Nile Virus-infected cells. J Virol 2007;81(17):9551–5.
29. Arias CF, Preugschat F, Strauss JH. Dengue 2 virus NS2B and NS3 form a stable complex that can cleave NS3 within the helicase domain. Virology 1993;193(2): 888–99.
30. Benarroch D, Selisko B, Locatelli GA, et al. The RNA helicase, nucleotide 5'-triphosphatase, and RNA 5'-triphosphatase activities of dengue virus protein NS3 are Mg^{2+}-dependent and require a functional Walker B motif in the helicase catalytic core. Virology 2004;328(2):208–18.
31. Chambers TJ, Grakoui A, Rice CM. Processing of the yellow fever virus nonstructural polyprotein: a catalytically active NS3 proteinase domain and NS2B are required for cleavages at dibasic sites. J Virol 1991;65(11):6042–50.
32. Chambers TJ, Weir RC, Grakoui A, et al. Evidence that the N-terminal domain of nonstructural protein NS3 from yellow fever virus is a serine protease responsible for site-specific cleavages in the viral polyprotein. Proc Natl Acad Sci U S A 1990;87(22):8898–902.
33. Falgout B, Pethel M, Zhang YM, et al. Both nonstructural proteins NS2B and NS3 are required for the proteolytic processing of dengue virus nonstructural proteins. J Virol 1991;65(5):2467–75.

34. Zhang L, Mohan PM, Padmanabhan R. Processing and localization of Dengue virus type 2 polyprotein precursor NS3-NS4A-NS4B-NS5. J Virol 1992;66: 7549–54.
35. Li H, Clum S, You S, et al. The serine protease and RNA-stimulated nucleoside triphosphatase and RNA helicase functional domains of dengue virus type 2 NS3 converge within a region of 20 amino acids. J Virol 1999;73(4):3108–16.
36. Nestorowicz A, Chambers TJ, Rice CM. Mutagenesis of the yellow fever virus NS2A/2B cleavage site: effects on proteolytic processing, viral replication, and evidence for alternative processing of the NS2A protein. Virology 1994; 199(1):114–23.
37. Warrener P, Tamura JK, Collett MS. RNA-stimulated NTPase activity associated with yellow fever virus NS3 protein expressed in bacteria. J Virol 1993;67(2):989–96.
38. Egloff MP, Benarroch D, Selisko B, et al. An RNA cap (nucleoside-2'-O-)-methyltransferase in the flavivirus RNA polymerase NS5: crystal structure and functional characterization. EMBO J 2002;21(11):2757–68.
39. Issur M, Geiss BJ, Bougie I, et al. The flavivirus NS5 protein is a true RNA guanylyltransferase that catalyzes a two-step reaction to form the RNA cap structure. RNA 2009;15(12):2340–50.
40. Ray D, Shah A, Tilgner M, et al. West Nile virus 5'-cap structure is formed by sequential guanine N-7 and ribose 2'-O methylations by nonstructural protein 5. J Virol 2006;80(17):8362–70.
41. Chu PW, Westaway EG. Characterization of Kunjin virus RNA-dependent RNA polymerase: reinitiation of synthesis in vitro. Virology 1987;157(2):330–7.
42. Grun JB, Brinton MA. Characterization of West Nile virus RNA-dependent RNA polymerase and cellular terminal adenylyl and uridylyl transferases in cell-free extracts. J Virol 1986;60(3):1113–24.
43. Guyatt KJ, Westaway EG, Khromykh AA. Expression and purification of enzymatically active recombinant RNA-dependent RNA polymerase (NS5) of the flavivirus Kunjin. J Virol Methods 2001;92(1):37–44.
44. Miller S, Krijnse-Locker J. Modification of intracellular membrane structures for virus replication. Nat Rev Microbiol 2008;6(5):363–74.
45. Mackenzie JM, Jones MK, Young PR. Immunolocalization of the dengue virus nonstructural glycoprotein NS1 suggests a role in viral RNA replication. Virology 1996;220:232–40.
46. Mackenzie JM, Jones MK, Westaway EG. Markers for trans-Golgi membranes and the intermediate compartment localize to induced membranes with distinct replication functions in flavivirus-infected cells. J Virol 1999;73:9555–67.
47. Welsch S, Miller S, Romero-Brey I, et al. Composition and three-dimensional architecture of the dengue virus replication and assembly sites. Cell Host Microbe 2009;5(4):365–75.
48. Westaway EG, Mackenzie JM, Kenney MT, et al. Ultrastructure of Kunjin virus-infected cells: colocalization of NS1 and NS3 with double-stranded RNA, and of NS2B with NS3, in virus-induced membrane structures. J Virol 1997;71(9): 6650–61.
49. Roosendaal J, Westaway EG, Khromykh A, et al. Regulated cleavages at the West Nile virus NS4A-2K-NS4B junctions play a major role in rearranging cytoplasmic membranes and Golgi trafficking of the NS4A protein. J Virol 2006; 80(9):4623–32.
50. Mackenzie JM, Kenney MT, Westaway EG, et al. West Nile virus strain Kunjin NS5 polymerase is a phosphoprotein localized at the cytoplasmic site of viral RNA synthesis. J Gen Virol 2007;88:1163–8.

51. Hoenen A, Liu W, Kochs G, et al. West Nile virus-induced cytoplasmic membrane structures provide partial protection against the interferon-induced antiviral MxA protein. J Gen Virol 2007;88(Pt 11):3013–7.
52. Lorenz IC, Kartenbeck J, Mezzacasa A, et al. Intracellular assembly and secretion of recombinant subviral particles from tick-borne encephalitis virus. J Virol 2003;77(7):4370–82.
53. Mackenzie JM, Westaway EG. Assembly and maturation of the flavivirus Kunjin virus appear to occur in the rough endoplasmic reticulum and along the secretory pathway, respectively. J Virol 2001;75(22):10787–99.
54. Hase T, Summers PL, Eckels KH, et al. An electron and immunoelectron microscopic study of dengue-2 virus infection of cultured mosquito cells: maturation events. Arch Virol 1987;92:273–9.
55. Guirakhoo F, Heinz FX, Mandl CW, et al. Fusion activity of flaviviruses: comparison of mature and immature (prM-containing) tick-borne encephalitis virions. J Gen Virol 1991;72(Pt 6):1323–9.
56. Yu IM, Zhang W, Holdaway HA, et al. Structure of the immature dengue virus at low pH primes proteolytic maturation. Science 2008;319:1834–7.
57. Li L, Lok SM, Yu IM, et al. The flavivirus precursor membrane-envelope protein complex: structure and maturation. Science 2008;319(5871):1830–4.
58. Rosen L. [Transovarial transmission of arboviruses by mosquitoes]. Med Trop (Mars) 1981;41(1):23–9 [in French].
59. Rosen L. Overwintering mechanisms of mosquito-borne arboviruses in temperate climates. Am J Trop Med Hyg 1987;37(Suppl 3):69S–76S.
60. Monath TP. Facing up to re-emergence of urban yellow fever. Lancet 1999; 353(9164):1541.
61. Bres PL. A century of progress in combating yellow fever. Bull World Health Organ 1986;64(6):775–86.
62. Monath TP. Yellow fever as an endemic/epidemic disease and priorities for vaccination. Bull Soc Pathol Exot 2006;99(5):341–7.
63. Monath TP. Yellow fever: an update. Lancet Infect Dis 2001;1(1):11–20.
64. Brunette GW, Kozarsky PE, Magill AJ, et al. CDC health information for international travel 2010. Elsevier; 2009. [Online].
65. Briand S, Beresniak A, Nguyen T, et al. Assessment of yellow fever epidemic risk: an original multi-criteria modeling approach. PLoS Negl Trop Dis 2009;3:e483.
66. Onyango CO, Ofula VO, Sang RC, et al. Yellow fever outbreak, Imatong, southern Sudan. Emerg Infect Dis 2004;10(6):1063–8.
67. Robertson SE, Hull BP, Tomori O, et al. Yellow fever: a decade of reemergence. JAMA 1996;276(14):1157–62.
68. Bryant JE, Holmes EC, Barrett AD. Out of Africa: a molecular perspective on the introduction of yellow fever virus into the Americas. PLoS Pathog 2007; 3(5):e75.
69. World Health Organisation. Yellow fever vaccine. WHO position paper. Wkly Epidemiol Rec 2003;78(40):349–59.
70. Monath TP. Yellow fever: Victor, Victoria? Conqueror, conquest? Epidemics and research in the last forty years and prospects for the future. Am J Trop Med Hyg 1991;45(1):1–43.
71. Nasidi A, Monath TP, DeCock K, et al. Urban yellow fever epidemic in western Nigeria 1987. Trans R Soc Trop Med Hyg 1989;83:401–6.
72. Barrett AD, Higgs S. Yellow fever: a disease that has yet to be conquered. Annu Rev Entomol 2007;52:209–29.

258   Gardner & Ryman

73. Monath TP, Cetron MS. Prevention of yellow fever in persons traveling to the tropics. Clin Infect Dis 2002;34(10):1369–78.
74. Monath TP. Treatment of yellow fever. Antiviral Res 2008;78(1):116–24.
75. Klotz O, Belt TH. The pathology of the liver in yellow fever. Am J Pathol 1930;6:663–88.
76. De Brito T, Siqueira SA, Santos RT, et al. Human fatal yellow fever. Immunohistochemical detection of viral antigens in the liver, kidney and heart. Pathol Res Pract 1992;188(1-2):177–81.
77. Quaresma JA, Barros VL, Pagliari C, et al. Revisiting the liver in human yellow fever: virus-induced apoptosis in hepatocytes associated with TGF-beta, TNF-alpha and NK cells activity. Virology 2006;345(1):22–30.
78. ter Meulen J, Sakho M, Koulemou K, et al. Activation of the cytokine network and unfavorable outcome in patients with yellow fever. J Infect Dis 2004;190(10):1821–7.
79. Khaiboullina SF, Rizvanov AA, Holbrook MR, et al. Yellow fever virus strains Asibi and 17D-204 infect human umbilical cord endothelial cells and induce novel changes in gene expression. Virology 2005;342(2):167–76.
80. Monath TP, Barrett AD. Pathogenesis and pathophysiology of yellow fever. Adv Virus Res 2003;60:343–95.
81. Monath TP. Yellow fever: a medically neglected disease. Report on a seminar. Rev Infect Dis 1987;9(1):165–75.
82. Huggins JW, Hsiang CM, Cosgriff TM, et al. Prospective, double-blind, concurrent, placebo-controlled clinical trial of intravenous ribavirin therapy of hemorrhagic fever with renal syndrome. J Infect Dis 1991;164(6):1119–27.
83. Arroyo JI, Apperson SA, Cropp CB, et al. Effect of human gamma interferon on yellow fever virus infection. Am J Trop Med Hyg 1988;38(3):647–50.
84. Barrett AD. Yellow fever vaccines. Biologicals 1997;25(1):17–25.
85. Monath TP. Yellow fever vaccine. Expert Rev Vaccines 2005;4(4):553–74.
86. Monath TP, Cetron MS, McCarthy K, et al. Yellow fever 17D vaccine safety and immunogenicity in the elderly. Hum Vaccin 2005;1(5):207–14.
87. Reinhardt B, Jaspert R, Niedrig M, et al. Development of viremia and humoral and cellular parameters of immune activation after vaccination with yellow fever virus strain 17D: a model of human flavivirus infection. J Med Virol 1998;56(2):159–67.
88. Niedrig M, Lademann M, Emmerich P, et al. Assessment of IgG antibodies against yellow fever virus after vaccination with 17D by different assays: neutralization test, haemagglutination inhibition test, immunofluorescence assay and ELISA. Trop Med Int Health 1999;4(12):867–71.
89. Poland JD, Calisher CH, Monath TP, et al. Persistence of neutralizing antibody 30-35 years after immunization with 17D yellow fever vaccine. Bull World Health Organ 1981;59(6):895–900.
90. Palmer DR, Fernandez S, Bisbing J, et al. Restricted replication and lysosomal trafficking of yellow fever 17D vaccine virus in human dendritic cells. J Gen Virol 2007;88(Pt 1):148–56.
91. Querec T, Bennouna S, Alkan S, et al. Yellow fever vaccine YF-17D activates multiple dendritic cell subsets via TLR2, 7, 8, and 9 to stimulate polyvalent immunity. J Exp Med 2006;203:413–24.
92. Barba-Spaeth G, Longman RS, Albert ML, et al. Live attenuated yellow fever 17D infects human DCs and allows for presentation of endogenous and recombinant T cell epitopes. J Exp Med 2005;202(9):1179–84.
93. Hacker UT, Erhardt S, Tschöp K, et al. Influence of the IL-1Ra gene polymorphism on in vivo synthesis of IL-1Ra and IL-1beta after live yellow fever vaccination. Clin Exp Immunol 2001;125:465–9.

94. Hacker UT, Jelinek T, Erhardt S, et al. In vivo synthesis of tumor necrosis factor-alpha in healthy humans after live yellow fever vaccination. J Infect Dis 1998; 177(3):774–8.

95. Bonnevie-Nielsen V, Heron I, Monath TP, et al. Lymphocytic 2',5'-oligoadenylate synthetase activity increases prior to the appearance of neutralizing antibodies and immunoglobulin M and immunoglobulin G antibodies after primary and secondary immunization with yellow fever vaccine. Clin Diagn Lab Immunol 1995;2(3):302–6.

96. Roers A, Hochkeppel HK, Horisberger MA, et al. MxA gene expression after live virus vaccination: a sensitive marker for endogenous type I interferon. J Infect Dis 1994;169(4):807–13.

97. Co MD, Terajima M, Cruz J, et al. Human cytotoxic T lymphocyte responses to live attenuated 17D yellow fever vaccine: identification of HLA-B35-restricted CTL epitopes on nonstructural proteins NS1, NS2b, NS3, and the structural protein E. Virology 2002;293(1):151–63.

98. van der Most RG, Harrington LE, Giuggio V, et al. Yellow fever virus 17D envelope and NS3 proteins are major targets of the antiviral T cell response in mice. Virology 2002;296(1):117–24.

99. Hahn CS, Dalrymple JM, Strauss JH, et al. Comparison of the virulent Asibi strain of yellow fever virus with the 17D vaccine strain derived from it. Proc Natl Acad Sci U S A 1987;84(7):2019–23.

100. Wang E, Ryman KD, Jennings AD, et al. Comparison of the genomes of the wild-type French viscerotropic strain of yellow fever virus with its vaccine derivative French neurotropic vaccine. J Gen Virol 1995;76(Pt 11):2749–55.

101. Xie H, Ryman KD, Campbell GA, et al. Mutation in NS5 protein attenuates mouse neurovirulence of yellow fever 17D vaccine virus. J Gen Virol 1998;79(Pt 8): 1895–9.

102. dos Santos CN, Post PR, Carvalho R, et al. Complete nucleotide sequence of yellow fever virus vaccine strains 17DD and 17D-213. Virus Res 1995;35(1): 35–41.

103. Galler R, Post PR, Santos CN, et al. Genetic variability among yellow fever virus 17D substrains. Vaccine 1998;16(9-10):1024–8.

104. Ryman KD, Ledger TN, Campbell GA, et al. Mutation in a 17D-204 vaccine substrain-specific envelope protein epitope alters the pathogenesis of yellow fever virus in mice. Virology 1998;244(1):59–65.

105. Ryman KD, Xie H, Ledger TN, et al. Antigenic variants of yellow fever virus with an altered neurovirulence phenotype in mice. Virology 1997;230(2):376–80.

106. Dunster LM, Wang H, Ryman KD, et al. Molecular and biological changes associated with HeLa cell attenuation of wild-type yellow fever virus. Virology 1999; 261(2):309–18.

107. McArthur MA, Suderman MT, Mutebi JP, et al. Molecular characterization of a hamster viscerotropic strain of yellow fever virus. J Virol 2003;77(2):1462–8.

108. Fatal viral encephalitis following 17D yellow fever vaccine inoculation. Report of a case in a 3-year-old child. JAMA 1966;198(6):671–2.

109. Merlo C, Steffen R, Landis T, et al. Possible association of encephalitis and 17D yellow fever vaccination in a 29-year-old traveller. Vaccine 1993;11(6):691.

110. Schoub BD, Dommann CJ, Johnson S, et al. Encephalitis in a 13-year-old boy following 17D yellow fever vaccine. J Infect 1990;21(1):105–6.

111. Centers for Disease Control and Prevention (CDC). Adverse events associated with 17D-derived yellow fever vaccination—United States, 2001-2002. MMWR Morb Mortal Wkly Rep 2002;51(44):989–93.

112. From the Centers for Disease Control and Prevention. Adverse events associated with 17D-derived yellow fever vaccination—United States, 2001-2002. JAMA 2002;288(20):2533–5.
113. Belsher JL, Gay P, Brinton M, et al. Fatal multiorgan failure due to yellow fever vaccine-associated viscerotropic disease. Vaccine 2007;25(50):8480–5.
114. Chan RC, Penney DJ, Little D, et al. Hepatitis and death following vaccination with 17D-204 yellow fever vaccine. Lancet 2001;358(9276):121–2.
115. Gerasimon G, Lowry K. Rare case of fatal yellow fever vaccine-associated viscerotropic disease. South Med J 2005;98(6):653–6.
116. Martin M, Tsai TF, Cropp B, et al. Fever and multisystem organ failure associated with 17D-204 yellow fever vaccination: a report of four cases. Lancet 2001; 358(9276):98–104.
117. Vasconcelos PF, Luna EJ, Galler R, et al. Serious adverse events associated with yellow fever 17DD vaccine in Brazil: a report of two cases. Lancet 2001; 358(9276):91–7.
118. Struchiner CJ, Luz PM, Dourado I, et al. Risk of fatal adverse events associated with 17DD yellow fever vaccine. Epidemiol Infect 2004;132(5):939–46.
119. Hayes EB. Acute viscerotropic disease following vaccination against yellow fever. Trans R Soc Trop Med Hyg 2007;101(10):967–71.
120. Global Advisory Committee on Vaccine Safety, 12-13 December 2007. Wkly Epidemiol Rec 2008;83(4):37–44.
121. WHO. Requirements for yellow fever vaccine. World Health Organ Tech Rep Ser 1998;872(Annex 2):30–68.
122. Pugachev KV, Guirakhoo F, Monath TP. New developments in flavivirus vaccines with special attention to yellow fever. Curr Opin Infect Dis 2005;18(5):387–94.

Human Ehrlichiosis and Anaplasmosis

Nahed Ismail, MD, PhD[a],*, Karen C. Bloch, MD, MPH[b],
Jere W. McBride, PhD[c]

KEYWORDS

• Ehrlichiosis • Epidemiology • Immunity • Pathogenesis
• Diagnosis • Treatment

Human ehrlichiosis and anaplasmosis are acute febrile tick-borne diseases caused by various members of the genera *Ehrlichia* and *Anaplasma* (Anaplasmataceae). Human monocytotropic ehrlichiosis (HME) was first reported in the United States in 1987, but during the ensuing 20 years it has become the most prevalent life-threatening tick-borne disease in the United States. Ehrlichiosis and anaplasmosis are becoming more frequently diagnosed as the cause of human infections, as animal reservoirs and tick vectors have increased in number and humans have inhabited areas where reservoir and tick populations are high.

Ehrlichia chaffeensis, the etiologic agent of HME, is an emerging zoonosis that causes clinical manifestations ranging from a mild febrile illness to a fulminant disease characterized by multiorgan system failure. The primary tick vector of HME is the Lone star tick (*Amblyomma americanum*). *Anaplasma phagocytophilum* causes human granulocytotropic anaplasmosis (HGA), previously known as human granulocytotropic ehrlichiosis (HGE). *A. phagocytophilum* is transmitted by *Ixodes scapularis*, which also transmits agents that cause Lyme disease and babesiosis.

HME and HGA have similar clinical presentations including fever, headache, leukopenia, thrombocytopenia, and elevated liver enzymes. Symptoms typically begin a median of 9 days following tick bite, with the majority of patients seeking medical attention within the first 4 days of illness. Neurologic manifestations are most frequently reported with HME. This article reviews recent advances in the understanding of ehrlichial diseases related to microbiology, epidemiology, diagnosis, pathogenesis, immunity, and treatment of the 2 prevalent tick-borne diseases found in the United States, HME and HGA.

This work was supported by the NIH/NCRR-RCMI fund (5G12RR003032).
[a] Department of Pathology and Department of Microbiology and Immunology, Meharry Medical College, 1005 Dr D.B. Todd Boulevard, Nashville, TN 37208, USA
[b] Infectious Disease Department, Vanderbilt University, School of Medicine, 1211 Medical Center Drive, Nashville, TN 37232, USA
[c] Department of Pathology, Center for Biodefense and Emerging Infectious Diseases, University of Texas Medical Branch, 301 University Boulevard, Galveston, TX 77555, USA
* Corresponding author.
E-mail address: nismail@mmc.edu

MICROBIOLOGY

The agents of human tick-borne ehrlichiosis include *Anaplasma* (formerly *Ehrlichia*) *phagocytophilum, Ehrlichia chaffeensis, Ehrlichia ewingii,* and recently reported *Ehrlichia canis* (**Table 1**). These pathogens are members of the family Anaplasmataceae, in the order Rickettsiales, and they are classified as α-proteobacteria.[1–4] The evolutionary relationships determined by 16S ribosomal RNA gene (*rrs*) and *groESL* comparisons indicate that *Ehrlichia* and *Anaplasma* spp share a common ancestor with other obligate intracellular pathogens such as *Wolbachia, Neorickettsia, Orientia,* and *Rickettsia*.[3–7] In addition to causing human disease, *Ehrlichia* species are important veterinary pathogens. Canine ehrlichiosis, first described in 1935 in Africa, is caused by *E. canis* and is transmitted by the Brown Dog tick, *Rhipicephalus sanguineus*.[6,7] *E. ewingii,* an agent that is transmitted by *Amblyomma americanum,* infects granulocytes and causes human ehrlichiosis ewingii.[8–10] Recent phylogenetic studies have concluded that the economically important veterinary pathogen *Ehrlichia* (formerly *Cowdria*) *ruminantium* (described in 1925) belongs to the genus *Ehrlichia* (**Fig. 1**).[10–16]

Agents of human tick-borne ehrlichioses are small (approximately 0.4–1.5 μm), obligately intracellular gram-negative bacteria that replicate in membrane-bound compartments inside host granulocytes (*A. phagocytophilum* and *E. ewingii*) or mononuclear phagocytes (*E. chaffeensis* and *E. canis*) (**Fig. 2**).[17,18] Ehrlichiae replicate within the host vacuoles forming microcolonies called morulae, derived from the Latin word "morus" for mulberry.[18–20] All *Ehrlichia* species pathogenic for humans can be cultivated in cell culture except *E. ewingii* (**Fig. 3**).

Ehrlichia and *Anaplasma* exist intracellularly in 2 morphologically distinct ultrastructural forms, dense-cored cells (DC) (0.4–0.6 μm) and reticulate cells (RC) (0.4–0.6 μm by 0.7–1.9 μm) (**Fig. 4**).[20] DCs are smaller and have an electron-dense chromatin, whereas the larger RCs have uniformly dispersed nucleoid filaments and ribosomes. In vitro kinetic analyses have shown that DC ehrlichiae predominate during the first 24 hours post infection, suggesting that DC forms are critical for bacterial adhesion and internalization. By 48 hours post infection, RC forms of ehrlichiae that divide by binary fission predominate. At 72 hours after infection, the RC ehrlichiae mature into dense-cored cell forms, correlating with the time when DC ehrlichiae are released to begin a new cycle (see **Fig. 4**).[21,22] Consistent with their life cycle, DC and RC forms of ehrlichiae differentially express 2 tandem repeat containing proteins (TRP); TRP120 and TRP47. The TRP47 is a secreted effector protein that interacts with numerous host cell proteins involved in cell signaling, transcriptional regulation, and vesicle trafficking.[23–26]

Ehrlichia and *Anaplasma* species have relatively small genomes (0.8–1.5 Mb) that have undergone several types of reductive evolutionary processes as they have lost redundant genes and developed dependence on the host cell for necessary functions.[27] *Ehrlichia* have a small subsets of genes associated with host-pathogen interactions, including tandem repeat containing proteins and ankyrin repeat proteins. Other common features of the *Ehrlichia* genomes include low GC content and high proportion of noncoding sequences. *E. chaffeensis* and *A. phagocytophilum* also have genes for synthesis of all nucleotides, vitamins, and cofactors.[27]

Ehrlichia and *Anaplasma* have the characteristic gram-negative cell wall structure, but lack important cell membrane components including lipopolysaccharide and peptidoglycan.[28] However, the ehrlichial cell wall is rich in cholesterol, which is derived from the host cell and seems to be important for ehrlichial survival and entry into mammalian cells. Recent study has demonstrated that *A. phagocytophilum* exploits host cell cholesterol derived from the low-density lipoprotein receptor (LDLR) mediated uptake pathway and LDLR regulatory system, to accumulate cholesterol in their inclusions to facilitate replication.[29] In addition to the possible role of cholesterol in supporting bacterial cell wall and promoting internalization, it is possible that cholesterol-rich cell walls may also function as ligands for stimulation of innate and acquired immune responses. In support of this conclusion, a recent report showed that heat-killed *Ehrlichia muris* are recognized by mouse CD1d-restricted natural killer T cells, which recognize lipids and glycolipid.[30]

E. chaffeensis, *E. ewingii*, *E. canis*, and *A. phagocytophilum* have immunodominant outer membrane proteins, which are members of Pfam PF01617 and constitute the OMP-1/MSP2/P44 families.[21,31–38] Evaluation of different *E. chaffeensis* isolates demonstrated a differential expression of p28/30-Omp proteins in infected macrophages and tick cell cultures. In infected macrophages, the dominant *E. chaffeensis* expressed proteins are the products of the p28-Omp19 and -20 genes.[39,40] In cultured tick cells derived from *E. chaffeensis* vector, *Amblyomma americanum* and nonvector (*Ixodes scapularis*) ticks, *E. chaffeensis* expression consists only of the p28-Omp 14 protein.[39,40] It is postulated that this differential expression of proteins within the p28/p30-Omp locus may be critical for the adaptation of *Ehrlichia* species to their different hosts (mammals and ticks). These observations support the long evolutionary relationship between the bacterium, its vector, and its niche within host monocytes. How differential expression of these proteins provides an advantage to the organism within these extremely different environments is not known. Thus, in vivo investigations of ehrlichial infection in animal models and natural tick vectors will be necessary to determine in vivo the biologic significance of these in vitro observations. To this end, a recent study by Ganta and colleagues[41] determined that C57BL/6 mice have different responses to infection depending on the source of the inoculum. ISE6 tick cell derived *Ehrlichia* inoculated into mice results in a more persistent infection, which includes relapses of increasing bacterial load. On the other hand, the *A. phagocytophilum* genome has 3 *omp-1*, 1 *msp2*, 2 *msp2* homologues, 1 *msp4*, and 113 *p44* loci belonging to the OMP-1/MSP2/P44 superfamily.[36–39] P44 plays a role in the binding of *A. phagocytophilum* to surfaces of neutrophils, and in antigenic variation and evasion of host immune responses. The *P44s* are diverse, include several paralogues (*p44-1* to *p44-65*) expressed in mammals and ticks, and confer antigenic environmental adaptation, especially during tick transmission.[36–39]

As mentioned above *Ehrlichiae* also express several secreted ankyrin, tandem repeat,[23–25,27,42–44] and putative lipoptoteins[28,29,34] that are major targets of the humoral immune response. Several genes code for major immunoreactive proteins of *E. chaffeensis*, including ankyrin (200 kDa) and tandem repeat containing proteins (120-, 47- and 32-kDa proteins).[23–25] These proteins contain major antibody eptiopes that are molecularly distinct and elicit strong species-specific host immune responses. The TRP47 has recently linked with host-pathogen interactions that suggest a complex network of interactions between TRP47 and the host (**Fig. 5**).[25] Another major immunoreactive protein includes TRP32 (variable-length polymerase chain reaction [PCR] target protein) *E. chaffeensis*, which has one conformational and one continuous epitope within the 90-bp TRs.[24] TRP32 repeats vary in number among *E. chaffeensis* isolates; hence, it has been used as a molecular target for differentiation of *E. chaffeensis* isolates.[24]

Ehrlichia and *Anaplasma* also contain genes for type IV secretion systems, which are structures known to use a complex of transmembrane proteins, and a pilus to mediate the translocation of macromolecules across the cell envelopes of both gram-negative and gram-positive bacteria.[27,45–47] Genes for Type IV

Table 1
Ehrlichiae and Anaplasmae species causing medical and veterinary diseases

Genus	Human or Animal Disease	Target Cells	Geographic Distribution	Vector	Reservoir
1. Ehrlichia					
Ehrlichia chaffeensis	Human monocytic ehrlichiosis (HME)	Monocytes/ macrophages	Southeast, south central, and Midwest states	Lone star tick Amblyomma	Deer
Ehrlichia canis	Canine ehrlichiosis, HME	Monocytes/ macrophages	Southeast, south central, and Midwest states	Rhipicephalus	Dogs
Ehrlichia ewingii	Human ewingii ehrlichiosis (HEE)	Neutrophils	Southeast, south central, and Midwest states	Lone star tick Amblyomma Dermacentor variabilis	Dogs, deer
Ehrlichia muris	Murine monocytic ehrlichiosis, possibly HME	Monocytes/ macrophages	Unknown	Ticks (Ixodes persulcatus, Haemaphysalis flava)	Apodemus mice, vole
Ehrlichia ruminantium	Heartwater in cattle	Monocytes/ macrophages endothelium	Africa	Lone star tick Amblyomma	Cattle, sheep, goats

2. Anaplasma					
Anaplasma marginale	Bovine anaplasmosis	Erythrocytes	Unknown	Unknown	Cattle, wild ruminants
Anaplasma phagocytophilum	Human granulocytic anaplasmosis (HGA)	Neutrophils	Northeastern and north central states and northern California	Ixodes	White-footed mice, wood rats, mice, horses, dogs, cats, sheep, cattle, white-tailed deer
3. Neorickettsia					
Neorickettsia helminthoeca	No human infection	Monocytes/macrophages	Unknown	Fish	Dogs
Neorickettsia sennetsu	Human infection Infectious mononucleosis like syndrome	Monocytes/macrophages	Unknown	Ticks (*Boophilus, Rhipicephalus,* and others)	No animal reservoir
Neorickettsia risticii	No human infection Causes rickettsial disease in horses	Macrophages, enterocytes, ticks (*Ixodes persulcatus, Haemophysalis flava*) mast cells	Unknown	Trematode larvae	Horse

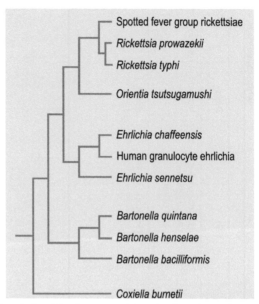

Fig. 1. Phylogenetic relationships between rickettsias based on 16S rRNA gene sequences. (*From* Mason PR, Kelly PJ. Rickettsia and rickettsia-like organisms. In: Cohen and Powderly, editors. Infectious diseases. 2nd edition. Mosby; 2004. Chapter 235; with permission.)

secretion are cotranscribed with genes for enzymes, such as superoxide dismutase (*sodB*), which catabolize reactive oxygen species. However, whether these enzymes are secreted by type IV secretion complexes needs to be investigated. Of note, among the genes that encode the classic type IV secretion system, VirB is common to all *Ehrlichia* species and has been associated with secretion of toxins.[45–47] One substrate, AnkA of *A. phagocytophilum*, of the type IV secretion system, has been identified. AnkA is secreted into host cell cytoplasm where it interacts with host cell tyrosine kinase Abl and phosphatase SHP-1, and eventually is transported into the host cell nucleus. There it interacts with nuclear chromatin and appears to target gene regulatory regions.[42–44] Other virulence genes, such as those that encode two-components regulatory systems, have also been described and studied, and seem to be involved in intracellular survival by inhibiting lysosomal fusion. Further comparison of ehrlichial genomes will provide insight and facilitate investigations of bacterial virulence factors, disease pathogenesis, and mechanisms of immune modulation, and will provide targets for vaccines or new antimicrobial therapies.

EPIDEMIOLOGY
Epidemiology of HME

HME was first described in 1986, and now more than 2300 cases have been reported to the Centers for Disease Control and Prevention (CDC) in the past 19 years.[48–50] Although the average incidence of HME in the United States is estimated at 0.7 cases per million population, this incidence is based on passive surveillance and is likely a significant underestimation of the actual disease incidence (**Fig. 6**A). Active surveillance in endemic areas has suggested rates of HME of 100 to 200 cases per population of 100,000.[49,50] The true incidence of human infection with *E. chaffeensis* is likely

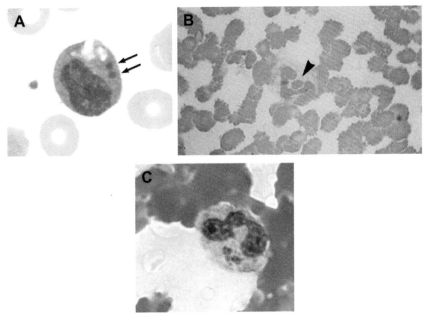

Fig. 2. Peripheral blood leukocytes containing ehrlichial morula in patients with human monocytic ehrlichiosis (A) and human granulocytic anaplasmosis (B and C). (A, B) A morula (arrow) containing Ehrlichia chaffeensis in a monocyte in patient with HME. (B, C) A morula (arrowhead) containing Anaplasma phagocytophilum in a neutrophil in patient with HGA. Wright stains, original magnifications ×1,200. (A: From Walker DH, Dumler JS. Ehrlichia chaffeensis (human monocytotropic ehrlichiosis), Anaplasma phagocytophilum (human granulocytotropic anaplasmosis), and other Ehrlichiae. In: Mandell, Bennett, Dolin, editors. Principles and practice of infectious diseases. 6th edition. Churchill Livingstone; 2005. Chapter 190; with permission. B: From Siberry GK, Dumler JS. Ehrlichiosis and anaplasmosis. In: Kliegman, editor. Nelson textbook of pediatrics. 18th edition. Saunders; 2007. Chapter 228; with permission. C: Courtesy of J.S. Dumler, MD, Baltimore, MD.

to be much higher, as two-thirds of the infections are either asymptomatic or minimally symptomatic.[51–57] A seroprevalence study found that 20% of the children residing in endemic areas had detectable antibody to E. chaffeensis, without prior history of clinical disease.[56,57]

Similar to other tick-borne diseases, the distribution of the arthropod vectors and vertebrate reservoirs correlates with the human disease incidence.[58,59] States with the highest reported rates of HME include Mississippi, Oklahoma, Tennessee, Arkansas, and Maryland (Fig. 6B).[60] The dominant zoonotic cycle of E. chaffeensis involves a reservoir of many persistently infected white-tailed deer (Odocoileus virginianus) and the tick vector, Amblyomma americanum, prevalent throughout the southeast and south central United States (Fig. 7A).[61–64] Other reservoirs such as dogs and coyotes, and other tick vectors including Ixodes pacificus,[65] Ixodes ricinus,[66] Haemophysalis yeni,[67] Amblyomma testudinarium, Amblyomma maculatum, and Dermacentor variabilis[67] may also have a limited role in human transmission. Similar to other ticks, Amblyomma ticks have 3 feeding stages (larval, nymph, and adult); each developmental stage feeds only once. Trans-stadial (ie, larva-nymph-adults) transmission of Ehrlichia occurs during nymph and adult feeding stages because larvae are

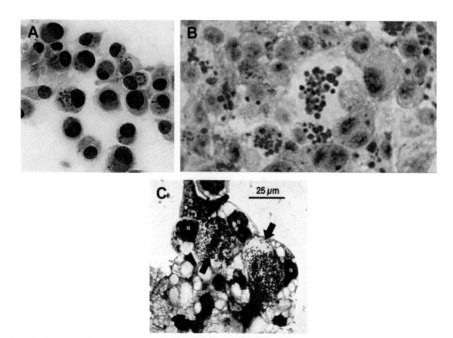

Fig. 3. Light microscopic picture of canine monocytes (DH82) are heavily infected in vitro with *E. chaffeensis* (*A*) and *E. canis* (*B*). Typical ehrlichial inclusions (morulae) are present inside the cytoplasm of infected cells (Giemsa staining, original magnification ×200). (*C*) Giemsa-stained ISE6 cells infected with *A. phagocytophilum* strain isolated from a female *I. scapularis* tick. *Anaplasma* organisms exist in large intracellular vacuoles (*arrow*). N, host cell nucleus. (*A: Courtesy of* N. Ismail. *B: From* Mason PR, Kelly PJ. *Rickettsia* and *Rickettsia*-like organisms. In: Cohen and Powderly, editors. Infectious diseases. 2nd edition. Mosby; 2004. Chapter 235; with permission. *C: From* Massung RF, Levin ML, Munderloh UG, et al. Isolation and propagation of the Ap-variant 1 strain of *Anaplasma phagocytophilum* in a tick cell line. J Clin Microbiol 2007;45(7):2138–43; with permission.)

uninfected. In contrast to *Rickettsia* spp, *Ehrlichia* are not maintained by trans-ovarial transmission (**Fig. 7B**).

There have been case reports of patients coinfected with both *E. chaffeensis* and *R. rickettsii*, which, although spread by different tick vectors, share a common geographic distribution.[68] Among cases of HME reported to the CDC between 2001 and 2002, 61% were male, and 95% of cases self-identified as Caucasian.[60] The median age for infection was 53 years; however, the age-specific incidence was highest in the group aged 70 years and older. Although cases were reported year-round, the greatest number of cases occurred during the period of May through August, corresponding to periods of abundant tick populations and human outdoor recreation.

Epidemiology of HGA

In the early 1990s, patients from Michigan and Wisconsin with a tick bite history experiencing a febrile illness similar to HME were described.[69,70] These cases were distinguishable by the presence of inclusion bodies in granulocytes rather than monocytes, causing this syndrome initially to be termed human granulocytic ehrlichiosis or HGE. The disease has recently been renamed human granulocytic anaplasmosis, or HGA, after phylogenetic analysis reclassified *Ehrlichia phagocytophilum* as a member of the genus *Anaplasma*.[70,71]

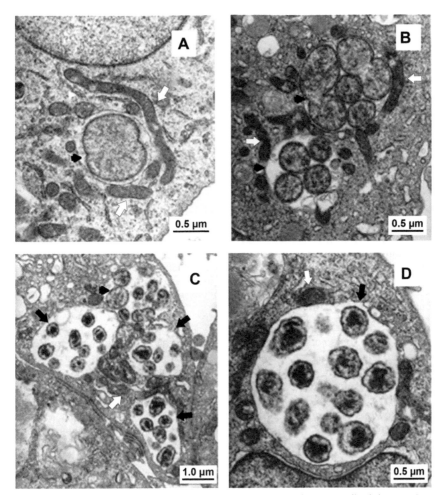

Fig. 4. Electron micrographs of *E. chaffeensis* interaction with DH82 cells. (*A*) At 24 hours post infection, a single reticulate cell (RC) is divided by binary fission (*black arrowhead*). (*B*) At 48 hours post infection, 2 morulae (*black arrowheads*) contain RC. (*C*) At 72 hours post infection, *Ehrlichia* have matured into dense core (DC). Three morulae contain DC (*black arrows*), and one morula contains RC (*black arrowhead*). (*D*) High-power micrograph of a morula containing DC at 72 hours post infection. Mitochondria surrounding morulae are indicated by white arrows. (*From* Zhang JZ, Popov VL, Gao S, et al. The developmental cycle of *Ehrlichia chaffeensis* in vertebrate cells. Cell Microbiol 2006;9(3):610–18; with permission.)

More than 2900 cases of HGA have been reported to the CDC between 1994 and 2005, with the annual number of cases of HGA exceeding that of HME at an estimated annual incidence of 1.6 cases per million in the United States. The highest annual incidence rates of HGA in the United States have been reported in Connecticut (14–16 cases/100,000 population), Wisconsin (24–58 cases/100,000 population), and New York state (2.7/100,000) (**Fig. 8**).[62] Active surveillance in endemic areas has identified incidence rates of more than 50 cases per 100,000 population.[71–73] As with *E. chaffeensis*, serosurveillance studies suggest that asymptomatic disease is common.[72,73]

A. phagocytophilum is transmitted by *I. scapularis* (**Fig. 9**A) in New England and north-central United States, *I. pacificus* (**Fig. 9**B) in the western United States, *I. ricinus*

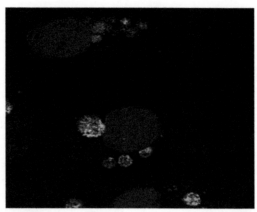

Fig. 5. *Ehrlichia* TR47: ultrastructure and confocal microscopy. Differential expression of TRP47 (*red*) on dense-cored *E. chaffeensis* cultured in vitro (DH82 cells) as visualized using 3-color scanning laser confocal fluorescent microscopy. *E. chaffeensis* infected cells were dually stained with rabbit anti-*Ehrlichia* disulfide bond formation protein (Dsb) (green Alexa Fluor 488), and mouse anti-*E chaffeensis* TRP47 (red Alexa Fluor 568). Host cell nuclei were counterstained with 4′,6′-diamidino-2-phenylindole, dihydrochloride (DAPI), and images merged. (*Courtesy of* W. McBride.)

in Europe, and *I. persulcatus* in Asia. *I. scapularis* is also the tick vector for *Borrelia burgdorferi*, *Babesia microti*, and tick-borne encephalitis viruses, and therefore approximately 10% of patients with HGA have serologic evidence of coinfection with Lyme disease or babesiosis.[74] The reservoir for *A. phagocytophilum* is primarily small mammals such as the White-footed mouse (*Peromyscus leucopus*); Dusky-footed Wood rats (*Neotoma fuscipes*), or others such as such as *Apodemus, Microtus*, or *Clethrionymus* species, with humans serving as dead-end hosts.[70] Transmission of *A. phagocytophilum* from tick-mammalian reservoir to humans is similar to that of *E. chaffeensis*.

Demographic characteristics of HGA patients are similar to HME patients. The median age is 51 years, with more than 95% of cases are reported in Caucasians, with a slight male predominance.[60] Cases occur year-round, with a peak incidence during June and July, perhaps reflecting the shorter arthropod season in these northern states or the relative importance of the nymphal stage of *Ixodes* ticks in disease transmission. Given the ubiquity of the tick vector, it is not surprising that cases of HGA have been confirmed worldwide, including Europe and Asia (China, Siberian Russia, and Korea) (**Fig. 10**).

Epidemiology of Human Ewingii Ehrlichiosis

Ehrlichia ewingii was exclusively a canine pathogen until a series of 4 human cases of *E. ewingii* infection were described in 1999.[5,8,9] The epidemiology of human ewingii ehrlichiosis (HEE) remains poorly defined due to the lack of a specific serologic assay for this organism and the absence of a dedicated reporting system for this infection. Most infections reported to date have occurred in patients with human immunodeficiency virus (HIV),[5,8,9] or who were immunosuppressed following organ transplantation.[75] *A. americanum*, the primary vector for *E. chaffeensis*, is also the primary vector for *E. ewingii*. Most cases of HEE have been reported in Tennessee, Missouri, and Oklahoma. However, *E. ewingii* infection in deer and dogs has been described

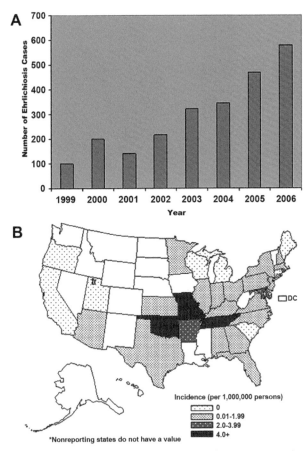

Fig. 6. (*A*) Number of ehrlichiosis cases caused by *E. chaffeensis* reported to CDC by State Health Department from 1999 to 2006. (*B*) Average reported annual incidence of human monocytic ehrlichiosis, United States, 2001 to 2002, by state and nationwide. (*From* Centers for Disease Control and Prevention. Tickborne rickettsial diseases. Available at http://www. cdc.gov/ticks/index.html.)

throughout the range of the Lone star tick, suggesting that human infection with this pathogen might be more widespread than is currently documented.[70]

CLINICAL PRESENTATION
General Clinical Features of HME

HME is a more severe disease than HGA or HEE, with 42% of cases requiring hospitalization, and a case fatality rate of 3%.[1,3,49–52,63] The median age of patients with either infection is approximately 50 years, and slightly more males (57%–61%) are infected than females. Up to 17% of patients develop life-threatening complications, although severe disease and death are more common in immunocompromised patients.[5,19,60] HME can be fatal in immunocompetent patients and be manifest as a multisystem disease resembling toxic or septic shock syndrome, or Rocky Mountain spotted fever, except for the infrequent occurrence of rash.[76–78] Other life-threatening manifestations include cardiovascular failure, aseptic meningitis, hemorrhage, hepatic insufficiency or failure, interstitial pneumonia, and adult respiratory distress

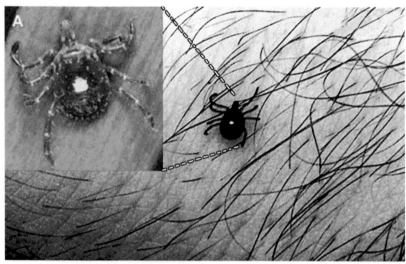

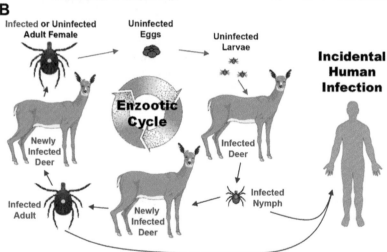

Fig. 7. (*A*) Lone Star tick, *Amblyomma americanum*, which transmits the agent of human monocytic ehrlichiosis. (*B*) Life cycle of monocytotropic *E. chaffeensis*. (*Courtesy of* KC Bloch; *open access data from* Centers for Disease Control and Prevention.)

syndrome.[77–80] The severity of the disease is greater in elderly and immunocompromised patients; however, HME can be fatal even in immunocompetent patients. Several studies have reported an association between the use of sulfonamide antibiotics and severe manifestations of *Ehrlichia*.[51,81] Whether this represents a causal relationship is unknown. A study of HME among transplant patients found no difference in severity of illness among patients taking prophylactic sulfa-antibiotics.[51,75]

Fever is an almost universal symptom (97%), followed by headaches (80%), myalgias (57%), and arthralgias (41%).[47–49,72] A skin eruption is relatively common among children with HME, occurring in 66% of pediatric cases compared with 21% of adults.[49,50] A rash is present in 10% of cases of HME and can be maculopapular, petechial, or be characterized by diffuse erythroderma,[78] but typically spares the face,

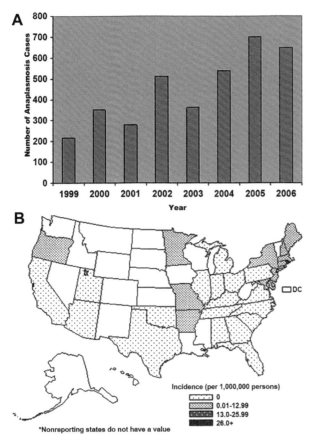

Fig. 8. (*A*) Number of ehrlichiosis cases caused by *A. phagocytophilum* reported to CDC by State Health Department from 1999 to 2006. (*B*) Average reported annual incidence of human monocytic ehrlichiosis, United States, 2001 to 2002, by state and nationwide. (*Data from* Centers for Disease Control and Prevention.)

palms, and soles of the feet. Nausea, vomiting, abdominal pain, and cough are variably present. Gastrointestinal symptoms such as nausea, vomiting, diarrhea, and anorexia are sometimes reported in the course of HME, mainly in children. Other frequently observed signs and symptoms in children and pregnant women with HME are altered mental status and abdominal pain that can be severe, mimicking acute appendicitis.

Although the clinical manifestations of *E. chaffeensis* infection are nonspecific, laboratory abnormalities provide important diagnostic clues. A prospective cohort study of patients in an endemic area presenting with a febrile illness following a tick bite found a significantly lower white blood cell (WBC) (mean 4.6×10^9 cells/L), neutrophil (mean 2.6×10^9 cells/L), and platelet count (mean 172×10^9 cells/L) among patients with HME than noninfected patients, and elevated transaminase levels were present in 83% of cases.[70] In pediatric patients, mild hyponatremia has been reported in 50% of the cases,[49,50,70] but this finding has been less frequently noted among infected adults.

Neurologic Features of HME

The most frequent neurologic manifestation of HME is meningitis or meningoencephalitis. Central nervous system involvement is identified in approximately 20% of

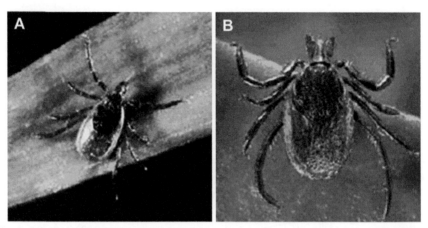

Fig. 9. (*A*) Black-legged tick, *Ixodes scapularis*, which transmits the agent of human granulocytic ehrlichiosis and Lyme disease. (*B*) Western black-legged tick, *Ixodes scapularis*, which transmits the agent of human granulocytic ehrlichiosis. (*From* Centers for Disease Control and Prevention. Tickborne rickettsial diseases. Available at http://www.cdc.gov/ticks/index.html.)

patients with HME,[80] and in some cases may be associated with seizures and coma. Uncommon complications include cranial nerve palsy, with onset after initiation of effective antimicrobial therapy being reported.[77–80] Long-term neurologic sequelae in children are uncommon, but include cognitive delays, fine motor impairment, and persistent foot drop. Subjective neurocognitive deficits following meningoencephalitis have also been reported in adults.[70,80–85]

Among patients with HME who undergo lumbar puncture, cerebrospinal fluid (CSF) pleocytosis is identified in approximately 60%.[80] Although most samples have a lymphocytic predominance, a neutrophilic or mixed picture is found in a third of cases.[80] The CSF WBC count is typically less than 100 cells/mm^3, and protein may be mildly elevated. Morulae are rarely identified in CSF monocytes by Giemsa stain.[1,78–80] Radiographic imaging may be normal, or may show leptomeningeal enhancement. Bilateral medial temporal lobe enhancement has been reported for a case with PCR evidence of *E. chaffeensis* and *A. phagocytophilum* coinfection.[86] Electroencephalography may show nonspecific slowing.[80] Although pathologic review of brain tissue from patients with HME neurologic dysfunction is limited, one study reported atypical lymphoid infiltration of the leptomeninges and Virchow-Robin space, with sparing of the brain parenchyma, whereas others have not shown central nervous system (CNS) pathology.[80]

General Clinical Features of HGA

HGA resembles HME with respect to the frequency of fever, headache, and myalgias, but rash is uncommon, noted in less than 10% of patients.[42,48,73,79] As with HME, leukopenia, thrombocytopenia, and elevations in transaminases are important clues to the diagnosis. HGA tends to be a less severe illness than HME, although life-threatening complications including acute respiratory distress syndrome, acute renal failure, and hemodynamic collapse have been reported.

Neurologic Features of HGA

CNS involvement is uncommon in HGA, with meningoencephalitis reported in only approximately 1% of cases.[86,87] In contrast, several different peripheral nervous

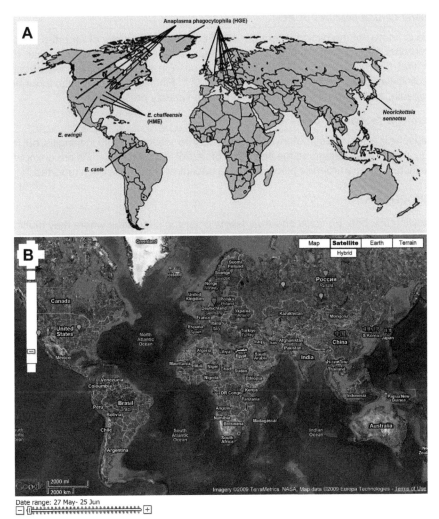

Fig. 10. (*A*) Worldwide distribution of *Ehrlichia* and *Anaplasma*. HGA, human granulocytic anaplasmosis; HME, human monocytic ehrlichiosis. (*B*) Global health map shows worldwide distribution of HGA and HME marked by yellow dots. (*A: From* Raoult D. Rickettsioses. In: Goldman, editor. Cecil medicine. 23rd edition. Saunders; 2007. Chapter 348; with permission. *B: From* "Worldwide Outbreak of *Ehrlichia*" tracking map. Available at: http://www. healthmap.com. Accessed June 15, 2009; with permission.)

system manifestations have been described, including brachial plexopathy, cranial nerve palsies, demyelinating polyneuropathy,[1,86,87] and bilateral facial nerve palsy,[86,87] for which recovery of neurologic function may be delayed over several months. As the geographic distribution of *B. burgdorferi* is similar to *A. phagocytophila*, patients should be tested for coinfection because Lyme disease has similar neurologic manifestations. Although the cause of neurologic dysfunction in HGA is not yet known, it is thought to be due to complicating opportunistic infections, or concomitant coinfection with *B. burgdorferi*. Lumbar puncture is performed less frequently for HGA than HME. Reported CSF abnormalities include lymphocytic pleocytosis and moderate elevation in proteins.[85–87]

General Clinical Features of HEE

Little is known of the clinical spectrum of HEE due to the paucity of reported cases. Symptoms appear to be similar to those described for HME and HGA. Despite the fact that the majority of HEE infections have been in immunocompromised hosts, the clinical manifestations appear to be milder.[75,82] Findings of leukopenia, thrombocytopenia, and abnormal liver function tests are variably present.[75,82]

Neurologic Features of HEE

Headache is a frequent symptom in HEE, and may be associated with meningitis, but the frequency of this finding and the spectrum of neurologic manifestations are unknown. One instance of neutrophilic pleocytosis in a patient with HEE has been reported.[8]

PATHOGENESIS

Following tick bite, *Ehrlichia* and *Anaplasma* enter the circulation where they multiply within their target cell monocytes/macrophages and polymorphonuclear leukocytes, respectively. *Ehrlichia* and *Anaplasma* enter through receptor-mediated endocytosis via a glycophosphoinositol anchored receptor within caveolae or lipid rafts. *Ehrlichiae* were found to localize exclusively within endosomes that avoid phagolysosomal pathways.[88] *Ehrlichia* and *Anaplasma* multiply within endosomes, ultimately reprogramming host cell defense mechanisms and processes to facilitate their survival.

Pathogenesis of HME

Following entry into mononuclear phagocytes, *E. chaffeensis* inhibits phagolysosome fusion involving genes controlled by a two-component regulatory system. *E. chaffeensis* also suppresses and induces host genes to facilitate their intracellular survival.[88–90] Microarray analysis of THP-1 cells infected with *E. chaffeensis* revealed down-regulation of Th1 cytokines such as IL-12 and IL-18, which are important inducers of adaptive Th1-mediated immune responses, and genes such as SNAP 23 (synaptosomal-associated protein, 23 kDa), Rab5A (member of RAS oncogene family), and STX16 (syntaxin 16), which are involved in membrane trafficking while up-regulating apoptosis inhibitors and cell cyclins.[90] An immunoreactive, secreted 200-kDa ankyrin protein (Ank200) of *E. chaffeensis* has recently been shown to be translocated to the host cell nucleus, where it binds gene regulatory regions within *Alu* elements and is thought to play a role in host cell gene regulation.[25] *E. chaffeensis* also circumvents host defenses by inhibiting the signal transduction pathway (Jak/Stat) of interferon-γ–mediated antiehrlichial activity, and increasing transferrin receptor delivery of iron to the ehrlichial vacuole. In vitro studies have shown at *E. chaffeensis* downregulates surface expression of Toll-like receptors (TLR)-2 and -4 as well as CD14 on infected monocytes, and inhibits activation of several transcription factors that are involved in the induction of proinflammatory innate immune responses.[89,90] The mechanism by which down-regulation of TLR-2 and -4 benefits survival within the macrophage is not understood, as pathogen-associated molecular patterns (PAMPs) have not been identified in ehrlichiae, and as mentioned earlier the traditional ligands for these receptors, peptidoglycan and lipopolysaccharide, which activate TLR-2 and -4, respectively, are not present in the bacterium.[28] However it is postulated that loss of traditional PAMPs in *Ehrlichia* genome may allow them to persist within their tick vectors, without inducing strong innate defenses that are normally elicited by these patterns.[91]

Studies with *E. muris* a mildly virulent *Ehrlichia* species have demonstrated that activation of innate lymphocytes such as natural killer T cells (NKT) occurs in a manner that is independent of TLRs, but dependent on CD1d expression on antigen-presenting cells such as the dendritic cells. Although NKT stimulation by *Ehrlichia* results in the production of interferon (IFN)-γ and elimination of intracellular ehrlichiae,[30] they also contribute to the development of *Ehrlichia*-induced toxic shocklike syndrome in murine models of fatal monocytic ehrlichiosis.[92]

Frequent pathologic findings of HME include granuloma formation, myeloid hyperplasia, and megakaryocytosis in the bone marrow.[77–79,86] Some patients develop erythrophagocytosis and plasmacytosis, suggesting a compensatory response. Other pathologic findings in patients with severe HME include focal hepatocellular necrosis; hepatic granulomas; cholestasis; splenic and lymph node necrosis; diffuse mononuclear phagocyte hyperplasia of the spleen, liver, lymph node, and bone marrow; perivascular lymphohistiocytic infiltrates of various organs including kidney, heart, liver, meninges, and brain; and interstitial mononuclear cell pneumonitis.[77,93,94] The severe pathology and multiorgan involvement in severe and fatal HME in immunocompetent patients is thought to be related to dysregulation of the host immune response that leads to tissue damage and, eventually, multi-system organ failure.[95] This conclusion is based on the finding that in fatal disease in the form of toxic shock-like syndrome, uninfected hepatocytes undergo apoptosis without evidence of ehrlichial infection.[77,93,94] Analysis of hepatic tissues from autopsy cases in immunocompetent patients with HME similarly showed lymphohistiocytic foci, centrilobular or coagulation necrosis, Kupffer cell hyperplasia, and marked monocytic infiltration, whereas *Ehrlichia*-infected cells are rarely identified.[77,78,93,94] In contrast, an overwhelming ehrlichial burden in the organs was observed in HME patients who are immunocompromised due to other infections such as HIV or chemotherapy.[77,93] The hypothesis that severe and fatal *Ehrlichia*-induced toxic shock-like syndrome is due to an immunopathologic mechanism is supported by studies in murine models of fatal ehrlichiosis, in which lethal ehrlichial infection with virulent *Ehrlichia* species named *Ixodes ovatus Ehrlichia* (IOE)[96,97] resulted in a progressive, fatal ehrlichiosis that mimics toxic shocklike syndrome.[98] Characteristic of this disease in murine models of fatal monocytotropic ehrlichiosis include focal hepatic necrosis and apoptosis, compared with formation of granuloma in animal models of mild monocytotropic ehrlichiosis (**Fig. 11**), liver dysfunction marked by elevated liver enzymes (aspartate aminotransferase and alanine aminotransferase), significant leukopenia and lymphopenia, and CD4+ T-cell apoptosis.[98–101] Further analysis indicated that severe and fatal primary HME in animals is due to the early overproduction of proinflammatory cytokines (eg, tumor necrosis factor [TNF]-α) and anti-inflammatory interleukin (IL)-10 cytokines. Of note, CD8+ T cells seem to play a pathogenic role in HME whereby fatal disease is correlated with significant expansion of cytotoxic CD8+ T-cell producing TNF-α and IFN-γ. Absence of CD8+ T cells in animals infected with virulent *Ehrlichia* species resulted in protection against fatal disease, decreased tissue injury, normal CD4+ T cell populations, and increased protective CD4+ Th1 responses, which suggest that CD8+ T cells mediate lymphopenia and tissue damage in fatal HME in an immunocompetent host.[100] Consistent with the pathogenic role of CD8+ T cells in fatal murine ehrlichiosis, Dierberg and Dumler[102] reported a significantly greater amount of hemophagocytosis (macrophage activation) and an increased number of CD8+ cells associated with low bacterial burden in the lymph nodes of patients who died of HME (**Fig. 12**). Thus, both human and animal model data suggest that organ pathology and fatal disease is indeed due to immune-mediated pathology.

Pathogenesis of HGA

A. phagocytophilum is observed predominantly in neutrophils in the peripheral blood and tissues from infected individuals. *A. phagocytophilum* has the unique ability to

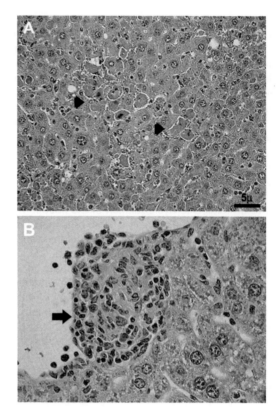

Fig. 11. (*A*) Hepatic histopathology in the murine model of fatal monocytic ehrlichiosis caused by systemic infection with virulent monocytic *Ehrlichia* (IOE). Hematoxylin-eosin (H&E) staining shows extensive focal necrosis and apoptosis of hepatocytes (*arrows*). (*B*) Hepatic histopathology in the murine model of mild monocytic ehrlichiosis caused by infection with mildly virulent *Ehrlichia muris*. H&E staining shows formation of well-formed granuloma (*arrowhead*). (*From* Ismail N, Soong L, McBride JW, et al. Overproduction of TNF-alpha by CD8+ type-1 cells and down-regulation of IFN-gamma production by CD4+ Th1 cells contribute to toxic shock-like syndrome in an animal model of fatal monocytotropic ehrlichiosis. J Immunol 2004;172(3):1786–800; with permission.)

selectively survive and multiply within cytoplasmic vacuoles of polymorphonuclear leukocyte cells by delaying their apoptosis through upregulation of antiapoptotic bcl-2 family member bfl-1 (A1), and blocking anti-FAS (CD95/Apo-1)-induced programmed cell death of human neutrophils.[103,104] A. phagocytophilum uses multiple evasion strategies to inhibit neutrophil antimicrobial functions.[105,106] Some studies have suggested that one of the mechanisms by which A. phagocytophilum avoids the toxic effects of neutrophils is its ability to inhibit the fusion of the lysosomes with the cytoplasmic vacuoles, and by arresting or inhibiting other signaling pathways related to respiratory burst.[103–108] The mechanism by which A. phagocytophilum inhibits phagosome-lysosome fusion remains to be elucidated. A. phagocytophilum seems to modulate host cell gene transcription through AnkA, a secreted protein that is transported to the infected host cell nucleus through binding to protein-DNA complexes in neutrophil nuclei.[109] Further studies are required to establish the effects of AnkA binding on neutrophil functions. The molecular basis by which

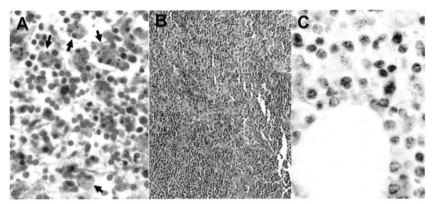

Fig. 12. (*A*) Hemophagocytosis (*arrows*) in lymph nodes from a patient with HME (H&E; original magnification ×240). (*B*) High cellularity in lymph node from patient with HME (original magnification ×64). (*C*) Immunohistochemical staining of lymph nodes from patient with HME shows typical low bacterial burden (immunoperoxidase with hematoxylin counterstain; original magnification ×240). (*From* Dierberg KL, Dumler JS. Lymph node hemophagocytosis in rickettsial diseases: a pathogenetic role for CD8 T lymphocytes in human monocytic ehrlichiosis (HME)? BMC Infect Dis 2006;6:121; with permission; open access article distributed under the terms of the Creative Commons Attribution License. Available at: http://creativecommons.org/licenses/by/2.0.)

A. phagocytophilum affects the respiratory burst of granulocytes was shown to be due to the down-regulation of gp91^{phox} and rac2, 2 important components of nicotinamide adenine dinucleotide phosphate-oxidase.[106,108] Another study paradoxically showed that infection with *A. phagocytophilum* induced protracted degranulation in human neutrophils,[110] which was attributed to inflammatory tissue injury. In addition, *A. phagocytophilum* up-regulates the production of chemokine IL-8 as well as proinflammatory cytokines. This increased proinflammatory activity and chemokines may facilitate the recruitment of additional host neutrophil cells and localized tissue injury when neutrophils are unable to generate effective antimicrobial responses.[111]

Pathologic findings in patients with HGA and animal models include normocellular or hypercellular bone marrow, erythrophagocytosis, hepatic apoptosis and periportal lymphohistiocytic infiltrates, focal splenic necrosis, and mild interstitial pneumonitis and pulmonary hemorrhage.[77,93,94] Similar to HME, HGA hematologic abnormalities include marked leukopenia and thrombocytopenia. Although the immune mechanisms that account for severe and fatal HGA are not completely understood, there is some evidence of immunosuppression in patients with HGA.[77,85,87,89] This conclusion is supported by the high number of fatal cases due to secondary opportunistic infections and organ failures.[79] The mechanism by which this immune suppression occurs in HGA is not yet completely defined.

REINFECTION AND IMMUNITY
HME

Immunity to primary *E. chaffeensis* infection in humans has not been investigated, but comparative murine models have provided some insight. A role for cell-mediated immunity has been suggested based on the severity of *E. chaffeensis* infection in HIV-infected patients and the lymphoproliferative responses observed in patients following recovery from HME.[52,54,84,112] However, the relative importance of cell-mediated and humoral immunity has not been firmly established.[113] Studies using murine models have suggested that protective immunity during primary and secondary ehrlichial infection is mediated by cellular immunity, mainly CD4$^+$ T cells producing IFN-γ (ie, Th1 cells).[98–101,114–117] IFN-γ production by CD4$^+$ Th1 cells likely leads to macrophage activation and induction of bactericidal mechanisms such as production of reactive oxygen species, which in turn lead to bacterial elimination.[115–117] In addition to IFN-γ, murine studies have shown that proinflammatory cytokines such as IL-12p40 and TNF-α are also important factors in the clearance of *Ehrlichia* and protection. Humoral immunity seems to also play a role in protection against *Ehrlichia* infection, as evidenced by significant seroconversion in patients who recover from disease. In murine studies, *Ehrlichia*-specific antibodies, mainly IgG2a (Th1-dependent Ig subclass), protect SCID mice from severe *E. chaffeensis* infection.[98,117,118]

It is unknown whether patients that recover from HME are immune or susceptible to reinfection. Such evidence is limited to a single report of reinfection with a genetically distinct *E. chaffeensis* strain in a liver transplant recipient receiving immunosuppressive therapy.[119] In murine studies, the development of heterologous protection model of ehrlichiosis has provided a mechanism to investigate immunity, including memory immune responses.[98,120] These studies indicate that prior infection of immunocompetent mice with *E. muris* causes persistent asymptomatic infection in mice and strong cell-mediated immune responses (**Fig. 11**B), and protects against secondary infection with highly virulent *Ehrlichia* species (IOE) that cause fatal disease in uninfected hosts.[98,120] Heterologous protection against *Ehrlichia* is associated with minimal tissue injury, development of well-defined granulomas, expansion of IFN-γ producing effector memory CD4$^+$ and CD8$^+$ type-1 cells, and substantial production of *Ehrlichia*-specific IgG2a antibodies. Vaccines are currently unavailable for HME.

HGA

At present, little is known about immunity following an *A. phagocytophilum* infection. Although infection may result in long-term immunity, there have been rare reports of laboratory-confirmed reinfection. Thus, individuals who live in endemic areas and are at risk of exposure to infected ticks should be vigilant about avoiding tick bites and other tick-borne pathogens. Similar to immunity against *E. chaffeensis*, protective immunity against *A. phagocytophilum* is mediated by cellular and humoral immune mechanisms.[27,73] It is generally believed that individuals who develop high titer antibodies are protected against reinfection; patients previously infected with *A. phagocytophilum* develop high titer antibodies that may last for as long as 3 years. Whether this persistence of antibodies is due to persistent infection or reinfection is not clearly determined. It is similarly not known if previous infection of human leads to antigen-specific memory T- and B-cell responses that protect the individual against reinfection. Vaccines are currently unavailable for HGA.

DIAGNOSIS
HME and HGA

Diagnosis of HME and HGA rests primarily on clinical suspicion due to the limited availability of rapid diagnostic tests such as PCR, and the absence of detectable serum antibodies at the time of clinical presentation (4 days after the onset of clinical illness).[19,112] The prognosis worsens if treatment is not administered or delayed[5,49,50,70,112] and therefore, it is important that empiric therapy with doxycycline be started for any patient with compatible clinical and laboratory findings. Initial diagnosis of ehrlichiosis can be based on nonspecific biochemical and hematological findings. However, confirmatory tests should be performed at different intervals after the onset of illness.

Hematologic and Biochemical Abnormalities

Presumptive diagnosis of HME is based on clinical manifestation, clues from medical history such as history of tick bite and outdoor activities, and specific laboratory abnormalities. Pancytopenias are a hallmark laboratory feature of HME early in the course of the illness.[121] Anemia occurs within 2 weeks of illness and influences 50% of patients. Mild to moderate leukopenia with largest decline in lymphocyte population is observed in approximately 60% to 70% of patients during the first week of illness.[49,50,70] Of note, during convalescence a significant increase in lymphocyte count, that is, relative and absolute lymphocytosis, is seen in most patients and is characterized predominantly by the expansion of activated $\gamma\delta$ T cells.[113] Marked thrombocytopenia is one of the pathognomonic findings in HME, which is usually detected in 70% to 90% of patients during their illness. Mildly or moderately elevated hepatic transaminase levels are detected in approximately 90% of patients associated with increased levels of alkaline phosphatase and bilirubin in some patients. Mild to moderate hyponatremia has been reported in as many as 50% of adult patients and 70% of pediatric patients.[50,70,112]

Other laboratory abnormalities that occur in severe disease are specific to the organ involved. Examples are increased serum creatinine, lactate dehydrogenase, creatine phosphokinase, and amylase, electrolyte abnormalities including hypocalcemia, hypomagnesemia, hypophosphatemia, prolonged prothrombin times, increased levels of fibrin degradation products, metabolic acidosis, profound hypotension, disseminated intravascular coagulopathy, hepatic and renal failure, adrenal insufficiency, and myocardial dysfunction.[47,48,73]

Specific Laboratory Diagnostic Tests

A diagnosis of HME can be confirmed by several laboratory methods. These tests include serologic detection of specific antibodies, detection of morulae in peripheral blood or in CSF leukocytes, detection of ehrlichial DNA by PCR of blood or CSF, direct detection of ehrlichiae in tissue samples by immunohistochemistry, and isolation of bacteria.

Serologic Testing

Serologic testing of IgM and IgG antibodies specific to *E. chaffeensis* using indirect immunofluorescence assay (IFA) is the "gold standard" and is the most frequently used confirmatory test for HME.[70,87,122] Paired sera collected during a 3- to 6-week interval represent the preferred specimens for serologic evaluation of HME. A single IgG antibody titer of at least 256, seroconversion from negative to positive antibody status (with a minimum titer of 64), and a 4-fold increase in titer during convalescence indicate HME when acute- and convalescent-phase samples are compared.[122,123] Although serology is one of major diagnostic criterion for ehrlichiosis, it has several limitations that should be considered such as: (1) IgG IFA test is negative in as many as 80% of patients during the first week of illness, and the IgM titers may also be uninformative at this time. Thus a negative serologic result for the acute-phase sample does not exclude the diagnosis; (2) A high rate of false-positive serology usually occurs due to cross-reactive antigens shared by *Ehrlichia* and *Anaplasma* that induce cross-reactive antibodies. Because of this cross-reactivity among ehrlichial species, sera should be tested against both *E. chaffeensis* and *A. phagocy-tophilum* antigens when ascribing a specific etiology; (3) Failure to seroconvert in some cases can be attributed to immune impairment; (4) Early treatment with a tetra-cycline-class antibiotic occasionally reduces or abrogates the antibody response to *E. chaffeensis*.[32,77,124]

Blood Smear Staining

Diagnosis of HME can be accomplished by the staining of blood smears from periph-eral blood, bone marrow, or CSF to detect morulae. Smears can be stained with Wright's, Diff-Quik, or Giemsa stains.[19,28] Although this method is rapid, it is relatively insensitive compared with other confirmatory tests, especially in immunocompetent patients in whom severe disease is usually associated with very low bacterial burden in blood and peripheral organs. Morulae are detected within monocytes in only about 3% of patients with HME. In contrast, blood smear is more useful for HGA diagnosis whereby 25% to 75% of patients have morulae in peripheral blood examinations, and sensitivity is highest during the first week of infection.[125,126]

Polymerase Chain Reaction Amplification

Due to its high specificity (60%–85%) and sensitivity (60%–85% for *E. chaffeensis* and 67%–90% for *A. phagocytophilum*) as well as rapid turnaround time, diagnosis of ehrli-chial infection by PCR has become the test of choice for confirming serology indicating HME and HGA.[125–127] PCR is the only definitive diagnostic test for *E. ewingii* infection because the bacteria is unculturable, although the sensitivity and specificity of this approach is unknown. Multiplex or multicolor testing capable of detecting several related etiologic agents in a single test has been described.[128] PCR of whole blood is commercially available, and allows rapid diagnosis of infection in up to 85% of cases.[125] Blood samples should be collected in ethylenediamine tetra-acetic acid or sodium citrate anticoagulants, and obtained before or at the initiation of therapy to increase sensitivity. However, because doxycycline treatment is highly effective at early stages of infection, treatment should start as soon as possible while waiting for laboratory results. PCR detection is particularly important for detection of ehrlichial infection at early stages when antibody levels are very low or undetectable. Although PCR of CSF may be positive, the sensitivity is lower than for whole blood, likely due to the significantly lower volume of infected cells.[2,4,125,126] Several conserved genes among different *Ehrlichia* isolates have been employed as PCR targets, including the *rrs* (16S rRNA) and groESL heat shock operon.[129] Other genes have been used, such as genus-specific disulfide bond formation protein gene (*dsb*), the *E. chaffeensis*-specific 120-kDa and TRP32 protein (VLPT) genes, and the 28-kDa outer membrane proteins (p28).[130]

Isolation

Similar to other infectious diseases, cultivation of *Ehrlichia* is the gold standard in diagnosis of HME and HGA; however, primary isolation may take up to several weeks. The sensitivity of *E. chaffeensis* isolation compared with PCR amplification is very low.[3,11,47] In contrast, the sensitivity of culture for detection of *A. phagocytophilum* can be equivalent to that of PCR and blood smear examination.[67] Similar to PCR amplification and blood smear examination, prior doxycycline treatment diminishes the sensitivity of culture to a greater degree. Due to lower sensitivity of this method, therapeutic decisions must often be based on a high index of clinical suspicion and laboratory evidence of the infection, such as PCR assays and peripheral blood smears.[67,72]

IMMUNOHISTOCHEMISTRY

Immunohistochemical (IHC) staining of the formalin fixed biopsy or autopsy tissues is another confirmatory method for diagnosis of *Ehrlichia* and *Anaplasma* infection. The IHC method is most useful in documenting the presence of organisms in patients before the initiation of antibiotic therapy or within the first 48 hours after antibiotic therapy has been initiated. IHC techniques also are available for diagnosing cases of ehrlichiosis and anaplasmosis from bone marrow biopsies and tissue obtained at autopsy of fatal cases, including the spleen, lymph nodes, liver, and lung.[49,50,77]

Diagnosis of HEE

A diagnosis of HEE is suggested by visualization of intracytoplasmic morulae in neutrophils in a patient with residence in or travel to an area of HME (rather than HGA) endemnicity. Morulae may be visualized in blood and, rarely, CSF.[8,9,11] Whereas there is no specific serologic assay for *E. ewingii*, there is significant serologic cross-reactivity to *E. chaffeensis*.[8,9] It is conceivable that in the absence of visualization of morulae in granulocytes or confirmatory PCR for *E. ewingii*, a proportion of cases meeting serologic criteria for HME actually represent HEE infection. A specific PCR for *E. ewingii* exists, but is limited to research laboratories. Similar to the PCR for *E. chaffeensis* and *A. phagocytophilum*, sensitivity is maximal early in the course of the illness, prior to antibiotic therapy.

Differential Diagnosis

The differential diagnosis of HME, HGA, and HEE at the early stages of the disease, when the symptoms and signs of disease are nonspecific and the patient presents with fever, headache, myalgia, and malaise, may include various viral syndromes, Rocky Mountain spotted fever, upper respiratory illness, urinary tract infection, and sepsis. If a history of tick bite and outdoor activities exists with these symptoms, the physician should consider other tick-borne febrile illnesses such as Rocky Mountain spotted fever, relapsing fever, tularemia, Lyme borreliosis, Colorado tick fever, and babesiosis.[50,122] CNS signs and symptoms with CSF pleocytosis suggest viral or bacterial meningoencephalitis. Other diseases that share clinical and laboratory findings of ehrlichial disease, particularly if patients presenting with rash, are meningococcemia, toxic shock syndrome, murine typhus, Q fever, typhoid fever, leptospirosis, hepatitis, enteroviral infection, influenza, bacterial sepsis, endocarditis, Kawasaki disease, collagen-vascular diseases, and immune thrombocytopenic purpura.[70]

TREATMENT

Most patients with HME or HGA respond well to tetracyclines if administrated early in illness. In vitro antimicrobial susceptibility testing has shown an excellent sensitivity of all *Ehrlichia* and *Anaplasma* species to doxycycline. In vivo, doxycycline is preferred over tetracycline because it has fewer side effects and better patient tolerance.[87,131] Doxycycline remains the treatment of choice in pediatric patients, despite the risk of dental discoloration in this age group.[132] This drug is bacteriostatic in its activity against rickettsial organisms.

Pregnant patients with ehrlichial infection represent a particular challenge, as doxycycline is contraindicated. In this population, as well as in patients with a specific contraindication to doxycycline, rifampin (adults: 300 mg twice daily; children under 45.4 kg [100 lb] 10 mg/kg twice daily) may be substituted.[133–135] In vitro susceptibility testing has shown that *E. chaffeensis* is resistant to representatives of most classes of antibiotics including aminoglycosides (gentamicin), fluoroquinolones (ciprofloxacin), penicillins (penicillin), macrolides and ketolides (erythromycin and telithromycin), and sulfa-containing drugs (cotrimoxazole).[85] Chloramphenicol is an alternative drug that has been considered for treatment of HGA or HME. However, this drug is associated with various side effects and might require monitoring of blood indices, and therefore is no longer available in the oral form in the United States.

Treatment of HME

Doxycycline is the recommended treatment for HME. Response to treatment is typically rapid, and fever persisting longer than 72 hours after initiation of treatment strongly suggests an alternative diagnosis. The recommended dose of doxycycline is 100 mg per dose administered twice daily (orally or intravenously) for adults or 2.2 mg/kg body weight per dose administered twice daily (orally or intravenously) for children weighing less than 45.4 kg (100 lb). Although no studies have specifically addressed duration of treatment, most authorities advocate continuing antibiotics for 3 to 5 days after defervescence,[87,132] and perhaps longer (eg, total of 10–14 days) if there is CNS involvement.[136]

Treatment of HGA

Therapeutic considerations for HGA are similar to HME, with doxycycline remaining the drug of choice for both pediatric and adult cases. If coinfection with *B. burgdorferi* is suspected based on characteristic skin findings or elevated antibodies, doxycycline should be continued for at least 10 days for adults.[137,138] In *B. burgdorferi* coinfected children younger than 8 years, doxycycline should be continued until the patient is afebrile for 3 days, with the remainder of the 14-day course completed with an alternative agent active against *B. burgdorferi* (eg, amoxicillin or cefuroxime axetil) to minimize the risk of dental discoloration.[10,11,47,70] Patients who fail to respond clinically to doxycycline monotherapy after 72 hours should be evaluated for an alternative diagnosis or the possibility of *Babesia* coinfection.

Treatment of HEE

There are no prospective studies evaluating treatment of *E. ewingii*; however, doxycycline is considered the treatment of choice in both adults and children. When therapy with this agent is started promptly, outcomes are uniformly excellent.[8,9,11] Considerations in dosing and administration of doxycycline are discussed in the section on HME management.

PREVENTION

Preventive antibiotic therapy for ehrlichial infection is not indicated for patients who have had recent tick bites and are not ill. Avoidance of tick bites and immediate removal of ticks remains the ultimate prevention approach. Individuals who live in endemic areas should wear light-colored clothes during outdoor activities, which allow the person to see crawling ticks.[139] Adults who are at high risk of getting bitten by ticks should apply Chemoprophylactic repellents such as DEET (*N,N*-diethyl-*m*-toluamide) to exposed skin that prevents tick attachment. Individuals should carefully inspect their body, hair, and clothes for ticks on return from potentially tick-infested areas, and should immediately remove any attached ones. Studies have shown that a period of 4 to 24 hours of infected ticks being attached to the host may be required before effective transmission of *Ehrlichia* and *Anaplasma* occur.[139–141] Therefore, immediate and complete removal of attached ticks is critical for prevention of transmission and infection.

ACKNOWLEDGMENTS

The authors thank Dr Veera Rajaratnam, Director of Scientific Publications and Grant Support at the Center for Women's Health Research, Meharry Medical College, for meticulously editing and expediting the article, and Christina Nelson for her graphics assistance.

REFERENCES

1. Dumler JS, Barbet AF, Bekker CP, et al. Reorganization of genera in the families rickettsiaceae and anaplasmataceae in the order rickettsiales: unification of some species of *Ehrlichia* with *Anaplasma*, Cowdria with *Ehrlichia* and *Ehrlichia* with Neorickettsia, descriptions of six new species combinations and designation of *Ehrlichia equi* and 'HGE agent' as subjective synonyms of *Ehrlichia phagocytophila*. Int J Syst Evol Microbiol 2001;51:2145–65.
2. Dawson JE, Anderson BE, Fishbein DB, et al. Isolation and characterization of an *Ehrlichia* sp. from a patient diagnosed with human ehrlichiosis. J Clin Microbiol 1991;29:2741–5.
3. Dumler JS, Bakken JS. Ehrlichial diseases of humans: emerging tick-borne infections. Clin Infect Dis 1995;20:1102–10.
4. Anderson BE, Dawson JE, Jones DC, et al. *Ehrlichia chaffeensis*, a new species associated with human ehrlichiosis. J Clin Microbiol 1991;29:2838–42.
5. Paddock CD, Liddell AM, Storch GA. Other causes of tick-borne ehrlichioses, including *Ehrlichia ewingii*. In: Goodman JL, Dennis DT, Sonenshine DE, editors. Tick-borne diseases of humans. Washington, DC: ASM Press; 2005. p. 258–67.
6. Perez M, Bodor M, Zhang C, et al. Human infection with *Ehrlichia canis* accompanied by clinical signs in Venezuela. Ann N Y Acad Sci 2006;1078:110–7.
7. Maeda K, Markowitz N, Hawley RC, et al. Human infection with *Ehrlichia canis*, a leukocytic *Rickettsia*. N Engl J Med 1987;316:853–6.
8. Buller RS, Arens M, Hmiel SP, et al. *Ehrlichia ewingii*, a newly recognized agent of human ehrlichiosis. N Engl J Med 1999;341:148–55.
9. Anderson BE, Greene CE, Jones DC, et al. *Ehrlichia ewingii* sp. nov., the etiologic agent of canine granulocytic ehrlichiosis. Int J Syst Bacteriol 1992;42: 299–302.
10. Bakken JS, Dumler JS, Chen SM, et al. Human granulocytic ehrlichiosis in the upper Midwest United States. A new species emerging? JAMA 1994;272:212–8.
11. Chen SM, Dumler JS, Bakken JS, et al. Identification of a granulocytotropic *Ehrlichia* species as the etiologic agent of human disease. J Clin Microbiol 1994;32: 589–95.
12. Pretzman C, Ralph D, Stothard DR, et al. 16S rRNA gene sequence of *Neorickettsia helminthoeca* and its phylogenetic alignment with members of the genus *Ehrlichia*. Int J Syst Bacteriol 1995;45:207–11.
13. Wen B, Rikihisa Y, Yamamoto S, et al. Characterization of the SF agent, an *Ehrlichia* sp. isolated from the fluke *Stellantchasmus falcatus*, by 16S rRNA base sequence, serological, and morphological analyses. Int J Syst Bacteriol 1996; 46:149–54.
14. Taylor MJ. *Wolbachia* endosymbiotic bacteria of filarial nematodes. A new insight into disease pathogenesis and control. Arch Med Res 2002;33:422–4.

15. Palmer GH, Brayton KA. Gene conversion is a convergent strategy for pathogen antigenic variation. Trends Parasitol 2007;23:408–13.
16. Frutos R, Viari A, Vachiery N, et al. *Ehrlichia ruminantium*: genomic and evolutionary features. Trends Parasitol 2007;23:414–9.
17. Rikihisa Y. The tribe ehrlichieae and ehrlichial diseases. Clin Microbiol Rev 1991; 4:286–308.
18. Rikihisa Y. Clinical and biological aspects of infection caused by *Ehrlichia chaffeensis*. Microbes Infect 1999;1:367–76.
19. Paddock CD, Sumner JW, Shore GM, et al. Isolation and characterization of *Ehrlichia chaffeensis* strains from patients with fatal ehrlichiosis. J Clin Microbiol 1997;35:2496–502.
20. Popov VL, Chen SM, Feng HM, et al. Ultrastructural variation of cultured *Ehrlichia chaffeensis*. J Med Microbiol 1995;43:411–21.
21. Ohashi N, Zhi N, Zhang Y, et al. Immunodominant major outer membrane proteins of *Ehrlichia chaffeensis* are encoded by a polymorphic multigene family. Infect Immun 1998;66:132–9.
22. Zhang JZ, Popov VL, Gao S, et al. The developmental cycle of *Ehrlichia chaffeensis* in vertebrate cells. Cell Microbiol 2007;9:610–8.
23. Doyle CK, Nethery KA, Popov VL, et al. Differentially expressed and secreted major immunoreactive protein orthologs of *Ehrlichia canis* and *E. chaffeensis* elicit early antibody responses to epitopes on glycosylated tandem repeats. Infect Immun 2006;74:711–20.
24. Luo T, Zhang X, Wakeel A, et al. A variable-length PCR target protein of *Ehrlichia chaffeensis* contains major species-specific antibody epitopes in acidic serine-rich tandem repeats. Infect Immun 2008;76:1572–80.
25. Wakeel A, Kuriakose JA, McBride JW. An *Ehrlichia chaffeensis* tandem repeat protein interacts with multiple host targets involved in cell signaling, transcriptional regulation, and vesicle trafficking. Infect Immun 2009;77: 1734–45.
26. Popov VL, Yu XJ, Walker DH. The 120-kDa outer membrane protein of *Ehrlichia chaffeensis*: preferential expression on dense-core cells and gene expression in *Escherichia coli* associated with attachment and entry. Microb Pathog 2000;28: 71–80.
27. Hotopp JC, Lin M, Madupu R, et al. Comparative genomics of emerging human ehrlichiosis agents. PLoS Genet 2006;2:e21.
28. Lin M, Rikihisa Y. *Ehrlichia chaffeensis* and *Anaplasma phagocytophilum* lack genes for lipid A biosynthesis and incorporate cholesterol for their survival. Infect Immun 2003;71:5324–31.
29. Xiong Q, Lin M, Rikihisa Y. Cholesterol-dependent *Anaplasma phagocytophilum* exploits the low-density lipoprotein uptake pathway. PLoS Pathog 2009;5: e1000329.
30. Mattner J, Debord KL, Ismail N, et al. Exogenous and endogenous glycolipid antigens activate NKT cells during microbial infections. Nature 2005;434: 525–9.
31. Yu XJ, Crocquet-Valdes P, Walker DH. Cloning and sequencing of the gene for a 120-kDa immunodominant protein of *Ehrlichia chaffeensis*. Gene 1997;184: 149–54.
32. Yu XJ, McBride JW, Diaz CM, et al. Molecular cloning and characterization of the 120-kilodalton protein gene of *Ehrlichia canis* and application of the recombinant 120-kilodalton protein for serodiagnosis of canine ehrlichiosis. J Clin Microbiol 2000;38:369–74.

33. Yu X, McBride JW, Zhang X, et al. Characterization of the complete transcriptionally active *Ehrlichia chaffeensis* 28 kDa outer membrane protein multigene family. Gene 2000;248:59–68.
34. Huang H, Lin M, Wang X, et al. Proteomic analysis of and immune responses to *Ehrlichia chaffeensis* lipoproteins. Infect Immun 2008;76:3405–14.
35. Park J, Choi KS, Dumler JS. Major surface protein 2 of *Anaplasma phagocytophilum* facilitates adherence to granulocytes. Infect Immun 2003;71:4018–25.
36. IJdo JW, Wu C, Telford SR, et al. Differential expression of the p44 gene family in the agent of human granulocytic ehrlichiosis. Infect Immun 2002; 70:5295–8.
37. Zhi N, Ohashi N, Rikihisa Y. Multiple p44 genes encoding major outer membrane proteins are expressed in the human granulocytic ehrlichiosis agent. J Biol Chem 1999;274:17828–36.
38. Caspersen K, Park JH, Patil S, et al. Genetic variability and stability of *Anaplasma phagocytophila* msp2(p44). Infect Immun 2002;70:1230–4.
39. Peddireddi L, Cheng C, Ganta RR. Promoter analysis of macrophage- and tick cell-specific differentially expressed *Ehrlichia chaffeensis* p28-Omp genes. BMC Microbiol 2009;9:99.
40. Ganta RR, Peddireddi L, Seo GM, et al. Molecular characterization of *Ehrlichia* interactions with tick cells and macrophages. Front Biosci 2009;14: 3259–73.
41. Ganta RR, Cheng C, Miller EC, et al. Differential clearance and immune responses to tick cell vs. macrophage culture-derived *Ehrlichia chaffeensis* in mice. Infect Immun 2006. DOI: 10.1128/IAI.01127-06.
42. Lin M, den Dulk-Ras A, Hooykaas PJ. *Anaplasma phagocytophilum* AnkA secreted by type IV secretion system is tyrosine phosphorylated by Abl-1 to facilitate infection. Cell Microbiol 2007;9:2644–57.
43. Caturegli P, Asanovich KM, Walls JJ, et al. an *Ehrlichia phagocytophila* group gene encoding a cytoplasmic protein antigen with ankyrin repeats. Infect Immun 2000;68:5277–83.
44. Park J, Kim KJ, Choi KS, et al. *Anaplasma phagocytophilum* AnkA binds to granulocyte DNA and nuclear proteins. Cell Microbiol 2004;6:743–51.
45. Christie PJ, Atmakuri K, Krishnamoorthy V, et al. Biogenesis, architecture, and function of bacterial type IV secretion systems. Annu Rev Microbiol 2005;59: 451–85.
46. Ohashi N, Zhi N, Lin Q, et al. Characterization and transcriptional analysis of gene clusters for a type IV secretion machinery in human granulocytic and monocytic ehrlichiosis agents. Infect Immun 2002;70:2128–38.
47. Dumler JS. *Anaplasma* and *Ehrlichia* infection. Ann N Y Acad Sci 2005;1063: 361–73.
48. Dumler JS, Barat NC, Barat CE, et al. Human granulocytic anaplasmosis and macrophage activation. Clin Infect Dis 2007;45:199–204.
49. Olano JP, Hogrefe W, Seaton B, et al. Clinical manifestations, epidemiology, and laboratory diagnosis of human monocytotropic ehrlichiosis in a commercial laboratory setting. Clin Diagn Lab Immunol 2003;10:891–6.
50. Olano JP, Masters E, Hogrefe W, et al. Human monocytotropic ehrlichiosis, Missouri. Emerg Infect Dis 2003;9:1579–86.
51. Peters TR, Edwards KM, Standaert SM. Severe ehrlichiosis in an adolescent taking trimethoprim-sulfamethoxazole. Pediatr Infect Dis J 2000;19:170–2.
52. Fishbein DB, Dawson JE, Robinson LE. Human ehrlichiosis in the United States, 1985–1990. Ann Intern Med 1994;120:736–43.

53. Harkess JR, Ewing SA, Crutcher JM, et al. Human ehrlichiosis in Oklahoma. J Infect Dis 1989;159:576–9.
54. Fishbein DB, Kemp A, Dawson JE, et al. Human ehrlichiosis: prospective active surveillance in febrile hospitalized patients. J Infect Dis 1989;160:803–9.
55. Carpenter CF, Gandhi TK, Kong LK, et al. The incidence of ehrlichial and rickettsial infection in patients with unexplained fever and recent history of tick bite in central North Carolina. J Infect Dis 1999;180:900–3.
56. Yevich SJ, Sanchez JL, DeFraites RF, et al. Seroepidemiology of infections due to spotted fever group rickettsiae and *Ehrlichia* species in military personnel exposed in areas of the United States where such infections are endemic. J Infect Dis 1995;171:1266–73.
57. Marshall GS, Jacobs RF, Schutze GE, et al. *Ehrlichia chaffeensis* seroprevalence among children in the southeast and south-central regions of the United States. Arch Pediatr Adolesc Med 2002;156:166–70.
58. Parola P, Davoust B, Raoult D. Tick- and flea-borne rickettsial emerging zoonoses [review]. Vet Res 2005;36:469–92.
59. Estrada-Peña A, Horak IG, Petney T. Climate changes and suitability for the ticks *Amblyomma hebraeum* and *Amblyomma variegatum* (Ixodidae) in Zimbabwe (1974–1999). Vet Parasitol 2008;151(2–4):256–67.
60. Demma LJ, Holman RC, McQuiston JH, et al. Human monocytic ehrlichiosis and human granulocytic anaplasmosis in the United States, 2001–2002. Ann N Y Acad Sci 2006;1078:118–9.
61. Anderson BE, Sims KG, Olson JG, et al. *Amblyomma americanum*: a potential vector of human ehrlichiosis. Am J Trop Med Hyg 1993;49:239–44.
62. Ewing SA, Dawson JE, Kocan AA, et al. Experimental transmission of *Ehrlichia chaffeensis* (Rickettsiales: Ehrlichieae) among white-tailed deer by *Amblyomma americanum* (Acari: Ixodidae). J Med Entomol 1995;32:368–74.
63. Lockhart JM, Davidson WR, Stallknecht DE, et al. Site-specific geographic *association between Amblyomma americanum* (Acari: Ixodidae) infestations and *Ehrlichia chaffeensis*-reactive (Rickettsiales: Ehrlichieae) antibodies in white-tailed deer. J Med Entomol 1996;33:153–8.
64. Lockhart JM, Davidson WR, Dawson JE, et al. Temporal association of *Amblyomma americanum* with the presence of *Ehrlichia chaffeensis* reactive antibodies in white-tailed deer. J Wildl Dis 1995;31:119–24.
65. Belongia EA. Epidemiology and impact of coinfections acquired from *Ixodes* ticks. Vector Borne Zoonotic Dis 2002;2:265–73.
66. MacLeod JR, Gordon WS. Studies in tick-borne fever of sheep. I. Transmission by the tick, *Ixodes ricinus*, with a description of the disease produced. Parasitology 1933;25:273–85.
67. Cao WC, Gao YM, Zhang PH, et al. Identification of *Ehrlichia chaffeensis* by nested PCR in ticks from Southern China. J Clin Microbiol 2000;38:2778–80.
68. Sexton DJ, Corey GR, Carpenter C, et al. Dual infection with *Ehrlichia chaffeensis* and a spotted fever group *Rickettsia*: a case report. Emerg Infect Dis 1998;4:311–6.
69. Walls JJ, Greig B, Neitzel DF, et al. Natural infection of small mammal species in Minnesota with the agent of human granulocytic ehrlichiosis. J Clin Microbiol 1997;35:853–5.
70. Chapman AS, Bakken JS, Folk SM, et al. Diagnosis and management of tick-borne rickettsial diseases: Rocky Mountain spotted fever, ehrlichioses, and anaplasmosis—United States: a practical guide for physicians and other

health-care and public health professionals. MMWR Recomm Rep 2006; 55(RR-4):1–27.

71. Bakken JS, Dumler JS. Human granulocytic ehrlichiosis. Clin Infect Dis 2000;31: 554–60.
72. Bakken JS, Krueth J, Wilson-Nordskog C, et al. Clinical and laboratory characteristics of human granulocytic ehrlichiosis. JAMA 1996;275:199–205.
73. Bakken JS, Dumler JS. Ehrlichiosis and anaplasmosis. Infect Med 2004;21: 433–51.
74. Nadelman RB, Horowitz HW, Hsieh T-C, et al. Simultaneous human granulocytic ehrlichiosis and Lyme borreliosis. N Engl J Med 1997;337:27–30.
75. Thomas LD, Hongo I, Bloch KC, et al. Human ehrlichiosis in transplant recipients. Am J Transplant 2007;7:1641–7.
76. Fichtenbaum CJ, Peterson LR, Weil GJ. Ehrlichiosis presenting as a life-threatening illness with features of the toxic shock syndrome. Am J Med 1993;95:351–7.
77. Walker DH, Dumler JS. Human monocytic and granulocytic ehrlichioses discovery and diagnosis of emerging tick-borne infections and the critical role of the pathologist. Arch Pathol Lab Med 1997;121:785–91.
78. Sehdev AE, Dumler JS. Hepatic pathology in human monocytic ehrlichiosis. *Ehrlichia chaffeensis* infection. Am J Clin Pathol 2003;119:859–65.
79. Marty AM, Dumler JS, Imes G, et al. Ehrlichiosis mimicking thrombotic thrombocytopenic purpura. Case report and pathological correlation. Hum Pathol 1995; 26:920–5.
80. Ratnasamy N, Everett ED, Roland WE, et al. Central nervous system manifestations of human ehrlichiosis. Clin Infect Dis 1996;23:314–9.
81. Brantley RK. Trimethoprim-sulfamethoxazole and fulminant ehrlichiosis [letter]. Pediatr Infect Dis J 2001;20:231.
82. Paddock CD, Folk SM, Shore GM, et al. Infections with *Ehrlichia chaffeensis* and *Ehrlichia ewingii* in persons coinfected with human immunodeficiency virus. Clin Infect Dis 2001;33:1586–94.
83. Everett ED, Evans KA, Henry RB, et al. Human ehrlichiosis in adults after tick exposure: diagnosis using polymerase chain reaction. Ann Intern Med 1994; 120:730–5.
84. Harkess JR. Ehrlichiosis. Infect Dis Clin North Am 1991;5:37–51.
85. Walker DH, Raoult D. *Rickettsia rickettsii* and other spotted fever group rickettsiae (Rocky Mountain spotted fever and other spotted fevers). In: Mandell GL, Bennett JE, Dolin R, editors. Mandell, Douglas, and Bennett's principles and practice of infectious diseases. 6th edition. Philadelphia: Churchill Livingstone; 2005. p. 2287–95.
86. Horowitz HW, Marks SJ, Weintraub M, et al. Brachial plexopathy associated with human granulocytic ehrlichiosis. Neurology 1996;46:1026–9.
87. Dumler JS, Madigan JE, Pusterla N, et al. Ehrlichioses in humans: epidemiology, clinical presentation, diagnosis, and treatment. Clin Infect Dis 2007;4:S45–51.
88. Rikihisa Y. *Ehrlichia* subversion of host innate responses. Curr Opin Microbiol 2006;9:95–101.
89. Lin M, Rikihisa Y. *Ehrlichia chaffeensis* downregulates surface toll-like receptors 2/4, CD14 and transcription factors PU.1 and inhibits lipopolysaccharide activation of NF-kB, ERK 1/2 and p38 MAPK in host monocytes. Cell Microbiol 2004;6: 175–86.
90. Zhang JZ, Sinha M, Luxon BA, et al. Survival strategy of obligately intracellular *Ehrlichia chaffeensis*: novel modulation of immune response and host cell cycles. Infect Immun 2004;72:498–507.

91. Mavromatis K, Doyle CK, Lykidis A, et al. The genome of the obligately intracellular bacterium *Ehrlichia canis* reveals themes of complex membrane structure and immune evasion strategies. J Bacteriol 2006;188:4015–23.
92. Stevenson H, Walker DH, Ismail N. Regulatory role of CD1d-restricted NKT cells in the induction of toxic shock-like syndrome in an animal model of fatal ehrlichiosis. Infect Immun 2008;76:1434–44.
93. Dumler JS, Brouqui P, Aronson J, et al. Identification of *Ehrlichia* in human tissue. N Engl J Med 1991;325:1109–10.
94. Dumler JS, Sutker WL, Walker DH. Persistent infection with *Ehrlichia chaffeensis*. Clin Infect Dis 1993;17:903–5.
95. Schutze GE, Buckingham SC, Marshall GS, et al. Human monocytic ehrlichiosis in children. Pediatr Infect Dis J 2007;26:475–9.
96. Shibata S, Kawahara M, Rikihisa Y, et al. New *Ehrlichia* species closely related to *Ehrlichia chaffeensis* isolated from *Ixodes ovatus* ticks in Japan. J Clin Microbiol 2000;38:1331–8.
97. Sotomayor E, Popov V, Feng HM, et al. Animal model of fatal human monocytotropic ehrlichiosis. Am J Pathol 2001;158:757–69.
98. Ismail N, Soong L, McBride JW, et al. Overproduction of TNF-a by CD8$^+$ type 1 cells and down-regulation of IFN-g production by CD4$^+$ Th1 cells contribute to toxic shock-like syndrome in an animal model of fatal monocytotropic ehrlichiosis. J Immunol 2004;172:1786–800.
99. Ismail N, Stevenson HL, Walker DH. Role of tumor necrosis factor alpha (TNF-alpha) and interleukin-10 in the pathogenesis of severe murine monocytotropic ehrlichiosis: increased resistance of TNF receptor p55- and p75-deficient mice to fatal ehrlichial infection. Infect Immun 2006;74:1846–56.
100. Ismail N, Crossley EC, Stevenson HL, et al. The relative importance of T cell subsets in monocytotropic ehrlichiosis: a novel effector mechanism involved in *Ehrlichia*-induced immunopathology in murine ehrlichiosis. Infect Immun 2007;75:4608–20.
101. Stevenson HL, Jordan JM, Peerwani Z, et al. An intradermal environment promotes a protective type-1 response against lethal systemic monocytotropic ehrlichial infection. Infect Immun 2006;74:4856–64.
102. Dierberg KL, Dumler JS. Lymph node hemophagocytosis in rickettsial diseases: a pathogenetic role for CD8 T lymphocytes in human monocytic ehrlichiosis (HME)? BMC Infect Dis 2006;6:121.
103. Klein MB, Miller JS, Nelson CM, et al. Primary bone marrow progenitors of both granulocytic and monocytic lineages are susceptible to infection with the agent of human granulocytic ehrlichiosis. J Infect Dis 1997;176:1405–9.
104. Yoshiie K, Kim HY, Mott J, et al. Intracellular infection by the human granulocytic ehrlichiosis agent inhibits human neutrophil apoptosis. Infect Immun 2000;68:1125–33.
105. Herron MJ, Nelson CM, Larson J, et al. Intracellular parasitism by the human granulocytic ehrlichiosis bacterium through the P-selectin ligand, PSGL-1. Science 2000;288:1653–6.
106. Carlyon JA, Chan WT, Galan J, et al. Repression of rac2 mRNA expression by *Anaplasma phagocytophila* is essential to the inhibition of superoxide production and bacterial proliferation. J Immunol 2002;169:7009–18.
107. Webster P, Ijdo JW, Chicoine LM, et al. The agent of human granulocytic ehrlichiosis resides in an endosomal compartment. J Clin Invest 1998;101:1932–41.
108. Banerjee R, Anguita J, Roos D, et al. Cutting edge: infection by the agent of human granulocytic ehrlichiosis prevents the respiratory burst by down-regulating gp91phox. J Immunol 2000;164:3946–9.

109. Choi KS, Garyu J, Park J, et al. Diminished adhesion of *Anaplasma phagocyto-philum*-infected neutrophils to endothelial cells is associated with reduced expression of leukocyte surface selectin. Infect Immun 2003;71:4586–94.

110. Choi KS, Webb T, Oelke M, et al. Differential innate immune cell activation and proinflammatory response in *Anaplasma phagocytophilum* infection. Infect Immun 2007;75:3124–30.

111. Klein MB, Hu S, Chao CC, et al. The agent of human granulocytic ehrlichiosis induces the production of myelosuppressing chemokines without induction of proinflammatory cytokines. J Infect Dis 2000;182:200–5.

112. Paddock CD, Childs JE. *Ehrlichia chaffeensis*: a prototypical emerging path-ogen. Clin Microbiol Rev 2003;16:37–64.

113. Caldwell CW, Everett ED, McDonald G, et al. Lymphocytosis of gamma/delta T cells in human ehrlichiosis. Am J Clin Pathol 1995;103:761–6.

114. Bitsaktsis C, Huntington J, Winslow G. Production of IFN-gamma by CD4 T cells is essential for resolving *Ehrlichia* infection. J Immunol 2004;172:6894–901.

115. Bitsaktsis C, Nandi B, Racine R, et al. T-cell-independent humoral immunity is sufficient for protection against fatal intracellular *Ehrlichia* infection. Infect Immun 2007;75:4933–41.

116. Bitsaktsis C, Winslow G. Fatal recall responses mediated by CD8 T cells during intracellular bacterial challenge infection. J Immunol 2006;177:4644–51.

117. Winslow GM, Yager E, Shilo K, et al. Antibody-mediated elimination of the obli-gate intracellular bacterial pathogen *Ehrlichia chaffeensis* during active infec-tion. Infect Immun 2000;68:2187–95.

118. Yager E, Bitsaktsis C, Nandi B, et al. Essential role for humoral immunity during *Ehrlichia* infection in immunocompetent mice. Infect Immun 2005;73:8009–16.

119. Liddell AM, Sumner JW, Paddock CD, et al. Reinfection with *Ehrlichia chaffeen-sis* in a liver transplant recipient. Clin Infect Dis 2002;34:1644–7.

120. Thirumalapura NR, Stevenson HL, Walker DH, et al. Protective heterologous immunity against fatal ehrlichiosis and lack of protection following homologous challenge. Infect Immun 2008;76:1920–30.

121. Paddock CD, Suchard DP, Grumbach KL, et al. Brief report: fatal seronegative ehrlichiosis in a patient with HIV infection. N Engl J Med 1993;329:1164–7.

122. Walker DH. Diagnosing human ehrlichioses: current status and recommenda-tions. ASM News 2000;66:287–91.

123. Childs JE, Sumner JW, Nicholson WL, et al. Outcome of diagnostic tests using samples from patients with culture-proven human monocytic ehrlichiosis: impli-cations for surveillance. J Clin Microbiol 1999;37:2997–3000.

124. Childs JE, McQuiston JH, Sumner JW, et al. Human monocytic ehrlichiosis due to *Ehrlichia chaffeensis*: how do we count the cases? In: Raoult D, Brouqui P, editors. Rickettsiae and rickettsial diseases at the turn of the third millennium. Paris: Elsevier; 1999. p. 287–93.

125. Standaert SM, Yu T, Scott MA, et al. Primary isolation of *Ehrlichia chaffeensis* from patients with febrile illnesses: clinical and molecular characteristics. J Infect Dis 2000;181:1082–8.

126. Tan HP, Dumler JS, Maley WR, et al. Human monocytic ehrlichiosis: an emerging pathogen in transplantation. Transplantation 2001;71:1678–80.

127. Anderson BE, Sumner JW, Dawson JE, et al. Detection of the etiologic agent of human ehrlichiosis by polymerase chain reaction. J Clin Microbiol 1992;30:775–80.

128. Doyle CK, Labruna MB, Breitschwerdt EB, et al. Detection of medically impor-tant *Ehrlichia* by quantitative multicolor TaqMan real-time polymerase chain reaction of the dsb gene. J Mol Diagn 2005;7:504–10.

129. Sumner JW, Nicholson WL, Massung RF. PCR amplification and comparison of nucleotide sequences from the groESL heat shock operon of *Ehrlichia* species. J Clin Microbiol 1997;35:2087–92.
130. Sumner JW, Childs JE, Paddock CD. Molecular cloning and characterization of the *Ehrlichia chaffeensis* variable-length PCR target: an antigen-expressing gene that exhibits interstrain variation. J Clin Microbiol 1999;37:1447–53.
131. Bakken JS, Dumler JS. *Ehrlichia* species. In: Yu VL, Merigan TC Jr, Barriere SL, editors. Antimicrobial therapy and vaccines. Baltimore (MD): The Williams & Wilkins Co; 1999. p. 546–54.
132. American Academy of Pediatrics. *Ehrlichia* infections (human ehrlichioses). In: Pickering LK, Baker CJ, Overturf GD, et al, editors. 2003 Red book: report of the committee on infectious diseases. 26th edition. Elk Grove Village (IL): American Academy of Pediatrics, Committee on Infectious Diseases; 2003. p. 266–9.
133. Walker DH, Sexton DJ. *Rickettsia rickettsii*. In: Yu VL, Merigan TC Jr, Barriere SL, editors. Antimicrobial therapy and vaccines. Baltimore (MD): Williams & Wilkins; 1999. p. 562–8.
134. Smith Sendev AE, Sehdev PS, Jacobs R, et al. Human monocytic ehrlichiosis presenting as acute appendicitis during pregnancy. Clin Infect Dis 2002;35: e99–102.
135. Buitrago MI, IJdo JW, Rinaudo P, et al. Human granulocytic ehrlichiosis during pregnancy treated successfully with rifampin. Clin Infect Dis 1998;27:213–6.
136. Hongo I, Bloch KC. *Ehrlichia* infection of the central nervous system. Curr Treat Options Neurol 2006;8:179–84.
137. Klein MB, Nelson CM, Goodman JL. Antibiotic susceptibility of the newly cultivated agent of human granulocytic ehrlichiosis: promising activity of quinolones and rifamycins. Antimicrob Agents Chemother 1997;41:76–9.
138. Wormser GP, Dattwyler RJ, Shapiro ED, et al. The clinical assessment, treatment, and prevention of Lyme disease, human granulocytic anaplasmosis, and babesiosis: clinical practice guidelines by the Infectious Diseases Society of America. Clin Infect Dis 2006;43:1089–134.
139. Katavolos P, Armstrong PM, Dawson JE, et al. Duration of tick attachment required for transmission of granulocytic ehrlichiosis. J Infect Dis 1998;177: 1422–5.
140. des Vignes F, Piesman J, Heffernan R, et al. Effect of tick removal on transmission of *Borrelia burgdorferi* and *Ehrlichia phagocytophila* by *Ixodes scapularis* nymphs. J Infect Dis 2001;183:773–8.
141. Needham GR. Evaluation of five popular methods of tick removal. Pediatrics 1985;75:997–1002.

Prion Diseases

Sriram Venneti, MD, PhD

KEYWORDS
- Creutzfeldt-Jakob disease • Prion diseases
- Rapidly progressive dementia
- Transmissible spongiform encephalopathies

Prion diseases are disorders affecting the central nervous system caused by alterations in the conformation of the cellular prion protein. They can be sporadic, hereditary, or acquired and usually present with myoclonus and rapidly progressive dementia in human patients. This article discusses the epidemiology, pathogenesis, diagnosis, and laboratory testing of prion diseases with a primary focus on Creutzfeldt-Jakob disease (CJD).

DISCUSSION

Prion diseases are a group of neurologic disorders caused by alterations in the conformation of prion proteins resulting in fatal neurodegeneration.[1] They are also referred to as "transmissible spongiform encephalopathies" because of the infectious nature of disease and the characteristic spongiform degeneration in the brain. Prion diseases that affect humans are listed in **Table 1**. CJD is the prototype prion disease and can be sporadic (sCJD), familial (fCJD), acquired through iatrogenic sources (iCJD), or by ingestion of contaminated meat from infected cows (variant form [vCJD]).[2] Other prion diseases include kuru, Gerstmann-Straussler-Scheinker (GSS), and fatal familial insomnia (FFI).[1] Kuru is a disease of historical importance and was noted in the tribes of New Guinea caused by ingestion of the brains of the deceased as a part of funeral rituals.[3] Prion diseases also occur naturally in animals (**Table 2**).[4] Of the animal diseases, bovine spongiform encephalopathy (BSE) is the only disease conclusively transmitted to humans to date resulting in vCJD.[4]

MICROBIOLOGY

The term "prion" stands for "*p*roteinatious *in*fectious particle that lacks *n*ucleic acid." This term was coined by Stanley Prusiner[5] to reflect the unique biology of this disease in that the "infectious agent" is a protein and unlike viruses without nucleic acids (also

Division of Neuropathology, Department of Pathology and Laboratory Medicine, Hospital of the University of Pennsylvania, 3400 Spruce Street, 6.093 Founders Building, Philadelphia, PA 19104, USA
E-mail address: Sriram.Venneti@uphs.upenn.edu

Clin Lab Med 30 (2010) 293–309
doi:10.1016/j.cll.2009.11.002
0272-2712/10/$ – see front matter © 2010 Elsevier Inc. All rights reserved.
labmed.theclinics.com

Table 1
Prion diseases in humans

Year of Description	Clinical Illness	Mode of Disease
1920	Creutzfeldt-Jakob disease	Familial, sporadic, and transmitted (mainly iatrogenic)
1928	Gerstmann-Straussler-Scheinker	Familial, genetic
1941	Kuru	Transmitted
1986	Fatal familial insomnia	Familial, genetic
1995	New variant of Creutzfeldt-Jakob disease	Transmitted

referred to as the "protein only" hypothesis). The complex pathogenesis of these disorders including transmissibility, familial, and sporadic forms of disease can be explained based on the prion hypothesis.[5] The definition of two isoforms of the prion protein is essential to understand the prion hypothesis (**Figs. 1–3**)[5]: PrP^C is the normal cellular isoform of the prion protein, predominantly α-helical in structure (see **Fig. 1**) and ubiquitously expressed but enriched in the nervous system; PrP^{Sc} is the disease-causing or transmitting isoform of the prion protein that is sporadically mutated, familialy inherited, or transmitted from a source and predominantly β-helical in structure (see **Fig. 1**).

The prion protein gene encoding PrP^C is termed $PRPN$ and is located on the short arm of chromosome 20 (see **Fig. 2**).[6] PrP^{Sc} is thought to propagate in mammals by binding to PrP^C and converting it to PrP^{Sc} by a process that is not completely understood.[5] This conversion involves the transformation of the α-helical structure of PrP^C into a β-helical structure of PrP^{Sc} and is the key event in disease initiation and progression (see **Fig. 3**).[5] The β-helical structure of PrP^{Sc} makes it resistant to proteinase K digestion and more prone to aggregate in the form of β-pleated sheets in the brain.[5,6] These aggregates are toxic to neurons resulting in irreversible neurodegeneration.[5,6]

Table 2
Prion diseases in animals

Year of Description	Animal	Disease	Known Transmission to Humans
1732	Sheep and goats	Scrapie	No
1947	Mink	Transmissible mink encephalopathy	No
1967	Elk and deer	Chronic wasting disease	No
1986	Cattle	Bovine spongiform encephalopathy	Yes
1986	Antelopes, bison	Exotic ungulate spongiform encephalopathy	No
1990	Domestic cats and captive large cats	Feline spongiform encephalopathy	No
1996	Captive nonhuman primates	Zoo primate spongiform encephalopathy	No

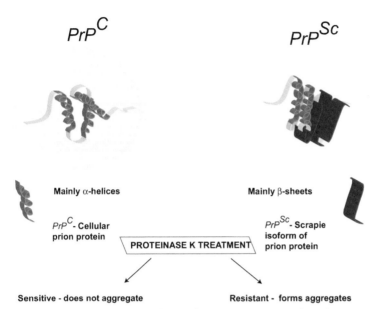

PrP^C

PrP^{Sc}

Mainly α-helices

PrP^C- Cellular
prion protein

PROTEINASE K TREATMENT

Mainly β-sheets

PrP^{Sc}- Scrapie
isoform of
prion protein

Sensitive - does not aggregate

Resistant - forms aggregates

Fig. 1. Normal and disease-related isoforms of the prion protein. The prion protein in its native configuration is designated PrP^C (cellular prion protein). PrP^{Sc} (SC stands for "scrapie" isoform) is the disease-related isoform of the prion protein. The polypeptide chains of PrP^C and PrP^{Sc} are identical in composition but differ in three-dimensional structure. The structure of PrP^C is predominantly α-helical (*blue coils*). PrP^C does not form aggregates and is readily degraded by proteinase K. The tertiary structure of PrP^{Sc} is predominantly β-helical (*red sheets*), which makes it prone to aggregation and resistant to proteinase K treatment.

Prion diseases are unique in that the infectious agent is devoid of nucleic acids and encoded by a host chromosomal gene. Although PrP^{Sc} is predominantly β-helical, PrP^{Sc} can exist in a variety of conformations, each of which is associated with a specific disease. How a specific disease-associated PrP^{Sc} conformation is imparted to the nascent PrP^C or how each of the prion diseases is caused by a specific PrP^{Sc} conformation is not understood.[5] Further, tertiary and quaternary structures of PrP^{Sc} are hypothesized to influence the rapidity of disease development and the distribution of neuropathology in the brain leading investigators to postulate that the PrP^{Sc} may carry strain-specific information.[7]

EPIDEMIOLOGY

CJD is the most common of all the prion diseases and can be classified into sporadic, iatrogenic, familial, and variant forms depending on the cause of disease (**Fig. 4**). sCJD represents approximately 85% of all human prion diseases (the rare diseases FFI and GSS constitutive approximately 1%).[8] Sporadic disease is a defined by ruling out detectable infectious and familial causes. sCJD presents with an annual incidence of one case per million people and is responsible for 1 in every 10,000 deaths. sCJD is found worldwide and is a disease of older ages (median age 68 years) affecting males and females equally.[8] fCJD constitutes 10% to 15% of all prion disease and is caused by inherited mutations in the prion protein gene.[8]

The transmissible forms of CJD are vCJD and iCJD and constitute less than 5% of all prion diseases (see **Fig. 4**).[8] In 1995 a new form of CJD began to appear in the

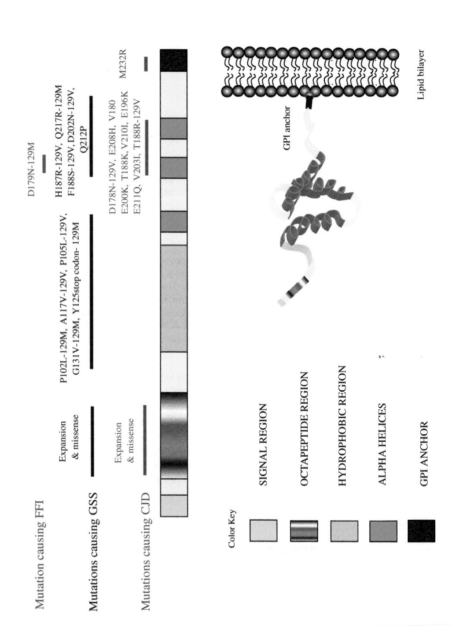

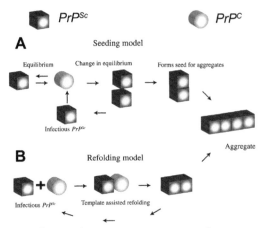

Fig. 3. Conversion of PrP^C to PrP^{Sc}. The conversion of PrP^C (*spheres*) to PrP^{Sc} (*cubes*) is a complex phenomenon that is not entirely understood. Two main theories are proposed to explain how this conversion occurs. The first is the seeding model (*A*), which proposes that the conversion of PrP^C to PrP^{Sc} is a reversible process with an equilibrium favoring PrP^C under normal circumstances. With the introduction of infectious PrP^{Sc}, this equilibrium is altered favoring the PrP^{Sc} conformation. PrP^{Sc} then forms "seeds" causing further conversion of endogenous PrP^C to PrP^{Sc} leading to the formation of aggregates. An alternate theory is the refolding model (*B*) wherein infectious PrP^{Sc} recruits and converts PrP^C to PrP^{Sc} using its β-helical confirmation as a template. The converted PrP^{Sc} recruits more PrP^C creating a vicious cycle leading to PrP^{Sc} aggregation. (*Adapted from* Aguzzi A, Montrasio F, Kaeser PS. Prions: health scare and biological challenge. Nat Rev Mol Cell Biol 2001;2:118–26; with permission.)

United Kingdom. This disease affected younger age groups (median age 28 years) compared with the classic sCJD and was termed "new variant CJD."[2,9] Evidence from epidemiologic, pathologic, and biochemical studies strongly suggested that this form of CJD is caused by human consumption of cattle products derived from animals infected with BSE.[2,6,9] vCJD has killed more than 200 people worldwide (**Fig. 5**). Three cases of documented vCJD are reported in the United States as of June 2008 (**Fig. 6A**). Two of these cases can be traced to previous residents of the United Kingdom and the third to a previous resident from Saudi Arabia (from the Center for Disease and Control http://www.cdc.gov/ncidod/dvrd/vcjd and the National Prion Disease Pathology Surveillance Center http://www.cjdsurveillance.com). vCJD peaked in the United Kingdom during the years 2000 to 2003 and shows declining incidence possibly because of public health measures taken to prevent contaminated food products from entering the human food chain (**Fig. 6B**).

Fig. 2. Illustration of the normal structure of PrP^C. The mature human PrP^C protein contains 208 amino acids. At the extreme N-terminus is a signal peptide (*green*). Missense mutations and expansions in the octapeptide region (*gray striped*) result in familial forms of CJD (fCJD) and GSS. A hydrophobic core (*orange*) and three α-helices (*blue*) are present. A glycosyl-phosphatidylinositol anchor (GPI) (*purple*) is attached to the C-terminus of PrP^C that helps link (*red sphere*) it to the extracellular membrane (lipid bilayer). Mutations in the various domains resulting in fCJD (*red*), GSS (*blue*), and FFI (*green*) are indicated above. (*Adapted from* Aguzzi A, Montrasio, Kaeser PS. Prions: health scare and biological challenge. Nat Rev Mol Cell Biol 2001;2:118–26; with permission.)

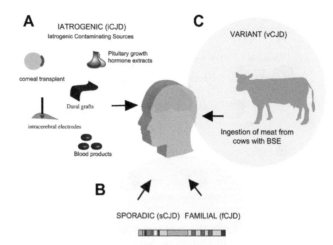

Fig. 4. Forms of CJD. CJD can be classified into four different groups based on etiology. The sporadic form of CJD (sCJD) accounts for more than 85% of all human prion diseases and is defined by exclusion of detectable infectious and familial causes (4B). Familial CJD (fCJD) caused by inherited mutations in the prion protein gene constitutes 10% of all prion disease (4B). The most common mutation is a change from glutamic acid to lysine at position 200 (E200K). The transmissible forms of CJD include iatrogenic CJD (iCJD, 6A) and the variant form of CJD (vCJD, 6C), which together constitute less than 5% of all prion diseases. iCJD (6A) is caused when *PrP*^Sc contaminated human tissue is introduced into patients by blood products, corneal transplants, dural grafts, intracerebral electrodes, and cadaveric human growth hormone. vCJD (6C) develops as a result of the consumption of meat derived from cows with bovine spongiform encephalopathy (BSE).

iCJD is relatively rare and is caused by the introduction of *PrP*^Sc in contaminated human tissue, such as blood products; corneal transplants; dural grafts; intracerebral electrodes; and cadaveric human growth hormone (now replaced by recombinant human growth hormone).[10] Kuru is a historical disease that was caused by ritualistic ingestion of brain tissue noted among the tribes of New Guinea.[3] Kuru has disappeared following cessation of ritualistic cannibalism.[3]

CLINICAL PRESENTATION

The clinical presentation of prion diseases in humans depends on the specific disease entity. The major clinical symptoms in each of these diseases are summarized in **Table 3**. The clinical presentation of CJD is discussed in more detail.

CJD usually begins with nonspecific prodromal symptoms that span several weeks to months, such as fatigue, headache, changes in appetite and sleep, weight loss, and depression.[11–13] Patients in early stages may show changes in behavioral and emotional affect, delusions and hallucinations, memory loss, visual disturbances, and ataxia.[11–13] The disease usually progresses rapidly with development of dementia and a characteristic myoclonic contraction that may be first evident as a striking startle response. The time from onset of disease to death is variable and ranges from 2 to 10 years. In approximately 10% of patients rapid progression in a matter of weeks may be seen.[11–13] Clinical distinction between sCJD and vCJD is of importance because the

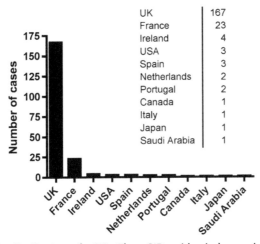

UK	167
France	23
Ireland	4
USA	3
Spain	3
Netherlands	2
Portugal	2
Canada	1
Italy	1
Japan	1
Saudi Arabia	1

Fig. 5. World-wide distribution of vCJD. The vCJD epidemic began in 1995 and mainly involves the United Kingdom and France. The Centers for Disease Control and Prevention reports three confirmed cases in the United States as of June 2008. Two of these cases were previous residents of the United Kingdom and the third was a previous resident of Saudi Arabia. (*Data from* the Centers for Disease Control and Prevention. Available at: http://www.cdc.gov/ncidod/dvrd/cjd.)

diagnosis of vCJD carries far greater public health implications. Although clinical spectra largely overlap and the two entities may not be entirely distinguishable until autopsy, some features may enable differentiating between sCJD and vCJD (**Table 4**).[14]

PATHOGENESIS

The pathogenesis of prion disease is variable and includes inheritable, sporadic, and transmitted causes (see **Table 3**). Although CJD and GSS have both sporadic and familial forms, FFI is familial and is caused by the D178N mutation.[8] The familial forms of all prion diseases (fCJD, GSS, and FFI) are inherited as autosomal-dominant disorders.[8] Polymorphisms at codon 129 of PRNP gene with either methionine or valine determine susceptibility and phenotypic expression of development of specific clinical forms of prion diseases. Homozygosity for methionine at position 129 (met/met at codon 129) predisposes to susceptibility and earlier age of onset of disease.[8,15] Further, the methionine or valine polymorphisms at codon 129 and protease resistance of PrP^{Sc} have been used to molecularly classify the disease variants of sCJD.[16]

The transmissible prion diseases are kuru, vCJD, and iCJD. vCJD is caused by the ingestion of contaminated meat derived from cows with BSE. PrP^{Sc} survives digestion and is hypothesized to be amplified by follicular dendritic cells and tingible body macrophages in gut-associated lymphatic tissue, such as Peyer patches (**Fig. 7**).[17] PrP^{Sc} eventually reaches draining lymphatics and the spleen by migrating follicular dendritic cells (see **Fig. 7**).[17] PrP^{Sc} is hypothesized to reach the brain by the sympathetic nervous system from lymphatic tissues (see **Fig. 7**).[17] PrP^{Sc} propagation in the brain causes it to accumulate and result in neurodegeneration.[18]

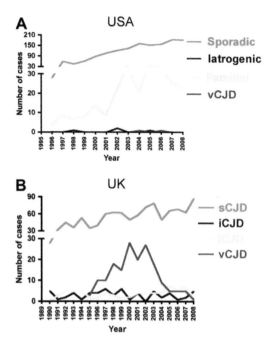

Fig. 6. Prion disease distribution in the United Kingdom and United States. (*A*) The distribution of all reported prion diseases (all forms of CJD, GSS, and FFI) in the United States from 1996 to 2008. Sporadic disease (*green*) represented 85% of all cases. Familial (*yellow*) and iatrogenic (*blue*) forms of disease represented 14.7% and 0.2% of all prion diseases, respectively. vCJD (*red*) was 0.1% of all cases (see **Fig. 5A**). (*Data from* National Prion Disease Pathology Surveillance Center. Available at: http://www.cjdsurveillance.com.) (*B*) Examining the various types of CJD reported in the United Kingdom best illustrates the epidemiology of CJD. sCJD (*green*) was the most prevalent disease representing approximately 78% of all CJD cases from 1989 to 2008. fCJD was 5%, iCJD was 4%, and vCJD was 13% of all CJD cases in this time period. (*Data from* The National Creutzfeldt-Jakob Disease Surveillance Unit. Available at: http://www.cjd.ed.ac.uk.) The trends in vCJD (*red*) between the two countries are of interest. vCJD peaked in 2000 and 2002 in the United Kingdom and two cases were reported each in 2004 and 2006 in the United States. The declining trend in vCJD in the United Kingdom is possibly reflective of stringent public health measures taken to prevent contaminated food products from entering the human food chain.

On autopsy the brain shows no gross abnormalities to cerebral atrophy in long-standing cases. The histopathologic features are striking and constitute the triad of spongiform degeneration (hence the name "[transmissible] spongiform encephalopathy"); loss of neurons; and gliosis (**Fig. 8A–D**).[5,19] An inflammatory response is conspicuously absent. Spongiform degeneration of the brain is characterized by the presence of many vacuoles ranging in size from 1 to 5 mm.[20] These changes are prominent in the basal ganglia, thalamus, cerebellum, and cortex.[5] Astrogliosis, although not specific to prion diseases, is always present and can be highlighted by an immunohistochemical stain for glial filament acidic protein (**Fig. 8E, F**). PrP^{Sc} accumulation in the form of β-sheets may lead to the formation of PrP amyloid plaques in approximately 10% of sCJD cases.[5] Immunostaining with antibodies against the prion protein can be used to highlight plaques (**Fig. 9**). Absence of staining

Table 3
Prion diseases in humans

Clinical Illness	Main Clinical Symptoms	Specific Feature
Kuru	Progressive tremors and ataxia	New Guinea tribes; ritualistic ingestion of brain tissue
Creutzfeldt-Jakob disease	Dementia and myoclonic jerking	Familial: autosomal-dominant Iatrogenic: accidental exposure to contaminated human tissues Sporadic New variant of CJD (vCJD) - Ingestion of contaminated meat from animals with BSE.
Gerstmann-Straussler-Scheinker	Cerebellar ataxia and spastic paraparesis	Sporadic Familial-genetic Autosomal dominant
Fatal familial insomnia	Progressive insomnia, autonomic dysfunction and dementia	Familial-genetic: autosomal-dominant

does not rule out the diagnosis of CJD.[5] Florid amyloid plaques are more abundant in vCJD compared with sCJD and show distinct morphologic features characterized by a dense central core of amyloid surrounded by vacuoles (flowerlike), illustrated in **Fig. 10.**[5,14]

DIAGNOSIS

The main diagnostic criteria for all forms of CJD are listed in **Table 5**.[13] The clinical diagnosis of prion diseases centers on the recognition of the group of major clinical characteristics (see **Table 4**). The clinical presentation of rapidly progressive dementia along with ataxia and myoclonus triggers a high suspicion of CJD and should prompt more detailed brain imaging, cerebrospinal fluid (CSF), and electroencephalogram studies.[12,13] Routine laboratory tests including CSF studies are within normal limits in prion diseases and any elevation of general indices, such as white blood cell counts, erythrocyte sedimentation rates, or CSF pleiocytosis should favor other etiologies.[12,13] CT scans of the brain may be nonspecific and relatively insensitive. MRI studies are more meaningful in the right clinical context and 70% to 90% of patients show cortical ribboning and/or increased intensity in the putamen and caudate nuclei on fluid-attenuated inversion-recovery sequences and diffusion-weighted MRI.[12,13] CSF may show increases in levels of the protein 14-3-3.[12,13] The electroencephalogram may be more valuable with the presence of characteristic high-voltage triphasic complexes. These changes are noted in only 60% of patients, however, and may not be present until more advanced stages of disease.[12,13] A definitive diagnosis of prion disease in the living subject is made only on a brain biopsy (or tonsil biopsy for vCJD).[12,13] In the United States all confirmed cases of CJD (and other prion diseases) must be reported to the Centers for Disease Control and Prevention and state health department. The International Classification of Diseases has classified prion diseases under the subheading of "slow virus infection and prion diseases of central nervous system" (code 046).

Table 4
Clinical features that distinguish vCJD from sCJD

Characteristic	Main Feature	sCJD	vCJD
Clinical features	Median age	68 y	28 y
	Median duration of illness	4 mo	13 mo
	Symptoms and signs	Dementia; early neurologic signs	Behavioral abnormalities, sensory symptoms and delayed neurologic signs
Clinical tests	Periodic triphasic sharp waves on electroencephalogram	Often present	Often absent
	Hyperintensity in posterior thalamus (pulvinar) in relation to the anterior putamen on brain imaging; called the "pulvinar sign"	Often absent	Present in >75% of cases
Laboratory tests	Presence of florid plaques on brain tissues including biopsy	Rare or absent	Present
	Immunohistochemistry for PrP^{Sc} in brain tissues	Variable accumulation	Marked accumulation of PrP^{Sc}
	Detectable PrP^{Sc} in lymphoid tissue including tonisillar biopsy	Not readily detected	Readily detected
	Codon 129 geneotype	Usually Met/Met	Polymorphism may be absent

Adapted from Belay E, Schonberger L. Variant Creutzfeldt-Jakob disease and bovine spongiform encephalopathy. Clin Lab Med 2002;22:849–62; with permission.

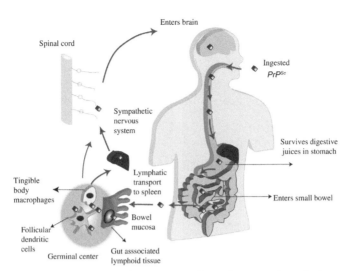

Fig. 7. Hypothesized mechanism of prion entry from the gastrointestinal tract into the nervous system. The exact process of entry of ingested PrP^{Sc} (*diamond*) from contaminated foods into the nervous system is not known. Recent studies have suggested that the immune system plays an important role. PrP^{Sc} survives digestive enzymes of the gastrointestinal tract and is taken up by gut-related lymphoid tissue, such as Peyer patches. Both follicular dendritic cells and tingible body macrophages present in germinal centers are thought to play a role in propagation of PrP^{Sc} in gut-associated lymphoid tissues. PrP^{Sc} is hypothesized to be taken up by the sympathetic nervous system either directly from these lymphoid tissues or after transport to the spleen. PrP^{Sc} may also be transported to draining lymph nodes and to more remote regions, such as the tonsils, by lymphatics (not illustrated). PrP^{Sc} is proposed to reach the brain by transport along the sympathetic nervous system.

DIFFERENTIAL DIAGNOSIS

Differential diagnosis of prion diseases includes a wide spectrum of neurologic disorders that may present with rapidly progressive dementia. Neurodegenerative disorders, such as Alzheimer's disease, dementia with Lewy bodies, frontotemporal dementias, corticobasal degeneration, and progressive supranuclear palsy, are high on the differential diagnosis.[12,13] These conditions may manifest with rapidly progressive dementia (usually slow progression) and overlapping clinical features, such as psychiatric, movement, behavioral, and cognitive abnormalities.[12,13] Depending on the clinical context several other neurologic conditions should also be considered, and Geschwind and colleagues[12,13] have organized these under the following subgroups: neurodegenerative, infectious, toxic and metabolic, autoimmune, vascular, and neoplastic conditions (**Table 6**). The diagnostic algorithm proposed by these authors is illustrated in **Fig. 11**.

THERAPY, PROGNOSIS, AND LONG-TERM OUTCOME

There are no current treatments for prion diseases and the prognosis is poor with invariable fatality with an average of 5 years between diagnosis and death.[21] Treatments with quniacrine (antimalarial), chlorpromazine (antipsychotic), amphotericin B (antifungal), acyclovir (antiviral), and pentosan polysulfate (anticoagulant) have been

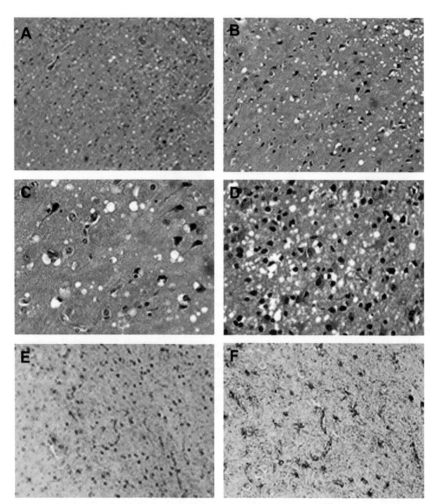

Fig. 8. (A–D) Neuropathology of prion diseases. Prion disorders are characterized by a triad of histopathologic features: spongiform degeneration, loss of neurons, and gliosis. No inflammatory response is present. Spongiform degeneration is illustrated from two different cases of sCJD. (A, B, and C, H&E stain) Images obtained from a brain biopsy specimen at ×5, ×20, and ×40 magnification, respectively. (D, H&E stain) Image from the frontal cortex of autopsy brain material obtained from a different patient at ×40 magnification. (*Courtesy of* Edward B. Lee, MD, PhD.) Both cases show vacuolar or spongiform changes (more prominent in D) in the neuropil. (E, F) Astrogliosis highlighted by an immunostain for glial fibrillary acidic protein (GFAP) from the first sample is represented at ×20 and ×40 magnifications, respectively.

used in human patients with no success.[21,22] Experimental therapies in cell culture and animal model that influence the interactions between PrP^C and PrP^{Sc}, modulating innate and adaptive immune system to enhance PrP^{Sc} elimination, and targeting the lymphatic system to decrease PrP^{Sc} generation show promise and may provide valuable insights in designing therapies in human subjects.[17,22–24] Genetic counseling of family members plays an important role in the familial forms of disease.

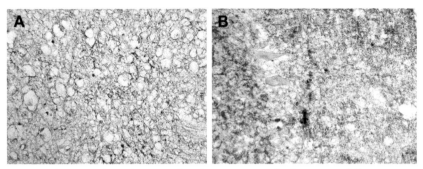

Fig. 9. (*A, B*) Immunohistochemistry for the prion protein from two different cases of sporadic CJD presented at ×20 and ×40 magnifications. PrP^{Sc} accumulation in the form of aggregates can be detected by immunohistochemistry using antibodies (antibody 3F4, mouse monoclonal) targeted against the prion protein. (*Courtesy of* Mark Cohen, MD, National Prion Disease Pathology Surveillance Center, Case Western Reserve University.)

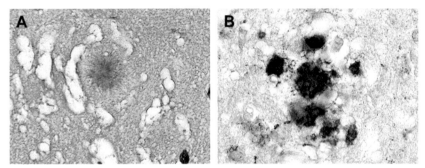

Fig. 10. (*A*) Florid plaques in prion diseases. PrP^{Sc} accumulation in the form of β-sheets may lead to the formation of *PrP* amyloid plaques in approximately 10% of sCJD cases (H&E stain presented at ×40 magnification). (*B*) An immunostain for the prion protein (antibody 34F) highlights the plaques (×40 magnification). Florid amyloid plaques are characteristic vCJD and are encountered very rarely in other forms of CJD. (*Courtesy of* Mark Cohen, MD, National Prion Disease Pathology Surveillance Center, Case Western Reserve University.)

Table 5 Diagnosis of CJD	
Features	**Clinical Features and Laboratory Test Result**
Possible CJD	Rapidly progressive dementia
	Myoclonus (may first present as exaggerated startle response)
	Ataxia and other motor abnormalities
	MRI with characteristic cortical rimming (sCJD) or pulvinar sign (vCJD)
	Increased cerebrospinal fluid levels of 14-3-3 protein
	Triphasic electroencephalogram complexes
	Family history (fCJD) or documented exposure (iCJD and vCJD)
Confirmed CJD	Mutations detected in PRNP gene (fCJD)
	Detectable PrP^{Sc} in brain biopsies or autopsy
	Detectable PrP^{Sc} in tonsillar biopsy (vCJD)

Data from Weller M, Aguzzi A. Prion diseases: Movement disorders reveal Creutzfeldt–Jakob disease. Nat Rev Neurol 2009;5:185–6.

Table 6
Differential diagnosis for prion diseases

Neurodegenerative	Alzheimer's disease
	Dementia with Lewy bodies
	Frontotemporal dementia
	Corticobasal dementia
	Progressive supranuclear palsy
Infectious	HIV-associated dementia
	Herpes encephalitis
	Progressive multifocal leukoencephalopathy
	Subacute sclerosing panencephalitis (young adults)
	Fungal infections (immunosuppression, central nervous system aspergillosis)
	Syphilis
	Parasites
	Lyme disease (rarely encephalopathy)
	Balamuthia
	Whipple disease
Toxic, metabolic	Vitamin B_{12} (cyanocobalamin) deficiency
	Vitamin B_1 (thiamine) deficiency
	Niacin deficiency
	Folate deficiency (dementia rare)
	Uremia
	Wilson disease
	Portosystemic encephalopathy
	Acquired hepatocerebral degeneration
	Porphyria
	Bismuth toxicity
	Lithium toxicity
	Mercury toxicity
	Arsenic toxicity
	Electrolyte abnormalities
Autoimmune	Hashimoto encephalopathy
	Paraneoplastic (autoimmune) limbic encephalopathy
	Nonparaneoplastic autoimmune abnormalities (eg, anti–voltage-gated potassium channel antibodies mediated)
	Lupus cerebritis
	Sarcoid
	Other central nervous system vasculitides
Endocrine	Thyroid disturbances
	Parathyroid abnormalities
	Adrenal diseases
Neoplastic	Nonautoimmune paraneoplastic conditions
	Primary central nervous system lymphoma
	Intravascular lymphoma
	Lymphomatoid granulomatosis
	Gliomatosis cerebri
	Metastases to central nervous system
Vascular	Stroke
	Hyperviscosity syndromes with polycythemia or monoclonal gammopathies
	Dural venous thrombosis
	Dural arteriovenous fistula

Data from Geschwind MD, Haman A, Miller BL. Rapidly progressive dementia. Neurol Clin 2007;25:783–807.

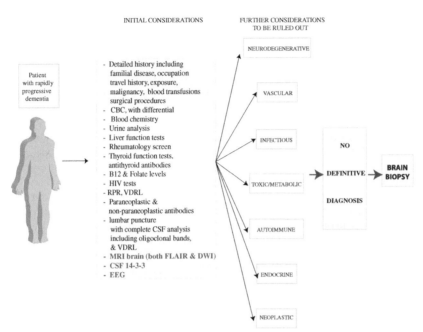

INITIAL CONSIDERATIONS

FURTHER CONSIDERATIONS
TO BE RULED OUT

NEURODEGENERATIVE

Patient
with rapidly
progressive
dementia

- Detailed history including
  familial disease, occupation
  travel history, exposure,
  malignancy, blood transfusions
  surgical procedures
- CBC, with differential
- Blood chemistry
- Urine analysis
- Liver function tests
- Rheumatology screen
- Thyroid function tests,
  antithyroid antibodies
- B12 & Folate levels
- HIV tests
- RPR, VDRL
- Paraneoplastic &
  non-paraneoplastic antibodies
- lumbar puncture
  with complete CSF analysis
  including oligoclonal bands,
  & VDRL
- MRI brain (both FLAIR & DWI)
- CSF 14-3-3
- EEG

VASCULAR

INFECTIOUS

TOXIC/METABOLIC

AUTOIMMUNE

ENDOCRINE

NEOPLASTIC

NO

DEFINITIVE

DIAGNOSIS

BRAIN
BIOPSY

Fig. 11. Clinical approach in a patient with rapidly progressive dementia. The differential diagnosis of a patient with rapidly progressive dementia is complex and a clinical algorithm proposed by Geshwind and colleagues is illustrated in **Fig. 11** and **Table 6**. Initial work-up should include delving deeper into the clinical history, comprehensive blood, urine, and cerebrospinal fluid analyses. Brain imaging including fluid-attenuated inversion-recovery and diffusion-weighted imaging, MRI, cerebrospinal fluid 14-3-3, and triphasic peaks on the electroencephalogram are suggestive but not diagnostic of prion diseases. Diseases that may manifest with dementia, especially other neurodegenerative disorders, should always be considered in the differential. Many diseases that may present with dementia, such as vascular, infectious diseases, toxic-metabolic disorders, endocrine and autoimmune abnormalities, and neoplasia (see **Table 6**) should be considered and ruled out. A brain biopsy should be performed when no definitive cause can be established. If vCJD is suspected a tonsil biopsy can be performed before a brain biopsy is attempted. (*Adapted from* Geschwind MD, Haman A, Miller BL. Rapidly progressive dementia. Neurol Clin 2007;25:783–807; with permission.)

LABORATORY TESTING RESULTS

Serologic tests for prion disease cannot be used in diagnosis, because the human body does not make antibodies to prion proteins. Conclusive diagnosis of prion diseases in the laboratory relies on the detection of PrP^{Sc}. The most common method of PrP^{Sc} detection relies on the biochemical differences between PrP^{Sc} and PrP^{C}. Limited proteolysis of PrP^{Sc} (using such agents as proteinase K) generates a smaller protease-resistant fragment (approximately 142 amino acids) termed "PrP 27–30." Under the same proteolytic conditions PrP^{C} is completely hydrolyzed. PrP 27–30 can then be detected by immunoassays, such as Western blotting. Monoclonal antibodies directed against the prion protein can be used in immunohistochemical assays in brain and tonsillar (for vCJD). Because PrP^{Sc} distribution in the brain is not uniform, however, absence of PrP^{Sc} aggregates in brain biopsies does not rule out prion disease.

The recent years have yielded many promising studies that can be applied to diagnosing prion diseases. Collinge and colleges report that precipitation of PrP^{Sc} from tissue homogenates using sodium phosphotungstic acid followed by Western blotting modified to increase sensitivity greatly enhanced detection levels of PrP^{Sc}.[25] The conformation-dependent immunoassay designed by Prusiner and colleges is independent of proteolysis and targets epitopes normally exposed in PrP^C but buried in PrP^{Sc} by using high-affinity antibodies.[26] Another assay is the protein misfolding cyclic amplification, which relies on detecting smaller PrP^{Sc} aggregates after sonification and disruption of larger aggregates into multiple smaller fragments.[27,28] This method shows a 6000-fold increase in sensitivity and was adapted in hamster models of prion diseases to detect PrP^{Sc} during early phases of infection.[28] It remains to be seen if this test can be modified for use in human subjects.

Apart from the identification of PrP^{Sc}, the ability to detect the infectivity of prions is of key importance. Infectivity has been tested using animal bioassays, which relies on the demonstration of formation of PrP^{Sc} after inoculation with the sample in transgenic animals that overexpress PrP^C.[10] The long incubation times and expense of such studies have led to the development of cell lines to test infectivity; however, these studies are yet to be adapted to routine laboratory evaluation. Other studies have focused on the detection of biomarkers in CSF and blood with the identification of potential candidate proteins, such as erythroid differentiation related factor and neuron-specific enolase.[10] These surrogate markers may not be specific, however, to the diagnosis of prion diseases. Although several promising leads are currently being actively pursued, the demonstration of PrP^{Sc} in tissues remains the definitive diagnostic test.

The National Prion Disease Pathology Surveillance Center based at Case Western Reserve University performs a variety of tests, such as immunohistochemistry and immunoblotting assays on biopsy and autopsy material, free of charge (http://www.cjdsurveillance.com).

SUMMARY

Prion diseases are a complex and fascinating set of diseases caused by conformation change of PrP^C, the native prion protein to PrP^{Sc}, the disease isoform. Prion diseases can develop from genetic, transmissible, or sporadic causes. They are invariably fatal and usually present with rapidly progressive dementia. Although brain imaging, CSF, and electroencephalogram studies have a role in diagnosis, conclusive diagnosis is made by the demonstration of PrP^{Sc} in tissue samples. There are no current effective treatments for prion diseases; however, several studies in animal models and cell culture systems offer promise in development of future therapies.

ACKNOWLEDGMENTS

The author would like to thank Clayton Wiley, MD, PhD and Mark Cohen, MD, for helpful comments. Sincere thanks are also expressed to Mark Cohen, MD, PhD and Edward Lee, MD, PhD, for providing histopathologic images.

REFERENCES

1. Prusiner SB. Shattuck lecture: neurodegenerative diseases and prions. N Engl J Med 2001;344(20):1516–26.
2. Mallucci G, Collinge J. Update on Creutzfeldt-Jakob disease. Curr Opin Neurol 2004;17(6):641–7.

3. Liberski PP, Brown P. Kuru: fifty years later. Neurol Neurochir Pol 2007;41(6): 548–56.
4. Sejvar JJ, Schonberger LB, Belay ED. Transmissible spongiform encephalopathies. J Am Vet Med Assoc 2008;233(11):1705–12.
5. Prusiner SB. Prions. Proc Natl Acad Sci U S A 1998;95(23):13363–83.
6. Aguzzi A, Sigurdson C, Heikenwaelder M. Molecular mechanisms of prion pathogenesis. Annu Rev Pathol 2008;3:11–40.
7. Aguzzi A, Heikenwalder M, Polymenidou M. Insights into prion strains and neurotoxicity. Nat Rev Mol Cell Biol 2007;8(7):552–61.
8. Aguzzi A, Baumann F, Bremer J. The prion's elusive reason for being. Annu Rev Neurosci 2008;31:439–77.
9. Prusiner SB. Prion diseases and the BSE crisis. Science 1997;278(5336):245–51.
10. Aguzzi A, Glatzel M. Prion infections, blood and transfusions. Nat Clin Pract Neurol 2006;2(6):321–9.
11. Johnson RT. Prion diseases. Lancet Neurol 2005;4(10):635–42.
12. Geschwind MD, Haman A, Miller BL. Rapidly progressive dementia. Neurol Clin 2007;25(3):783–807, vii.
13. Geschwind MD, Shu H, Haman A, et al. Rapidly progressive dementia. Ann Neurol 2008;64(1):97–108.
14. Belay ED, Schonberger LB. Variant Creutzfeldt-Jakob disease and bovine spongiform encephalopathy. Clin Lab Med 2002;22(4):849–62, v–vi.
15. Mead S, Poulter M, Uphill J, et al. Genetic risk factors for variant Creutzfeldt-Jakob disease: a genome-wide association study. Lancet Neurol 2009;8(1): 57–66.
16. Parchi P, Giese A, Capellari S, et al. Classification of sporadic Creutzfeldt-Jakob disease based on molecular and phenotypic analysis of 300 subjects. Ann Neurol 1999;46(2):224–33.
17. Aguzzi A, Sigurdson CJ. Antiprion immunotherapy: to suppress or to stimulate? Nat Rev Immunol 2004;4(9):725–36.
18. Harris DA, True HL. New insights into prion structure and toxicity. Neuron 2006; 50(3):353–7.
19. Prusiner SB. The prion diseases. Brain Pathol 1998;8(3):499–513.
20. DeArmond SJ, Prusiner SB. Prion protein transgenes and the neuropathology in prion diseases. Brain Pathol 1995;5(1):77–89.
21. Stewart LA, Rydzewska LH, Keogh GF, et al. Systematic review of therapeutic interventions in human prion disease. Neurology 2008;70(15):1272–81.
22. Weissmann C, Aguzzi A. Approaches to therapy of prion diseases. Annu Rev Med 2005;56:321–44.
23. DeArmond SJ, Prusiner SB. Perspectives on prion biology, prion disease pathogenesis, and pharmacologic approaches to treatment. Clin Lab Med 2003;23(1): 1–41.
24. Mallucci G, Collinge J. Rational targeting for prion therapeutics. Nat Rev Neurosci 2005;6(1):23–34.
25. Wadsworth JD, Joiner S, Hill AF, et al. Tissue distribution of protease resistant prion protein in variant Creutzfeldt-Jakob disease using a highly sensitive immunoblotting assay. Lancet 2001;358(9277):171–80.
26. Safar JG, Geschwind MD, Deering C, et al. Diagnosis of human prion disease. Proc Natl Acad Sci U S A 2005;102(9):3501–6.
27. Saborio GP, Permanne B, Soto C. Sensitive detection of pathological prion protein by cyclic amplification of protein misfolding. Nature 2001;411(6839):810–3.
28. Aguzzi A. Prion biology: the quest for the test. Nat Methods 2007;4(8):614–6.

Lyme Disease

Thomas S. Murray, MD, PhD, Eugene D. Shapiro, MD*

KEYWORDS

- Lyme disease • *Borrellia burdorferi* • Tick-borne infections
- Erythema migrans • Serologic testing • Misdiagnosis

OVERVIEW

Lyme disease, caused by the spirochete *Borrelia burgdorferi*, is the most common vector-borne disease in the United States. The clinical presentation varies depending on the stage of the illness and includes erthyma migrans, carditis, central nervous system disease, and arthritis. Regardless of the clinical presentation, most patients with Lyme disease have resolution of their clinical symptoms when treated with appropriate antimicrobials. Persistent symptoms after therapy are most often caused by misdiagnosis rather than treatment failure. Although Lyme disease is a public health concern, extensive publicity has resulted in a degree of anxiety about Lyme disease that is out of proportion to the actual morbidity that it causes.

MICROBIOLOGY

Lyme disease is caused by the spirochete, *B burgdorferi* sensu lato, a fastidious, microaerophilic bacterium that replicates slowly and requires special medium to grow in the laboratory (**Fig. 1**).[1] The organism has been subclassified into several genomospecies, including *B burgdorferi* sensu stricto, *B garinii*, *B afzelii*, and others. Different genomospecies seem to be associated with an increased likelihood of certain specific manifestations of Lyme disease; for example, *B burgdorferi* sensu stricto seems to have a prediction to cause arthritis (if not treated early), whereas *B garinii* seems to be associated with an increased risk of neurologic manifestations of Lyme disease. In the United States only *B burgdorferi* sensu stricto has been

---

This publication was supported in part by Clinical and Translational Science Awards grant numbers UL1 RR024139, KL2 RR024138, and K24RR022477 (EDS) from the National Center for Research Resources (NCRR) a component of the National Institutes of Health (NIH), and NIH Road map for Medical Research and K08 AI 071074 (TSM). Its contents are solely the responsibility of the authors and do not necessarily represent the official view of NCRR or NIH. Information on Re-engineering the Clinical Research Enterprise can be obtained from the NIH Web site.
Department of Pediatrics, School of Medicine, Yale University, 333 Cedar Street, PO Box 208064, New Haven, CT 06520-8064, USA
* Corresponding author.
E-mail address: Eugene.Shapiro@Yale.edu.

Clin Lab Med 30 (2010) 311–328
doi:10.1016/j.cll.2010.01.003
0272-2712/10/$ – see front matter © 2010 Elsevier Inc. All rights reserved.

labmed.theclinics.com

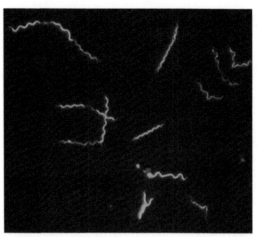

Fig. 1. *Borrellia burgdorferi*, infective bacterium of Lyme disease. The spirochete is stained with Syto 9 and visualized with fluorescent microscopy. (*Courtesy of* Sarojini Adusumilli.)

isolated from humans. In contrast, there is substantial variation in the genomospecies of *B burgdorferi* sensu lato isolated from humans in Europe.

EPIDEMIOLOGY

Most cases of Lyme disease in the United States occur in southern New England, southeastern New York, New Jersey, eastern Pennsylvania, eastern Maryland, Delaware, and parts of Minnesota, Wisconsin, and Michigan. More than three-quarters of these cases occur in fewer than 70 counties, an indication of the geographic limitation of the disease (**Fig. 2**).[2] Information about the true incidence of the disease is complicated by reliance on passive reporting of cases as well as by the high frequency of misdiagnosis.[3,4] In the most highly endemic areas of the United States, such as Connecticut, the incidence is about 0.5 cases/1000, but can be substantially higher in local areas. The incidence is highest in children 5 to 10 years of age, nearly twice as high as the incidence among adults.

In Europe, most cases occur in the Scandinavian countries and in central Europe (especially in Germany, Austria, and Switzerland), although cases have been reported throughout the region, including the United Kingdom (where many cases occur in the South Downs or New Forest areas).

B burgdorferi is transmitted by Ixodid ticks; in the United States, primarily by *Ixodes scapularis*, the deer tick (**Fig. 3**).[1] Ixodid ticks must be distinguished from other common endemic ticks such as the dog tick (**Fig. 4**). Other vectors include *Ixodes ricinus* (the sheep tick), *Ixodes persulcatus*, and *Ixodes pacificus* in Europe, Asia, and the Pacific coast of the United States, respectively. Ixodid ticks have a 2-year, 3-stage life cycle (**Fig. 5**). The larvae hatch in the early summer and are usually not infected with *B burgdorferi*. The tick may become infected at any stage of its life cycle by feeding on a host that is a natural reservoir for *B burgdorferi*, usually a small mammal such as the white-footed mouse (*Peromyscus leucopus*) (**Fig. 6**). The larvae overwinter and emerge the following spring in the nymphal stage, which is the stage of the tick that is most likely to transmit the infection.[5] Nymphs molt to become adults in the autumn. Adult females, which often spend the winter attached to large animals such as deer or

Reported Cases of Lyme Disease -- United States, 2008

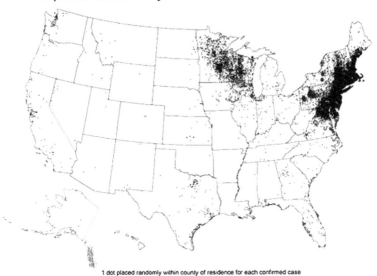

1 dot placed randomly within county of residence for each confirmed case

Fig. 2. Epidemiology of Lyme disease. The distribution of disease corresponds to the distribution of the *Ixodes* ticks that transmit *B burgdorferi*. (*Courtesy of* the Centers for Disease Control and Prevention.)

sheep (hence the names deer or sheep tick), lay their eggs the following spring before they die, and the 2-year life cycle begins again.

Several factors are associated with the risk of transmission of *B burgdorferi* from ticks to humans. First, the tick must be infected. The proportion of infected ticks varies

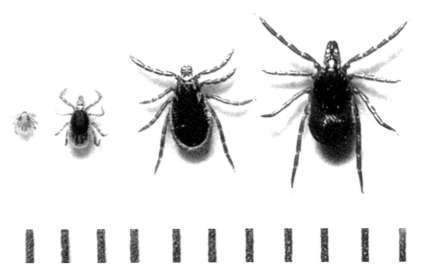

Fig. 3. Various stages of the life cycle of the deer tick *Ixodes scapularis*, the vector for Lyme disease in the northern United States. The larval stage is shown on the left, followed by the nymphal stage, the adult female, and the adult male on the right. Most infections are transmitted from ticks at the nymphal stage.

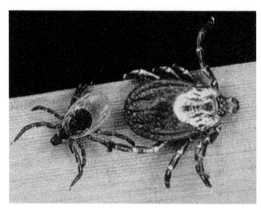

Fig. 4. A comparison of the deer tick *Ixodes scapularis*, on the left, with the dog tick *Dermacentor variabilis*, on the right. Typically, dog ticks are much larger than deer ticks.

greatly by geographic area and by the stage of the tick in its life cycle. Lyme disease is uncommon in the Pacific states because few *Ixodes pacificus* ticks are infected with *B burgdorferi*, in part because the serum of lizards, 1 of its major hosts, kills *B burgdorferi*.[6] By contrast, in highly endemic areas of southern New England rates of infection of *I scapularis* are approximately 2% for larvae, 15% to 30% for nymphs and 30% to 50% for adult ticks.[1]

There has been substantial variation in rates of infection of *Ixodes ricinus* in reports from various European countries, but approximate averages are 10% for nymphs and 20% for adult ticks.[7]

Based on studies with experimental animals, to transmit *B burgdorferi*, an infected tick generally must feed for 48 to 72 hours or longer.[8] These experimental findings were confirmed in a study in humans in which the risk of transmission from ticks (for which the duration of feeding could be assessed) to humans was 25% for nymphal ticks that had fed for at least 72 hours and 0% for nymphal ticks that had fed for less than 72 hours.[5] The bacteria live in the midgut of the tick, which needs to become engorged with blood (**Fig. 7**) before the bacteria migrate to the salivary glands and the saliva, through which the organism is injected into the host. Persons with occupational, recreational, or residential exposure to tick-infested fields, yards, or woodlands in endemic areas are at increased risk of developing Lyme disease.

CLINICAL PRESENTATION

The clinical manifestations of Lyme disease are classified into stages: early localized disease, early disseminated disease, and late disease (**Table 1**).[9,10] Erythema migrans, the manifestation of early localized disease, appears at the site of the tick bite, 3 to 30 days (typically within 7–14 days) after the bite. In the United States, erythema migrans (single or multiple) is found in about 90% of patients with objective evidence of infection with *B burgdorferi*.[11–13]

The lesion begins as a red macule or papule and expands for days to weeks to form a large, annular, erythematous lesion that is at least 5 cm and as much as 70 cm in diameter (median of 15 cm) (**Fig. 8**). Most often, the rash is uniformly erythematous or it may appear as a target lesion with variable degrees of central clearing (see **Fig. 8**). It can vary greatly in shape, and, occasionally, may have vesicular or necrotic areas in the center. Erythema migrans is usually asymptomatic but may be pruritic or

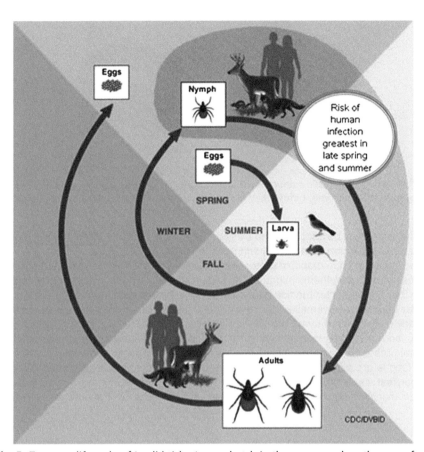

Fig. 5. Two-year life cycle of Ixodid ticks. Larvae hatch in the summer when they may feed on a small mammal infected with *B burgdorferi*. The larvae survive the winter and emerge the following spring as nymphs, when they are most likely to transmit infection. The nymphs molt to become adults in the autumn, attach to large animals during the winter, and the females lay eggs the following spring (CDC Open access photo). (*Courtesy of* the Centers for Disease Control and Prevention.)

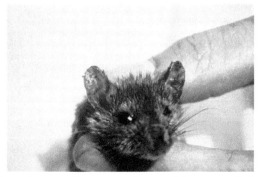

Fig. 6. The white-footed mouse (*Peromyscus leucopus*) is a reservoir for *Ixodes scapularis*. Note the large numbers of ticks attached to this mouse.

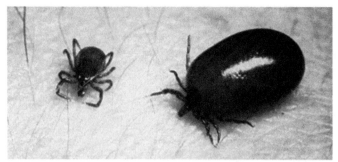

Fig. 7. An engorged *Ixodid scapularis* tick. Ticks become engorged after 48 to 72 hours. Ticks removed before this time, before they become engorged, rarely transmit Lyme disease.

painful, and it may be accompanied by systemic findings such as fever, malaise, headache, regional lymphadenopathy, stiff neck, myalgia, or arthralgia.

The most common manifestation of early disseminated Lyme disease in the United States is multiple erythema migrans. The secondary skin lesions, which usually appear from 3 to 5 weeks after the tick bite, consist of multiple annular erythematous lesions similar to, but usually smaller than, the primary lesion. Other common manifestations of early disseminated Lyme disease are cranial nerve palsies, especially facial nerve palsy, and meningitis (sometimes accompanied by papilledema and increased intracranial pressure). Systemic symptoms such as fever, myalgia, arthralgia, headache, and fatigue are also common in this stage of Lyme disease. Carditis, which usually is manifest as a prolonged PR interval or, sometimes, complete heart block, is a rare manifestation of early disseminated disease (**Fig. 9**). Patients may present

Table 1			
Clinical presentations and therapy for Lyme disease			
Disease Stage	**Clinical Manifestations**	**Treatment**	**Duration**
Early localized	Erythema migrans	Oral	14–21 days
Early disseminated	Multiple erythema migrans	Oral	14–21 days
	Isolated cranial nerve palsy	Oral	14–21 days
	Meningoradiculoneuritis		14–28 days
	Meningitis	Intravenous or oral	14–21 days
	Carditis		
	–Ambulatory	Oral	14–21 days
	–Hospitalized	Intravenous[a] followed by oral	14–21 days
	Borrelial lymphocytoma	Oral	14–21 days
Late	Arthritis	Oral	28 days
	Recurrent arthritis after oral therapy	Oral or intravenous	28 days or 14–28 days
	Encephalitis	Intravenous	14–28 days
	Acrodematitis chronica atrophicans	Oral	14–28 days

[a] At the time of discharge, the patient may receive oral medication to complete therapy.

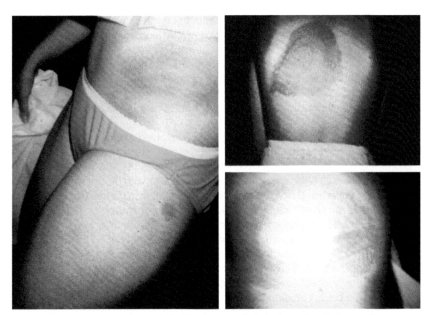

Fig. 8. Erythema migrans. This rash is the characteristic lesion of early Lyme disease. It may appear as a targetlike lesion with central clearing or may be erythematous throughout.

with fatigue, dizziness, or syncopal episodes. Although it occurs only rarely in the United States, borrelial lymphocytoma, an inflammatory infiltrate that typically occurs in the ear lobe or the breast, is seen with some frequency in patients with Lyme disease in Europe. Likewise, meningoradiculoneuritis (Bannwarth syndrome), a sometimes painful radiculopathy caused by Lyme disease, is far more common in Europe than in the United States.

The most common manifestation of late Lyme disease, which occurs weeks to months after the initial infection, is arthritis. The arthritis is usually monoarticular but

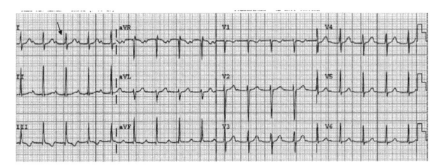

Fig. 9. Prolonged PR interval from Lyme carditis. This electrocardiogram was performed on a 9-year-old child from a Lyme endemic area with known tick exposures who presented with a history of fever, flulike symptoms, and syncope. His PR interval (shown by the arrow) was 0.548 (normal limits 0.12–0.2) consistent with first-degree heart block. He was admitted to the hospital and placed on ceftriaxone therapy. His symptoms improved after 3 days and he was discharged home on doxycycline to complete 21 days of antimicrobial therapy.

may also be oligoarticular and primarily affects the large joints, particularly the knee. Although the affected joint is typically swollen and somewhat tender, the intense pain associated with a septic arthritis is usually not present. However, Lyme arthritis can be difficult to distinguish from septic arthritis.[14] Encephalitis, encephalopathy, and polyneuropathy are also manifestations of late Lyme disease, but they are rare in children. Acrodematitis chronica atrophicans, a chronic sclerosing dermatitis, is an uncommon manifestation of Lyme disease in Europe but is virtually unknown in the United States.

Small numbers of case reports, most of which involved women with unrecognized and untreated Lyme disease during their pregnancies, suggested B burgdorferi may be transmitted across the placenta and that congenital Lyme disease was associated with poor outcomes.[15] Although spirochetes compatible with B burgdorferi were seen in pathologic specimens, B burgdorferi was never isolated in culture from any of these cases. Several subsequent studies, designed to assess the potential link between Lyme disease during pregnancy and congenital infection with B burgdorferi, found no documented B burgdorferi infections of either the fetus or the infant.[16] Additional studies found no difference in birth outcomes comparing seropositive and seronegative pregnant women.[17,18] Similarly, a survey of neurologists in endemic areas found no evidence of any credible cases of congenital Lyme disease.[19] Transmission of Lyme disease via breast feeding has also not been documented.

PATHOGENESIS

Information about the pathogenesis of Lyme disease comes from human studies and from animal models. B burgdorferi express outer surface proteins (Osps) that are important for survival in the tick and for infection in humans. OspA is required for B burgdorferi adherence to the tick midgut.[20,21] Its expression decreases during engorgement as the spirochete leaves the midgut for the salivary glands and subsequent injection into the mammalian host. During this period, the expression of OspC increases; it has been postulated that OspC plays a role in migration of and infection by the spirochete.[20] The spirochete's ability to spread through skin and other tissues may be facilitated by the binding of OspC to human plasminogen.[22] This dissemination from the site of the tick bite, via the bloodstream, produces the systemic systems that may be associated with early Lyme disease as well as the clinical manifestations of early disseminated and, ultimately, of late Lyme disease.

In humans with erythema migrans, infiltrates of macrophages and of T cells produce inflammatory and antiinflammatory cytokines.[23] There is also evidence that in disseminated infections, adaptive T-cell and B-cell responses in lymph nodes produce antibodies against many components of the spirochete.[24,25] During dissemination within humans, B burgdorferi attaches to certain host integrins[26,27] eliciting a proinflammatory response[28] that includes production of matrix glycosaminoglycans and extracellular matrix proteins,[29,30] which may explain the organism's tropisms for particular tissues (eg, collagen fibrils in the extracellular matrix in the heart, nervous system, and joints).[29]

Animal models have provided information about the clinical manifestations and immune response during early disseminated disease including neuroborreliosis and carditis. Studies in mice have clearly demonstrated the importance of inflammatory innate immune responses in controlling early disseminated Lyme disease.[31,32] After infection with B burgdorferi, mice that lack either toll-like receptor 2, a part of the innate immune system, or the toll-like receptor adaptor, MyD88, have higher bacterial loads and more severe arthritis than isogenic wild-type mice.[33,34] The role of complement in controlling infection has also been well described. Mice that lack C3 have increased numbers of spirochetes when infected; moreover, B burgdoferi produces specific proteins that inhibit complement activity, which facilitates infection.[20] A C3H mouse model of Lyme carditis has been developed in which cardiac infiltrates of macrophages and T cells produce inflammatory cytokines.[35] In these mice, the killing of spirochetes through cellular immune mechanisms seems to be the dominant factor in the resolution of cardiac disease.[36]

A nonhuman, primate, animal model of neuroborreliosis has been developed to try to better understand the spread of B burgdorferi within the nervous system.[37] In immunosuppressed monkeys with an exceptionally large inoculum of bacteria, B burgdorferi infiltrated the leptomeninges, the motor and sensory nerve roots, and the dorsal-root ganglia, but not the brain parenchyma.[38] B burgdorferi also infiltrated the perineurium (the connective tissue sheath surrounding each bundle of peripheral nerve fibers) in the peripheral nervous system of these monkeys.

Studies of patients with clinical manifestations of late disease, specifically Lyme arthritis, have confirmed observations in animals that the host immune response is important for the pathogenesis of disease. Synovial tissue from patients with Lyme arthritis typically shows synovial hypertrophy, vascular proliferation, and a marked mononuclear cell infiltrate. Sometimes pseudolymphoid follicles are present that resemble peripheral lymph nodes.[39] During acute Lyme arthritis, innate immune responses to B burgdorferi lipoprotein, as well as marked adaptive immune responses to many spirochetal proteins, are found.[40–42] Th-1 and Th-2 dependent cytokines are found in the joint fluid.[43,44] In addition, patients with Lyme arthritis typically have higher Borrelia-specific antibody titers than do patients with other manifestation of Lyme disease.[40,45] Some adult patients with Lyme arthritis, particularly those with HLA-DRB1 alleles, will develop a chronic, antibiotic treatment-resistant, autoimmune arthritis.[46,47]

DIAGNOSIS

The diagnosis of Lyme disease, especially in the absence of the characteristic rash, may be difficult, because the other clinical manifestations of Lyme disease are not specific. Even the diagnosis of erythema migrans may sometimes be difficult because the rash initially may be confused with nummular eczema, granuloma annulare, an insect bite, ringworm, or cellulitis. The rapid and prolonged (untreated, it lasts for weeks) expansion of erythema migrans helps to distinguish it from these other conditions.

The sensitivity of culture for B burgdorferi is only fair and special medium is required; moreover, it is necessary for patients to undergo an invasive procedure to obtain appropriate tissue or fluid for culture. Consequently, such tests are indicated only in rare circumstances. Diagnostic tests that are based on the identification of either antigens or DNA of B burgdorferi, including the polymerase chain reaction (PCR), have not been shown to be sufficiently accurate to be clinically useful under nonexperimental conditions. Although studies in research laboratories suggest that the PCR test is promising, contamination is a potential problem in commercial laboratories and an invasive procedure is still necessary to obtain appropriate material to test. Consequently, the confirmation of Lyme disease by the laboratory usually rests on the demonstration of antibodies to B burgdorferi in the patient's serum.

It is well documented that the sensitivity and specificity of antibody tests for Lyme disease vary substantially.[48] The accuracy and reproducibility of prepackaged commercial kits is much poorer than that of tests performed by reference laboratories that maintain tight quality control and regularly prepare the materials that are used in the test. Official recommendations from the Second National Conference on Serologic Diagnosis of Lyme Disease and from the Centers for Disease Control and Prevention are that clinicians use a 2-step procedure when ordering antibody tests for Lyme disease: first, a sensitive screening test, such as an enzyme-linked immunosorbent assay (ELISA) and, if that result is positive or equivocal, a Western immunoblot (a more specific test than the ELISA) to confirm the result.[10,49] If the ELISA result is negative, an immunoblot is not indicated. Immunoblots should not be ordered without ordering an ELISA simultaneously. The ELISA provides a quantitative estimate of the concentration of antibodies against *B burgdorferi*. The immunoblot provides information about the specificity of the antibodies; positive bands mean that antibodies against specific protein antigens of *B burgdorferi* are present. Most authorities require the presence of antibodies against at least either 2 (for IgM) or 5 (for IgG) specific proteins of *B burgdorferi* for the immunoblot to be considered positive (**Fig. 10**).[10,49] Antibody test results are not useful for the diagnosis of early localized Lyme disease. Only a minority of patients with single erythema migrans will have a positive test result because the rash usually develops before the antibodies are detectable. A diagnosis of Lyme disease should not be based on a positive IgM result alone in patients who have had symptoms for 4 weeks or more.[9]

MISDIAGNOSIS

It is critically important to understand that the predictive value of antibody test results, even of very accurate tests, is highly dependent on the prevalence of the infection

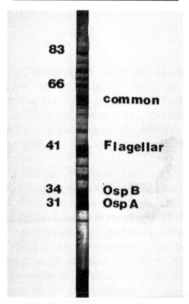

Fig. 10. IgG immunoblot used to aid in the diagnosis of Lyme disease. Immunoblots are indicated after a positive ELISA from a patient with a clinical syndrome consistent with Lyme disease. The criteria for a positive IgG immunoblot are the presence of 5 bands. In patients with erythema migrans, the immunoblot can initially be negative before the development of antibodies against *B burgdorferi*.

among patients who are tested (**Table 2**).[50] Antibody tests for Lyme disease should not be used as screening tests.[50,51] Unfortunately, because many lay persons (as well as physicians) have the erroneous belief that chronic nonspecific symptoms alone (eg, fatigue or arthralgia) may be manifestations of Lyme disease, patients with only nonspecific symptoms are frequently tested for Lyme disease. Lyme disease is the cause of the nonspecific symptoms in very few such patients, if any. However, because the specificity of even the best antibody tests for Lyme disease is nowhere near 100%, some of the test results in patients without specific signs or symptoms of Lyme disease will be falsely positive (see **Table 2**).[50,51] An erroneous diagnosis of Lyme disease is frequently made and such patients are often treated unnecessarily with antimicrobials.[52]

Clinicians should realize that even though a symptomatic patient has a positive serologic test result for antibodies to *B burgdorferi*, it is possible that Lyme disease may not be the cause of that patient's symptoms. In addition to the possibility that it is a false-positive result, the patient may have been infected with *B burgdorferi* previously, and the patient's current symptoms may be unrelated to that previous infection. Once serum antibodies to *B burgdorferi* develop, IgG and IgM may persist for many years despite adequate treatment and clinical cure of the illness.[53,54] There is no indication to recheck serology after therapy to determine the effectiveness of treatment. In addition, because some people who become infected with *B burgdorferi* never develop symptoms, in endemic areas there is a background rate of seropositivity among patients who have never had clinically apparent Lyme disease. Physicians should not routinely order antibody tests for Lyme disease for patients who have not been in endemic areas or for patients with only nonspecific symptoms.

DIFFERENTIAL DIAGNOSIS

The differential diagnosis of Lyme disease varies depending on the stage of disease. Erythema migrans, the rash of early Lyme disease, must be differentiated from inflammation associated with insect bites, nummular eczema, granuloma annulare, ringworm, and cellulitis. Other causes of carditis include viral agents, specifically Coxsackie enteroviruses. The differential diagnosis for arthritis is long and includes bacterial septic arthritis, rheumatologic, and oncologic processes.

Ixodes ticks may transmit other pathogens in addition to *B burgdorferi,* including *Babesia, Anaplasma,* other *Borrelia* species, and viruses.[1,10] These agents may be

Table 2				
Predictive value of serologic tests vary by disease prevalence				
Disease Prevalence	**Test Result**	**Disease Present**	**Disease Absent**	**Total**
1%	Positive	95	990	1085
	Negative	5	8910	8915
	Total	100	9900	10,000
	Predictive value	8.8%[a]	99.9%[b]	
10%	Positive	950	900	1850
	Negative	50	8100	8150
	Total	1000	9000	10,000
	Predictive value	51.4%[a]	99.4%[b]	

In each case the test is 95% sensitive and 90% specific.
[a] Predictive value of a positive test.
[b] Predictive value of a negative test.

transmitted either separately from or simultaneously with *B burgdorferi*. Patients should be evaluated for these organisms if they have physical or laboratory findings suggestive of these diseases.

TREATMENT

Guidelines for antimicrobial therapy for specific stages of Lyme disease have been published by the Infectious Disease Society of America (see **Table 1; Table 3**).[10] Early disease characterized by erythema migrans is best treated orally with doxycycline or amoxicillin for 14 days, although there is some evidence that 10 days of therapy may be adequate. Early disseminated disease diagnosed as either a localized cranial nerve palsy, multiple erythema migrans, or carditis in outpatients without complete heart block can also be treated with oral agents. Late disease, manifesting as arthritis, typically responds well to oral therapy with doxycycline or amoxicillin. Additional treatment with nonsteroidal antiinflammatory drugs may also provide symptomatic benefit to the patient.

Intravenous therapy with ceftriaxone is often used for Lyme meningitis. However, data from Europe shows that oral doxycycline is as effective as ceftriaxone for Lyme meningitis.[55] Another indication for ceftriaxone is myocarditis and heart block in symptomatic patients requiring hospitalization.[10] As symptoms improve, these patients can complete therapy with an oral agent.

Few clinical trials of treatment of Lyme disease have been conducted in children.[56] Most recommendations for the treatment of children are extrapolated from studies of adults. Children younger than 8 years of age should not be treated with doxycycline because it may cause permanent discoloration of their teeth. Patients who are treated with doxycycline should be alerted to the risk of developing dermatitis in sun-exposed areas while taking the medication. Cefuroxime is also approved for the treatment of Lyme disease and is an alternative for persons who cannot take doxycycline and who are allergic to penicillin. Azithromycin is less efficacious than other oral agents and should only be used when there is a clear contraindication to the preferred

Table 3
Antibiotic regimens for Lyme disease

	Treatment[a]	Adult Dose	Pediatric Dose
Oral therapy	**Doxycycline** (patients ≥8 y)	100 mg twice a day	4 mg/kg (up to 100 mg) twice a day
	Amoxicillin	500 mg three times a day	50 mg/kg (up to 500 mg) three times a day
	Cefuroxime axetil	500 mg twice a day	30 mg/kg (up to 500 mg) twice a day
Intravenous therapy	**Ceftriaxone**	2 g once a day	50–75 mg/kg (up to 2 g) once a day
	Cefotaxime	2 g every 8 h	150–200 mg/kg (up to 2 g) every 8 h
	Penicillin G	18–24 million U/d divided every 4 h	200,000–400,000 U/kg daily divided every 4 h (up to 18–24 million U/d)

[a] Most commonly used antibiotics are in bold type.

antimicrobials. There is little need to use newer agents because the results of treatment with either amoxicillin or doxycycline have been excellent.

Some patients may develop a Jarisch-Herxheimer reaction soon after treatment is initiated. The manifestations of this reaction are increased temperature, sweats, and myalgia. These symptoms resolve spontaneously within 24 to 48 hours, although administration of nonsteroidal antiinflammatory drugs is often beneficial. Antimicrobial treatment during a Jarisch-Herxheimer reaction should not be discontinued.

PROGNOSIS

The long-term prognosis for individuals who are treated with appropriate antimicrobial therapy for Lyme disease, regardless of the stage of the disease, is excellent. The most common reason for a lack of response to appropriate antimicrobial therapy for Lyme disease is misdiagnosis (ie, the patient does not have Lyme disease). Nonspecific symptoms (such as fatigue, arthralgia, or myalgia) may persist for several weeks even in successfully treated patients with early Lyme disease; their presence should not be regarded as an indication for additional treatment with antimicrobials. These symptoms usually respond to nonsteroidal antiinflammatory agents. Within a few months of completing the initial course of antimicrobial therapy, these vague nonspecific symptoms will usually resolve without additional antimicrobial therapy. For those unusual patients who have persistent symptoms more than 6 months after the completion of antimicrobial therapy, an attempt should be made to determine if these symptoms are the result of a postinfectious phenomenon or of another illness.

Klempner and colleagues[57] recently reported the results of 2 controlled trials of antibiotic treatment of adult patients with chronic musculoskeletal pain, neurocognitive symptoms, or both that persisted after antibiotic treatment of Lyme disease. One study included patients who were seropositive for IgG antibodies to B burgdorferi at the time of enrollment; the other study included patients who were seronegative. In both studies, patients were randomly assigned to receive either ceftriaxone administered intravenously for 30 days followed by doxycycline orally for 60 days or matching regimens with intravenous and oral placebos. There were no significant differences in the outcomes of patients treated with antibiotics compared with those treated with placebo among the seropositive or seronegative patients. Nearly 40% of subjects treated with placebo improved. These findings support earlier recommendations that such patients are best treated symptomatically rather than with prolonged courses of antibiotic therapy, which have been associated with serious adverse side effects.[58] Additional clinical studies of these patients confirm that the risks of long-term treatment far outweigh any possible benefits.[59]

PREVENTION OF LYME DISEASE

Reducing the risk of tick bites is 1 obvious strategy to prevent Lyme disease.[60] In endemic areas, clearing brush and trees, removing leaf litter and woodpiles, and keeping grass mowed may reduce exposure to ticks. Recent data showed that the application of acaricide to white-tailed deer prevented feeding by ticks, reducing the risk for tick-borne disease.[61] Application of pesticides to residential properties is effective in suppressing populations of ticks, but may be harmful to other wildlife and to people.

Tick and insect repellents that contain n,n-diethylmetatoluamide (DEET) applied to the skin provide additional protection, but require reapplication every 1 to 2 hours for maximum effectiveness. Serious neurologic complications in children from either frequent or excessive application of DEET-containing repellents have been reported, but they are rare and the risk is low when these products are used according to the instructions on the labels. Use of products with concentrations of DEET greater than 30% is not necessary and increases the risk of adverse effects. DEET should be applied sparingly only to exposed skin, but not to the face, hands, or skin that is either irritated or abraded. After returning indoors, skin that was treated should be washed with soap and water. Permethrin (a synthetic pyrethroid) is available in a spray for application to clothing only and is particularly effective because it kills ticks on contact.

Because most people (approximately 75%) who recognize that they were bitten by a tick remove the tick within 48 hours, the risk of Lyme disease from recognized deer tick bites is low (approximately 1%–3% in areas with a high incidence of Lyme disease). Indeed, the risk of Lyme disease is higher for unrecognized bites (because such ticks will feed for a longer time). People should be taught to inspect themselves and their children's bodies and clothing daily after possible exposure to Ixodid ticks. An attached tick should be grasped with fine-tipped tweezers as close to the skin as possible and removed by gently pulling the tick straight out. If some of the mouth parts remain embedded in the skin, they should be left alone, because they are usually extruded eventually; additional attempts to remove them often result in unnecessary damage to tissue and may increase the risk of local bacterial infection. Analysis of ticks to determine whether they are infected is not indicated because it is unclear how these test results correlate with the probability of human disease. No vaccine for Lyme disease is currently available.

A study of antimicrobial prophylaxis for tick bites among adults found that a single 200-mg dose of doxycycline was 87% effective in preventing Lyme disease, although the 95% confidence interval around this estimate of efficacy was wide (the lower bound was 25% or less, depending on the method used).[5] In that study, the only people who developed Lyme disease had been bitten by nymphal stage ticks that were at least partially engorged; the risk of Lyme disease in this group was 9.9% (among recipients of placebo), whereas it was 0% for bites by all larval and adult deer ticks. Unfortunately, the expertise to identify the species, stage, and degree of engorgement of a tick, and thereby to assess the degree of risk, is rarely available to the person who is bitten. Consequently, routine use of antimicrobial agents to prevent Lyme disease in persons who are bitten by a deer tick, even in highly endemic areas, is not generally recommended because the overall risk of Lyme disease is low (1%–3%), only doxycycline (which is not recommended for children <8 years of age) has been shown to be effective, and treatment of Lyme disease, if it does develop, is effective.[62]

SUMMARY

Lyme disease is caused by the spirochete *Borrelia burgdorferi,* injected into the blood stream after an infected tick has been attached for 48 to 72 hours. Lyme disease can manifest as early localized disease (erythema migrans), early disseminated disease (eg, meningitis or multiple erythema migrans), or late disease (large joint arthritis). The innate and adaptive immune systems contribute to the inflammatory response, which results in clinical symptoms. Regardless of the clinical presentation, most patients who are treated for Lyme disease with short courses of appropriate antibiotics do extremely well. Serologic testing for Lyme disease is imperfect and should be reserved for patients from endemic areas with a clinical syndrome and physical findings consistent with Lyme disease. Preventive measures such as checking for and removing ticks after extensive time outdoors, wearing of pants and long-sleeved shirts, and the application of tick repellant can potentially reduce the risk of Lyme disease for individuals with increased exposure to ticks.

REFERENCES

1. Shapiro ED, Gerber MA. Lyme disease. Clin Infect Dis 2000;31(2):533–42.
2. Centers for Disease Control and Prevention. Lyme disease – United States 2001–2002. MMWR Morb Mortal Wkly Rep 2004;53:365–9.
3. Steere AC, Taylor E, McHugh GL, et al. The overdiagnosis of Lyme disease. JAMA 1993;269(14):1812–6.
4. Reid MC, Schoen RT, Evans J, et al. The consequences of overdiagnosis and overtreatment of Lyme disease: an observational study. Ann Intern Med 1998; 128(5):354–62.
5. Nadelman RB, Nowakowski J, Fish D, et al. Prophylaxis with single-dose doxycycline for the prevention of Lyme disease after an *Ixodes scapularis* tick bite. N Engl J Med 2001;345(2):79–84.
6. Ullmann AJ, Lane RS, Kurtenbach K, et al. Bacteriolytic activity of selected vertebrate sera for *Borrelia burgdorferi sensu stricto* and *Borrelia bissettii*. J Parasitol 2003;89(6):1256–7.
7. Rauter C, Hartung T. Prevalence of *Borrelia burgdorferi* sensu lato genospecies in *Ixodes ricinus* ticks in Europe: a metaanalysis. Appl Environ Microbiol 2005; 71(11):7203–16.
8. Piesman J, Mather TN, Sinsky RJ, et al. Duration of tick attachment and *Borrelia burgdorferi* transmission. J Clin Microbiol 1987;25(3):557–8.
9. Steere AC. Lyme disease. N Engl J Med 2001;345(2):115–25.
10. Wormser GP, Dattwyler RJ, Shapiro ED, et al. The clinical assessment, treatment, and prevention of Lyme disease, human granulocytic anaplasmosis, and babesiosis: clinical practice guidelines by the Infectious Diseases Society of America. Clin Infect Dis 2006;43(9):1089–134.
11. Nadelman RB, Wormser GP. Lyme borreliosis. Lancet 1998;352(9127):557–65.
12. Gerber MA, Shapiro ED, Burke GS, et al. Lyme disease in children in southeastern Connecticut. Pediatric Lyme Disease Study Group. N Engl J Med 1996;335(17):1270–4.
13. Steere AC, Sikand VK, Meurice F, et al. Vaccination against Lyme disease with recombinant *Borrelia burgdorferi* outer-surface lipoprotein A with adjuvant. Lyme Disease Vaccine Study Group. N Engl J Med 1998;339(4):209–15.
14. Thompson A, Mannix R, Bachur R. Acute pediatric monoarticular arthritis; distinguishing Lyme arthritis from other etiologies. Pediatrics 2009;123:959–65.
15. Schlesinger PA, Duray PH, Burke BA, et al. Maternal-fetal transmission of the Lyme disease spirochete, *Borrelia burgdorferi*. Ann Intern Med 1985;103(1):67–8.
16. Cartter ML, Hadler JL, Gerber MA, et al. Lyme disease and pregnancy. Conn Med 1989;53(6):341–2.
17. Silver HM. Lyme disease during pregnancy. Infect Dis Clin North Am 1997;11(1): 93–7.
18. Strobino BA, Williams CL, Abid S, et al. Lyme disease and pregnancy outcome: a prospective study of two thousand prenatal patients. Am J Obstet Gynecol 1993;169(2 Pt 1):367–74.
19. Gerber MA, Zalneraitis EL. Childhood neurologic disorders and Lyme disease during pregnancy. Pediatr Neurol 1994;11(1):41–3.
20. Tilly K, Rosa PA, Stewart PE. Biology of infection with *Borrelia burgdorferi*. Infect Dis Clin North Am 2008;22:217–34.

21. Hovius JW, van Dam AP, Fikrig E. Tick-host-pathogen interactions in Lyme borreliosis. Trends Parasitol 2007;23(9):434–8.
22. Coleman JL, Gebbia JA, Piesman J, et al. Plasminogen is required for efficient dissemination of *B. burgdorferi* in ticks and for enhancement of spirochetemia in mice. Cell 1997;89(7):1111–9.
23. Mullegger RR, McHugh G, Ruthazer R, et al. Differential expression of cytokine mRNA in skin specimens from patients with erythema migrans or acrodermatitis chronica atrophicans. J Invest Dermatol 2000;115(6):1115–23.
24. Fikrig E, Feng W, Aversa J, et al. Differential expression of *Borrelia burgdorferi* genes during erythema migrans and Lyme arthritis. J Infect Dis 1998;178(4): 1198–201.
25. Krause A, Brade V, Schoerner C, et al. T cell proliferation induced by *Borrelia burgdorferi* in patients with Lyme borreliosis. Autologous serum required for optimum stimulation. Arthritis Rheum 1991;34(4):393–402.
26. Coburn J, Leong JM, Erban JK. Integrin alpha IIb beta 3 mediates binding of the Lyme disease agent *Borrelia burgdorferi* to human platelets. Proc Natl Acad Sci U S A 1993;90(15):7059–63.
27. Coburn J, Magoun L, Bodary SC, et al. Integrins alpha(v)beta3 and alpha5beta1 mediate attachment of Lyme disease spirochetes to human cells. Infect Immun 1998;66(5):1946–52.
28. Behera AK, Durand E, Cugini C, et al. *Borrelia burgdorferi* BBB07 interaction with integrin alpha3beta1 stimulates production of pro-inflammatory mediators in primary human chondrocytes. Cell Microbiol 2008;10(2):320–31.
29. Guo BP, Brown EL, Dorward DW, et al. Decorin-binding adhesins from *Borrelia burgdorferi*. Mol Microbiol 1998;30(4):711–23.
30. Probert WS, Johnson BJ. Identification of a 47 kDa fibronectin-binding protein expressed by *Borrelia burgdorferi* isolate B31. Mol Microbiol 1998;30(5): 1003–15.
31. Weis JJ, McCracken BA, Ma Y, et al. Identification of quantitative trait loci governing arthritis severity and humoral responses in the murine model of Lyme disease. J Immunol 1999;162(2):948–56.
32. Barthold SW, de Souza M. Exacerbation of Lyme arthritis in beige mice. J Infect Dis 1995;172(3):778–84.
33. Wooten RM, Ma Y, Yoder RA, et al. Toll-like receptor 2 is required for innate, but not acquired, host defense to *Borrelia burgdorferi*. J Immunol 2002;168(1): 348–55.
34. Liu N, Montgomery RR, Barthold SW, et al. Myeloid differentiation antigen 88 deficiency impairs pathogen clearance but does not alter inflammation in *Borrelia burgdorferi*-infected mice. Infect Immun 2004;72(6):3195–203.
35. Kelleher Doyle M, Telford SR 3rd, Criscione L, et al. Cytokines in murine Lyme carditis: Th1 cytokine expression follows expression of proinflammatory cytokines in a susceptible mouse strain. J Infect Dis 1998;177(1):242–6.
36. Barthold SW, Feng S, Bockenstedt LK, et al. Protective and arthritis-resolving activity in sera of mice infected with *Borrelia burgdorferi*. Clin Infect Dis 1997; 25(Suppl 1):S9–17.
37. Roberts ED, Bohm RP Jr, Lowrie RC Jr, et al. Pathogenesis of Lyme neuroborreliosis in the rhesus monkey: the early disseminated and chronic phases of disease in the peripheral nervous system. J Infect Dis 1998;178(3):722–32.
38. Cadavid D, O'Neill T, Schaefer H, et al. Localization of *Borrelia burgdorferi* in the nervous system and other organs in a nonhuman primate model of Lyme disease. Lab Invest 2000;80(7):1043–54.

39. Steere AC, Duray PH, Butcher EC. Spirochetal antigens and lymphoid cell surface markers in Lyme synovitis. Comparison with rheumatoid synovium and tonsillar lymphoid tissue. Arthritis Rheum 1988;31(4):487–95.
40. Akin E, McHugh GL, Flavell RA, et al. The immunoglobulin (IgG) antibody response to OspA and OspB correlates with severe and prolonged Lyme arthritis and the IgG response to P35 correlates with mild and brief arthritis. Infect Immun 1999;67(1):173–81.
41. Vincent MS, Roessner K, Sellati T, et al. Lyme arthritis synovial gamma delta T cells respond to *Borrelia burgdorferi* lipoproteins and lipidated hexapeptides. J Immunol 1998;161(10):5762–71.
42. Chen J, Field JA, Glickstein L, et al. Association of antibiotic treatment-resistant Lyme arthritis with T cell responses to dominant epitopes of outer surface protein A of *Borrelia burgdorferi*. Arthritis Rheum 1999;42(9):1813–22.
43. Gross DM, Steere AC, Huber BT. T helper 1 response is dominant and localized to the synovial fluid in patients with Lyme arthritis. J Immunol 1998;160(2): 1022–8.
44. Yin Z, Braun J, Neure L, et al. T cell cytokine pattern in the joints of patients with Lyme arthritis and its regulation by cytokines and anticytokines. Arthritis Rheum 1997;40(1):69–79.
45. Dressler F, Whalen JA, Reinhardt BN, et al. Western blotting in the serodiagnosis of Lyme disease. J Infect Dis 1993;167(2):392–400.
46. Steere AC, Levin RE, Molloy PJ, et al. Treatment of Lyme arthritis. Arthritis Rheum 1994;37(6):878–88.
47. Steere AC, Klitz W, Drouin EE, et al. Antibiotic-refractory Lyme arthritis is associated with HLA-DR molecules that bind a *Borrelia burgdorferi* peptide. J Exp Med 2006;203(4):961–71.
48. Shapiro ED. Lyme disease in children. Am J Med 1995;98(4A):69S–73S.
49. Centers for Disease Control and Prevention. Recommendations for test performance and interpretation from the Second National Conference on Serologic Diagnosis of Lyme Disease. MMWR Morb Mortal Wkly Rep 1995;44:590–1.
50. Seltzer EG, Shapiro ED. Misdiagnosis of Lyme disease: when not to order serologic tests. Pediatr Infect Dis J 1996;15(9):762–3.
51. Tugwell P, Dennis DT, Weinstein A, et al. Laboratory evaluation in the diagnosis of Lyme disease. Ann Intern Med 1997;127(12):1109–23.
52. Steere AC, Sikand VK. The presenting manifestations of Lyme disease and the outcomes of treatment. N Engl J Med 2003;348(24):2472–4.
53. Feder HM Jr, Gerber MA, Luger SW, et al. Persistence of serum antibodies to *Borrelia burgdorferi* in patients treated for Lyme disease. Clin Infect Dis 1992;15(5): 788–93.
54. Kalish RA, McHugh G, Granquist J, et al. Persistence of immunoglobulin M or immunoglobulin G antibody responses to *Borrelia burgdorferi* 10–20 years after active Lyme disease. Clin Infect Dis 2001;33(6):780–5.
55. Ljostad U, Skogvoll E, Eikeland R, et al. Oral doxycycline versus intravenous ceftriaxone for European Lyme neuroborreliosis: a multicentre, non-inferiority, double-blind, randomised trial. Lancet Neurol 2008;7(8):690–5.
56. Mullegger RR, Millner MM, Stanek G, et al. Penicillin G sodium and ceftriaxone in the treatment of neuroborreliosis in children – a prospective study. Infection 1991; 19(4):279–83.
57. Klempner MS, Hu LT, Evans J, et al. Two controlled trials of antibiotic treatment in patients with persistent symptoms and a history of Lyme disease. N Engl J Med 2001;345(2):85–92.

58. Ettestad PJ, Campbell GL, Welbel SF, et al. Biliary complications in the treatment of unsubstantiated Lyme disease. J Infect Dis 1995;171(2):356–61.
59. Feder HM Jr, Johnson BJ, O'Connell S, et al. A critical appraisal of "chronic Lyme disease". N Engl J Med 2007;357(14):1422–30.
60. Vazquez M, Muehlenbein C, Cartter M, et al. Effectiveness of personal protective measures to prevent Lyme disease. Emerg Infect Dis 2008;14(2):210–6.
61. Brei B, Brownstein JS, George JE, et al. Evaluation of the United States Department of Agriculture Northeast Area-wide Tick Control Project by meta-analysis. Vector Borne Zoonotic Dis 2009;9(4):423–30.
62. Shapiro ED. Doxycycline for tick bites – not for everyone. N Engl J Med 2001; 345(2):133–4.

Clostridium difficile

Scott Curry, MD*

KEYWORDS
- *Clostridium difficile* • Diarrhea • Toxigenic culture
- Asymptomatic

OVERVIEW

Since its discovery as the leading cause of antibiotic-associated diarrhea and colitis in 1978, *Clostridium difficile* infections have evolved from nuisance complications of antimicrobial therapy to severe, sometimes fatal, events that are the scourge of hospitals worldwide. Despite preliminary evidence that community-acquired disease exists, *C difficile* infection (CDI) remains the paradigm of a hospital-acquired infection. This article discusses the changing epidemiology, clinical presentation, and pathogenesis of CDI and highlights the ongoing challenges of its laboratory diagnosis, treatment, and relapse.

MICROBIOLOGY

C difficile is an obligate anaerobic, spore-forming, gram-positive rod first described in 1935 as *Bacillus difficilis* among the fecal flora of healthy infants.[1] The organism was recognized as the cause of what had previously been referred to as antibiotic-associated colitis in 1977.[2,3] *C difficile* was so named by Hall and O'Toole to reflect the difficulty with which it was isolated mostly attributable to its relatively slow growth (40–70 minutes doubling time) compared with most other members of the genus *Clostridium*.[1] Adding to this difficulty, *C difficile* is exquisitely aerointolerant during logarithmic growth phases when vegetative cells predominate,[4] making it difficult for clinical microbiology laboratories not equipped with anaerobic chambers to passage the organism before sporulation. However, culture of the organism has been unfairly perceived as difficult because various selective media have been developed to aid in the identification of the organism from stool specimens (**Fig. 1**).[5,6] These media capitalize on the ability of *C difficile* to ferment fructose and mannitol as well as alkalinize undefined media; these reactions occur because Stickland reactions play a central role in the organism's biosynthetic pathways.[7] Bile salts, particularly pure sodium taurocholate, have been shown to be vital to the germination of *C difficile* endospores in vitro and are included in many formulations of selective media.[8,9]

Division of Infectious Diseases, University of Pittsburgh School of Medicine, Pittsburgh, PA, USA
* Public Health ID Laboratory, 861 Scaife Hall, 3550 Terrace Street, Pittsburgh, PA 15261.
E-mail address: currysr@upmc.edu

Clin Lab Med 30 (2010) 329–342
doi:10.1016/j.cll.2010.04.001
0272-2712/10/$ – see front matter © 2010 Elsevier Inc. All rights reserved.

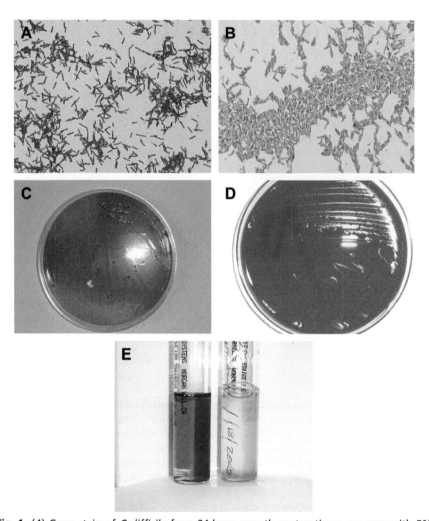

Fig. 1. (*A*) Gram stain of *C difficile* from 24-hour growth on trypticase soy agar with 5% sheep blood. The vegetative cell bodies are often gram negative during early growth; note the abundant subterminal endospores that do not swell the parent cell. (*B*) Malachite green stain of 48-hour growth of *C difficile*. The safranin counterstain renders vegetative cells pink, whereas the endospores stain green, revealing their ovoid shape. (*C*) A 48-hour growth of *C. difficile* on typical selective agar medium, *C difficile* basal agar with moxalactam and norfloxacin, CDMN, that uses norfloxacin and moxalactam as selective antibiotics to allow primary isolation from stool specimens. Other media use combinations of cycloserine and cefoxitin as selective antibiotics (cycloserine cefoxitin fructose agar). Neutral red is turned yellow by *C difficile* growth. (*D*) Typical appearance of *C difficile* colonies on trypticase soy agar with 5% sheep blood at 48 hours. Colonies are nonhemolytic. (*E*) A selective broth medium for isolation of *C difficile*, cycloserine cefoxitin mannitol broth with taurocholate and lysozyme. The tube at right shows turbidity and growth of *C difficile* at 24 hours, with obvious alkalinization of the neutral red indicator. The tube at left is a negative control.

Once isolated from human or animal specimens, *C difficile* can be passed anaero-bically to routine media, such as 5% sheep blood agar, in which it assumes its char-acteristic irregular ground-glass colonial morphology (**Fig. 2**). Colonies vary greatly in size, with more motile strains having maximum colony widths of 12 to 15 mm. Smaller colonies of *C difficile* can be difficult to distinguish from those of *Clostridium innoc-uum*, the next most frequently encountered species when working with human stool specimens, but biochemical confirmation with L-proline aminopeptidase activity on a spot disk test can provide rapid confirmation of suspect *C difficile*.[10]

The endospores of *C difficile* are resistant to heat, 70% ethanol used in hand san-itizers, and the quaternary ammonium detergents used as hospital and laboratory disinfectants, but sodium hypochlorite–based solutions are capable of inactivating spores.[11] The viability of *C difficile* endospores contaminating hospital environments declines with time but has no theoretical limit, a property that explains the persistence of *C difficile* in hospital environments.[12]

EPIDEMIOLOGY

Two risk factors have been traditionally considered the *sine qua non* for CDI: exposure to antimicrobials and to health care facilities. In addition, age greater than 65 years has been repeatedly associated with an increased risk of symptomatic infection.[13,14]

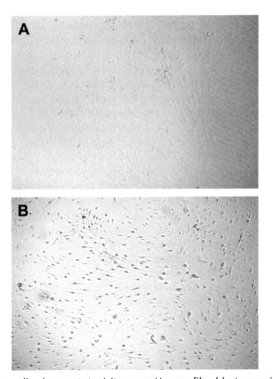

Fig. 2. (*A*) Negative cell culture cytotoxicity assay. Human fibroblasts remain spindle-shaped and in contact with each other. (*B*) Positive cell culture cytotoxicity assay revealing cyto-pathic effects of *C difficile* toxin B causing cell rounding and separation. (*Courtesy of* Ray Hariri, PhD.)

Beginning in 2000, however, CDI epidemiology changed dramatically, with an increase in disease incidence and severity, including fulminant colitis, colectomy, and death.[15–17] This epidemic has been reported worldwide, and C difficile incidence in US hospitals doubled from 1996 to 2003.[13] A newly emergent epidemic strain of C difficile, which was rarely encountered before 2000 and is now responsible for 30% to 50% of CDI cases, has been associated with this phenomenon.[16,17] The epidemic strain has been named NAP1 by pulsed-field gel electrophoresis, 027 by polymerase chain reaction (PCR) ribotyping, and BI by restriction endonuclease typing and is usually referred to as NAP1/BI/027 in recent literature.[18]

Only 3% to 15% of healthy, nonhospitalized adults are colonized with C difficile, and studies have shown that the colonization is transient.[19,20] In contrast, a prospective survey found that 26% of 428 hospitalized patients in a medical ward acquired C difficile. In this study, only 38% developed symptoms consistent with CDI by 11 months, indicating that 62% of patients who acquired C difficile were asymptomatically colonized.[21]

The silent reservoir of asymptomatically colonized patients has been implicated as a source of nosocomial CDI cases.[22] In a classic study by Clabots and colleagues,[22] 21% of all admissions to a single medical ward at a Veterans Affairs hospital were positive for C difficile carriage during a 9-month period. Of these, 86% were asymptomatic carriers. Nosocomial acquisition was observed in 41% of admissions. Molecular typing of recovered isolates revealed 19 instances of nosocomial transmission among asymptomatic patients. Nosocomial acquisition of the same strains was documented within the same hospital room separated in time by up to 24 weeks, suggesting that environmental contamination contributes to C difficile transmission and infection via spores. The study also documented transmission between pairs of patients who were in rooms far separated from each other, suggesting transmission of C difficile spores on the hands of health care workers to new ward admissions.[22] Based on these results, asymptomatic C difficile carriage from new admissions, mostly from other health care facilities, is a major source of incident CDI cases within hospitals.

Since 2005, severe C difficile disease has been reported in patients previously assumed to be at a low risk for CDI, including pregnant women and outpatients without known exposures to antimicrobials.[23] Population-based studies have been undertaken in Connecticut and Manitoba, which showed rates of community disease as 7.6 and 23.4 cases per 100,000 person-years, respectively.[24,25] These studies could not exhaustively exclude secondary exposures to health care facilities, such as visiting hospitalized relatives. However, even if these estimates of the incidence of community-acquired C difficile are accurate, they pale in comparison to incidence rates of hospital-acquired C difficile, which are expressed per 10,000 patient-days.

C difficile is also an important pathogen in livestock animals and has been found in retail meats and even in salads, leading to the speculation that community-onset CDI could be a zoonotic or food-borne infection.[26–37] However, thus far, the strains found in food and animals have been strains that are uncommon in human infections, and no clear epidemiologic link has been established between the food supply and CDI to date.

CLINICAL PRESENTATION

Asymptomatic carriers are by far the most prevalent group among those individuals who are culture-positive for toxigenic C difficile, representing 62% to 86% of hospitalized individuals with C difficile-positive stools in previous prospective studies.[21,22] Among those with symptomatic CDI, the disease manifests as anything from mild diarrhea to fulminant colitis. The onset of CDI is often considerably delayed, occurring up to 60 days (median 20.3 days) from the time of hospital discharge.[38] Observational evidence indicates that patients remain at risk for CDI for up to 12 weeks after exposure to antimicrobials.[39,40]

Few descriptive series of CDI have been published, but in the pre-2001 era, development of semiformed diarrhea more than 7 days after antimicrobial exposure was the most common presentation among a series of 43 inpatients.[41] Leukocytosis is a common feature of CDI, which has been found to be the most common cause for unexplained leukocytosis among inpatients and the fourth most common cause for leukocytosis overall.[42,43] Fever is seen in only 50% of cases, and bloody diarrhea is seen in a distinct minority of cases.[41] Rapid increases in leukocytosis, abdominal distension or pain, and sudden cessation of diarrhea are poor prognostic signs associated with development of severe colitis.[44]

PATHOGENESIS

The secretory diarrhea and colonic inflammation seen in CDI is attributable to the effects of 2 large toxins, toxin A (TcdA) and toxin B (TcdB), both encoded as part of the 19.6-kb pathogenicity locus (PaLoc) on the C difficile chromosome.[45–47] Toxin-negative strains of C difficile in which the entire PaLoc is replaced with a 115-bp sequence are common.[48] TcdA and TcdB, similar to other large clostridial toxins, glycosylate small guanosine triphosphatases in the Rho and Ras families when endocytosed into epithelial cells, leading to actin filament disassembly, disruption of tight junctions, and ultimately cell death.[49] Previous studies using pure TcdB and TcdA pointed to a synergistic role for the 2 toxins in CDI, but the recent ability to create gene knockouts in C difficile has led to the demonstration that TcdB is necessary and sufficient to cause disease in a hamster model.[50] This finding is concordant with the clinical observation that TcdA−TcdB+ C difficile strains are fully capable of causing human disease.[51–53]

In wild-type strains of C difficile, TcdA and TcdB are expressed only in late-logarithmic and stationary growth phases.[46,54] Toxin production is under the immediate control of 2 other proteins also encoded on the PaLoc, TcdR and TcdC, which serve as positive and negative regulators, respectively.[46,54–56] BI/NAP1/027 strains have been strongly associated with nonsense mutations in tcdC that lead to a truncated, dysfunctional TcdC and thus TcdB production at all phases of growth.[57,58] There is also in vitro evidence that BI/NAP1/027 strains produce more toxins than wild-type strains.[55,56,59]

C difficile also has potential virulence factors outside the PaLoc, including a binary toxin, encoded by two genes cdtA and cdtB, which is also common among BI/NAP1/027 strains.[60–62] Evidence for a role of CDT in CDI, however, is limited by the observation that CDT+TcdA−TcdB− strains are incapable of reproducing CDI in the hamster model[63] and that these strains have not yet been associated with human disease. Preliminary evidence also points to increased adherence to intestinal mucosa mediated by mutations in slpA, a surface layer protein, in BI/NAP1/027 strains of C difficile.[64] BI/NAP1/027 strains have an enhanced sporulation capacity compared with wild-type strains.[65] Antibiotic resistance, particularly to clindamycin, macrolides, fluoroquinolones, and rifampin, is also more common in the BI/NAP1/027 strains and leads to potentiation of the spread of the organism within hospitals where such antibiotics are in common use.[15,17,66]

DIAGNOSIS

Diagnosis of CDI remains one of the most vexing difficulties for hospital microbiology laboratories. The gold standard for diagnosis of CDI involves isolation of C difficile from stool by anaerobic culture followed by confirmation that the recovered isolate generates toxin, a process termed toxigenic culture (TC). TC takes up to 7 days and lacks specificity because of the large number of asymptomatically colonized individuals, and few hospital microbiology labs are equipped to perform it.

Cell culture cytotoxicity neutralization assays (CCCNAs) (see **Fig. 2**) remain the most sensitive test for CDI in clinical use. Patient stool is filtered and incubated with human fibroblast cells with and without *C difficile* antitoxin for up to 48 hours, and if the antitoxin-free well shows a cytopathic effect and the antitoxin well does not, the presence of *C difficile* toxin in stool is confirmed (see **Fig. 2**). Historically, CCCNA was 67% to 78% sensitive when compared with TC as the gold standard,[67,68] but over time such assays came to be regarded as a clinical gold standard in their own right to which more rapid assays were compared. More recent studies, however, confirm the imperfect sensitivity of CCCNA itself compared with TC.[69,70] This finding may reflect continued improvements in the selective media used in TC and the skill of the labs performing it.

Cell culture cytotoxicity assays have been replaced in 90% of hospital microbiology labs in North America and Europe by enzyme-linked immunosorbent assays (ELISAs) for TcdA or TcdA+TcdB because of their ease of use and rapid turnaround time of approximately 2 hours. However, ELISA suffers from a comparatively low sensitivity of 80% to 90% when compared with cell culture cytotoxicity,[68,71–73] and it is even less sensitive when compared with TC.

Clinicians and laboratories have struggled with the sensitivity issue for CDI in several ways. Repeated testing, that is, submission of multiple samples from the same patient within a short time frame, has a marginal return for ELISA and cell culture cytotoxicity assays and lacks sufficient negative predictive value to guide decisions about withholding empiric CDI therapy.[74–77] Various 2-step testing algorithms incorporating a rapid card test for *C difficile* common antigen (glutamate dehydrogenase) followed by backup testing of positives to confirm toxin production by ELISA or cell culture cytotoxicity have been devised,[78–80] but recent reports questioning the sensitivity of the common antigen screen have cast doubt on this strategy.[81,82]

The development of PCR testing for *C difficile* holds great promise in combining the relative sensitivity of cell culture cytotoxicity with the rapid turnaround time of ELISA. Most commercial and research assays have used *tcdB* and/or *tcdC* as their targets, thus excluding false-positive results from detection of nontoxigenic strains of *C difficile*. The performance characteristics of the assays published to date are summarized in **Table 1**. Although PCR-based assays could theoretically supersede the sensitivity of TC because of the ability to detect nonviable *C difficile*, to date the published data indicate that PCR has approximated the sensitivity of CCCNAs (see **Table 1**). PCR shares with TC an inability to distinguish the asymptomatic carrier state from CDI; the published specificities for the assay excluded solid stool specimens from testing. Labs that do not reject solid specimens for *C difficile* testing may expect a diminished specificity for CDI.

DIFFERENTIAL DIAGNOSIS

Presumed community-onset CDI should also be considered in the same scenarios in which *Campylobacter*, *Clostridium perfringens*, *Giardia* spp, and *Entamoeba histolytica* infections are entertained. *Salmonella* spp, *Shigella*, *E. coli* H7:O157 should also be entertained given the occasional presentation of CDI as bloody diarrhea. Clinicians should bear in mind that although *C difficile* is the leading infectious cause of diarrhea after antibiotics, 70% of postantibiotic diarrhea is simply a consequence of the

Table 1
Performance characteristics of PCR assays for detection of *C difficile* toxin genes in stool samples

Gene Target	Chemistry/ Manufacturer	Sensitivity	Specificity	PPV	NPV	Gold Standard	References
tcdB	Prodesse (Gen-Probe Prodesse, Waukesha, WI, USA)	77.3	99.2	99.2	99.4	TC	70
tcdB	BD GeneOhm (BD Diagnostics, LaJolla, CA, USA)	96.4	99.1	99.6	91.4	Composite[a]	83
tcdB	Cepheid (Sunnyvale, CA, USA)	97.1	93.0	72.3	99.4	CCCNA	84
tcdB	BD GeneOhm	88.5	95.4	88.5	95.4	TC	85
tcdB	BD GeneOhm	83.6	98.2	89.5	97.1	TC	69
tcdC	FRET	86	97	90	96	TC	73
tcdB	SYBR green	93.3	97.4	75.7	99.4	Composite[a]	86
tcdB	Taqman-FAM	87.1	96.5	60.0	99.2	CCCNA	87

Abbreviations: FRET, fluorescence resonance energy transfer probe; NPV, negative predictive value; PPV, positive predictive value; TC, toxigenic culture.
[a] Composite, CCCNA with TC used to resolve discrepant results.

antimicrobials themselves. Ischemic colitis and inflammatory bowel disease should always be on the differential diagnosis for acute and chronic diarrheal illnesses, and the latter has a unique association with CDI that is poorly understood.

Despite the foregoing, the differential diagnosis of hospital-onset diarrhea after 48 hours of admission virtually excludes all other infectious causes of diarrhea other than *C difficile*, and many hospital microbiology labs do not process routine stool cultures or parasite screens collected after 48 hours of hospitalization in immunocompetent patients.

TREATMENT, PROGNOSIS, AND LONG-TERM OUTCOME

Before the emergence of the BI/NAP1/027 strain, *C difficile* was often regarded as a self-limited disease so long as the inciting antimicrobial agents could be stopped. Early therapeutic trials sometimes contained placebo arms, and head-to-head comparisons of the 2 main *C difficile* antimicrobials, enteral vancomycin and metronidazole, failed to show superiority for either.[88] Metronidazole was generally recommended by expert guidelines as first-line therapy for reasons of cost and out of concern that widespread use of vancomycin would promote acquisition of vancomycin-resistant enterococci within hospitals. Post-2001, however, several observational reports indicated an increasing failure rate for metronidazole treatment, and a randomized, double-blind trial of metronidazole versus vancomycin showed superior response rates for vancomycin in a subset of patients with severe disease.[89] There are no randomized trials of parenteral therapy for patients with toxic megacolon or obstipation caused by severe CDI, a frequent circumstance in severe disease. Intravenous metronidazole in combination with vancomycin enemas is a common anecdotal combination, as is the recently reported tigecycline monotherapy used successfully for severe disease in several cases in the Netherlands.[90]

The choice of anti–*C difficile* antimicrobial, particularly in severe cases, is unlikely to be of critical importance for a toxin-mediated disease. Alternative therapies aimed at binding toxins using sequestrant polymers were initially promising but failed in phase 3 trials.[91] Probiotics, chiefly various formulations of *Lactobacillus* spp and *Saccharomyces boulardii*, attracted much initial attention as agents for primary prevention of CDI and for secondary prevention of recurrence, but the evidence for efficacy of these agents has been lacking and concerns about their safety in immunocompromised patients have led to a marked decrease in enthusiasm for their use.[92]

The prognosis for most patients with CDI remains favorable, but in the era of the BI/NAP1/027 strain predominance, adverse event rates for CDI (colectomy/death) reached as high as 44 of 253 (17.3%) for inpatients with hospital-acquired CDI at the University of Pittsburgh during a 2-year period.[15] A 30-day attributable mortality of 6.9% was observed in 20 hospitals in Quebec subsequently.[17] For patients who require colectomy, all-cause mortality is 50%.[44] *C difficile* thus remains a dire complication for hospitalized patients who develop severe disease.

IMMUNITY AND REINFECTION

The most troubling aspect of CDI is the high relapse rate of 25%, generally higher in elderly individuals, particularly those older than 65 years. Multiple relapses are a common occurrence in the same population group and have been strongly associated with a failure to demonstrate an anamnestic IgG response against TcdA.[93–97] Besides age and immune senescence, continued exposure to antibiotics is a powerful predictor of CDI relapse.[98] Efforts to devise a *C difficile* toxoid vaccine have met with initial success in individuals with multiple relapses,[99] but to date there are no published trials using vaccines for primary prevention of CDI. The debilitating effects of multiple CDI relapses have led to varying treatment approaches, all anecdotal, such as long, tapering courses of vancomycin,[100] courses of the nonabsorbable antibiotic rifaximin,[101] or even fecal bacteriotherapy (stool transplant) administered by enema or nasogastric tube.[102–104] Although reported response rates for fecal bacteriotherapy have been astonishingly good, there may be substantial publication bias, and the technique is difficult to make widespread or practical. A recent randomized, placebo-controlled trial of passive immunotherapy for recurrent CDI using monoclonal antibodies to TcdA and TcdB showed an 18% reduction in the absolute risk of recurrence.[105]

SUMMARY

C difficile has reemerged as a major hospital-acquired infection since 2001. The development of PCR-based testing holds substantial promise as a single clinical diagnostic test with sufficient sensitivity, specificity, and turnaround time to be entirely reliable for disease diagnosis in comparison to previously used tests. The importance of *C difficile* acquired outside the hospital environment remains an unknown factor and awaits further epidemiologic investigation. Treatment of CDI is currently limited to antimicrobials, which themselves alter the fecal flora and may exacerbate the problem of recurrent disease, but passive immunotherapy and vaccine strategies hold promise for a more rational therapy for this toxin-mediated disease.

REFERENCES

1. Hall I, O'Toole E. Intestinal flora in newborn infants with a description of a new pathogenic anaerobe, *Bacillus difficilis*. Am J Dis Child 1935;49:390–402.
2. Bartlett JG, Chang TW, Gurwith M, et al. Antibiotic-associated pseudomembranous colitis due to toxin-producing clostridia. N Engl J Med 1978;298(10):531–4.

3. Bartlett JG, Onderdonk AB, Cisneros RL, et al. Clindamycin-associated colitis due to a toxin-producing species of Clostridium in hamsters. J Infect Dis 1977;136(5):701–5.

4. Jump RL, Pultz MJ, Donskey CJ. Vegetative *Clostridium difficile* survives in room air on moist surfaces and in gastric contents with reduced acidity: a potential mechanism to explain the association between proton pump inhibitors and *C. difficile*-associated diarrhea? Antimicrob Agents Chemother 2007;51(8):2883–7.

5. Arroyo LG, Rousseau J, Willey BM, et al. Use of a selective enrichment broth to recover *Clostridium difficile* from stool swabs stored under different conditions. J Clin Microbiol 2005;43(10):5341–3.

6. Riggs MM, Sethi AK, Zabarsky TF, et al. Asymptomatic carriers are a potential source for transmission of epidemic and nonepidemic *Clostridium difficile* strains among long-term care facility residents. Clin Infect Dis 2007;45(8): 992–8.

7. Jackson S, Calos M, Myers A, et al. Analysis of proline reduction in the nosocomial pathogen *Clostridium difficile*. J Bacteriol 2006;188(24):8487–95.

8. Wilson KH. Efficiency of various bile salt preparations for stimulation of *Clostridium difficile* spore germination. J Clin Microbiol 1983;18(4):1017–9.

9. Wilson KH, Kennedy MJ, Fekety FR. Use of sodium taurocholate to enhance spore recovery on a medium selective for *Clostridium difficile*. J Clin Microbiol 1982;15(3):443–6.

10. Fedorko DP, Williams EC. Use of cycloserine-cefoxitin-fructose agar and L-proline-aminopeptidase (PRO Discs) in the rapid identification of *Clostridium difficile*. J Clin Microbiol 1997;35(5):1258–9.

11. Fawley WN, Underwood S, Freeman J, et al. Efficacy of hospital cleaning agents and germicides against epidemic *Clostridium difficile* strains. Infect Control Hosp Epidemiol 2007;28(8):920–5.

12. Kim KH, Fekety R, Batts DH, et al. Isolation of *Clostridium difficile* from the environment and contacts of patients with antibiotic-associated colitis. J Infect Dis 1981;143(1):42–50.

13. McDonald LC, Owings M, Jernigan DB. *Clostridium difficile* infection in patients discharged from US short-stay hospitals, 1996-2003. Emerg Infect Dis 2006; 12(3):409–15.

14. Zilberberg MD, Shorr AF, Kollef MH. Increase in adult *Clostridium difficile*-related hospitalizations and case-fatality rate, United States, 2000-2005. Emerg Infect Dis 2008;14(6):929–31. PMCID: 2600276.

15. Muto CA, Pokrywka M, Shutt K, et al. A large outbreak of *Clostridium difficile*-associated disease with an unexpected proportion of deaths and colectomies at a teaching hospital following increased fluoroquinolone use. Infect Control Hosp Epidemiol 2005;26(3):273–80.

16. McDonald LC, Killgore GE, Thompson A, et al. An epidemic, toxin gene-variant strain of *Clostridium difficile*. N Engl J Med 2005;353(23):2433–41.

17. Loo VG, Poirier L, Miller MA, et al. A predominantly clonal multi-institutional outbreak of *Clostridium difficile*-associated diarrhea with high morbidity and mortality. N Engl J Med 2005;353(23):2442–9.

18. Rupnik M, Wilcox MH, Gerding DN. *Clostridium difficile* infection: new developments in epidemiology and pathogenesis. Nat Rev Microbiol 2009;7(7): 526–36.

19. Nakamura S, Mikawa M, Nakashio S, et al. Isolation of *Clostridium difficile* from the feces and the antibody in sera of young and elderly adults. Microbiol Immunol 1981;25(4):345–51.

20. Ozaki E, Kato H, Kita H, et al. *Clostridium difficile* colonization in healthy adults: transient colonization and correlation with enterococcal colonization. J Med Microbiol 2004;53(Pt 2):167–72.

21. McFarland LV, Mulligan ME, Kwok RY, et al. Nosocomial acquisition of *Clostridium difficile* infection. N Engl J Med 1989;320(4):204–10.

22. Clabots CR, Johnson S, Olson MM, et al. Acquisition of *Clostridium difficile* by hospitalized patients: evidence for colonized new admissions as a source of infection. J Infect Dis 1992;166(3):561–7.

23. Centers for Disease Control and Prevention (CDC). Severe *Clostridium difficile*-associated disease in populations previously at low risk-four states, 2005. MMWR Morb Mortal Wkly Rep 2005;54(47):1201–5.

24. Centers for Disease Control and Prevention (CDC). Surveillance for community-associated *Clostridium difficile*–Connecticut, 2006. MMWR Morb Mortal Wkly Rep 2008;57(13):340–3.

25. Lambert PJ, Dyck M, Thompson LH, et al. Population-based surveillance of *Clostridium difficile* infection in Manitoba, Canada, by using interim surveillance definitions. Infect Control Hosp Epidemiol 2009;30(10):945–51.

26. Indra A, Lassnig H, Baliko N, et al. *Clostridium difficile*: a new zoonotic agent? Wien Klin Wochenschr 2009;121(3–4):91–5.

27. Jobstl M, Heuberger S, Indra A, et al. *Clostridium difficile* in raw products of animal origin. Int J Food Microbiol 2010;138(1–2):172–5.

28. Norman KN, Harvey RB, Scott HM, et al. Varied prevalence of *Clostridium difficile* in an integrated swine operation. Anaerobe 2009;15(6):256–60.

29. Rodriguez-Palacios A, Reid-Smith RJ, Staempfli HR, et al. Possible seasonality of *Clostridium difficile* in retail meat, Canada. Emerg Infect Dis 2009;15(5):802–5.

30. Rodriguez-Palacios A, Staempfli HR, Duffield T, et al. *Clostridium difficile* in retail ground meat, Canada. Emerg Infect Dis 2007;13(3):485–7. PMCID: 2725909.

31. Songer JG. The emergence of *Clostridium difficile* as a pathogen of food animals. Anim Health Res Rev 2004;5(2):321–6.

32. Songer JG. Clostridia as agents of zoonotic disease. Vet Microbiol 2010; 140(3–4):399–404.

33. Songer JG, Trinh HT, Killgore GE, et al. *Clostridium difficile* in retail meat products, USA, 2007. Emerg Infect Dis 2009;15(5):819–21.

34. Weese JS. *Clostridium difficile* in food–innocent bystander or serious threat? Clin Microbiol Infect 2010;16(1):3–10.

35. Weese JS, Avery BP, Rousseau J, et al. Detection and enumeration of *Clostridium difficile* spores in retail beef and pork. Appl Environ Microbiol 2009; 75(15):5009–11.

36. Weese JS, Reid-Smith RJ, Avery BP, et al. Detection and characterization of *Clostridium difficile* in retail chicken. Lett Appl Microbiol 2010;50(4):362–5.

37. Bakri MM, Brown DJ, Butcher JP, et al. *Clostridium difficile* in ready-to-eat salads, Scotland. Emerg Infect Dis 2009;15(5):817–8.

38. Kelly CP, Pothoulakis C, LaMont JT. *Clostridium difficile* colitis. N Engl J Med 1994;330(4):257–62.

39. Kutty PK, Benoit SR, Woods CW, et al. Assessment of *Clostridium difficile*-associated disease surveillance definitions, North Carolina, 2005. Infect Control Hosp Epidemiol 2008;29(3):197–202.

40. McDonald LC, Coignard B, Dubberke E, et al. Recommendations for surveillance of *Clostridium difficile*-associated disease. Infect Control Hosp Epidemiol 2007;28(2):140–5.

41. Manabe YC, Vinetz JM, Moore RD, et al. *Clostridium difficile* colitis: an efficient clinical approach to diagnosis. Ann Intern Med 1995;123(11):835–40.
42. Wanahita A, Goldsmith EA, Marino BJ, et al. *Clostridium difficile* infection in patients with unexplained leukocytosis. Am J Med 2003;115(7):543–6.
43. Wanahita A, Goldsmith EA, Musher DM. Conditions associated with leukocytosis in a tertiary care hospital, with particular attention to the role of infection caused by *Clostridium difficile*. Clin Infect Dis 2002;34(12):1585–92.
44. Dallal RM, Harbrecht BG, Boujoukas AJ, et al. Fulminant *Clostridium difficile*: an underappreciated and increasing cause of death and complications. Ann Surg 2002;235(3):363–72.
45. Soehn F, Wagenknecht-Wiesner A, Leukel P, et al. Genetic rearrangements in the pathogenicity locus of *Clostridium difficile* strain 8864–implications for transcription, expression and enzymatic activity of toxins A and B. Mol Gen Genet 1998;258(3):222–32.
46. Hundsberger T, Braun V, Weidmann M, et al. Transcription analysis of the genes tcdA-E of the pathogenicity locus of *Clostridium difficile*. Eur J Biochem 1997; 244(3):735–42.
47. Braun V, Hundsberger T, Leukel P, et al. Definition of the single integration site of the pathogenicity locus in *Clostridium difficile*. Gene 1996;181(1–2):29–38.
48. Cohen SH, Tang YJ, Silva J Jr. Analysis of the pathogenicity locus in *Clostridium difficile* strains. J Infect Dis 2000;181(2):659–63.
49. Voth DE, Ballard JD. *Clostridium difficile* toxins: mechanism of action and role in disease. Clin Microbiol Rev 2005;18(2):247–63.
50. Lyras D, O'Connor JR, Howarth PM, et al. Toxin B is essential for virulence of *Clostridium difficile*. Nature 2009;458(7242):1176–9.
51. Johnson S, Sambol SP, Brazier JS, et al. International typing study of toxin A-negative, toxin B-positive *Clostridium difficile* variants. J Clin Microbiol 2003; 41(4):1543–7.
52. Samra Z, Talmor S, Bahar J. High prevalence of toxin A-negative toxin B-positive *Clostridium difficile* in hospitalized patients with gastrointestinal disease. Diagn Microbiol Infect Dis 2002;43(3):189–92.
53. Moncrief JS, Zheng L, Neville LM, et al. Genetic characterization of toxin A-negative, toxin B-positive *Clostridium difficile* isolates by PCR. J Clin Microbiol 2000;38(8):3072–5.
54. Hammond GA, Lyerly DM, Johnson JL. Transcriptional analysis of the toxigenic element of *Clostridium difficile*. Microb Pathog 1997;22(3):143–54.
55. Dupuy B, Govind R, Antunes A, et al. *Clostridium difficile* toxin synthesis is negatively regulated by TcdC. J Med Microbiol 2008;57(Pt 6):685–9.
56. Matamouros S, England P, Dupuy B. *Clostridium difficile* toxin expression is inhibited by the novel regulator TcdC. Mol Microbiol 2007;64(5):1274–88.
57. Curry SR, Marsh JW, Muto CA, et al. tcdC genotypes associated with severe TcdC truncation in an epidemic clone and other strains of *Clostridium difficile*. J Clin Microbiol 2007;45(1):215–21.
58. MacCannell DR, Louie TJ, Gregson DB, et al. Molecular analysis of *Clostridium difficile* PCR ribotype 027 isolates from Eastern and Western Canada. J Clin Microbiol 2006;44(6):2147–52.
59. Warny M, Pepin J, Fang A, et al. Toxin production by an emerging strain of *Clostridium difficile* associated with outbreaks of severe disease in North America and Europe. Lancet 2005;366(9491):1079–84.
60. Rupnik M, Grabnar M, Geric B. Binary toxin producing *Clostridium difficile* strains. Anaerobe 2003;9(6):289–94.

61. Barbut F, Decre D, Lalande V, et al. Clinical features of *Clostridium difficile*-associated diarrhoea due to binary toxin (actin-specific ADP-ribosyltransferase)-producing strains. J Med Microbiol 2005;54(Pt 2):181–5.

62. McEllistrem MC, Carman RJ, Gerding DN, et al. A hospital outbreak of *Clostridium difficile* disease associated with isolates carrying binary toxin genes. Clin Infect Dis 2005;40(2):265–72.

63. Geric B, Carman RJ, Rupnik M, et al. Binary toxin-producing, large clostridial toxin-negative *Clostridium difficile* strains are enterotoxic but do not cause disease in hamsters. J Infect Dis 2006;193(8):1143–50.

64. Joost I, Speck K, Herrmann M, et al. Characterisation of *Clostridium difficile* isolates by *slpA* and *tcdC* gene sequencing. Int J Antimicrob Agents 2009; 33(Suppl 1):S13–8.

65. Akerlund T, Persson I, Unemo M, et al. Increased sporulation rate of epidemic *Clostridium difficile* Type 027/NAP1. J Clin Microbiol 2008;46(4):1530–3.

66. Curry SR, Marsh JW, Shutt KA, et al. High frequency of rifampin resistance identified in an epidemic *Clostridium difficile* clone from a large teaching hospital. Clin Infect Dis 2009;48(4):425–9.

67. Peterson LR, Olson MM, Shanholtzer CJ, et al. Results of a prospective, 18-month clinical evaluation of culture, cytotoxin testing, and culturette brand (CDT) latex testing in the diagnosis of *Clostridium difficile*-associated diarrhea. Diagn Microbiol Infect Dis 1988;10(2):85–91.

68. Walker RC, Ruane PJ, Rosenblatt JE, et al. Comparison of culture, cytotoxicity assays, and enzyme-linked immunosorbent assay for toxin A and toxin B in the diagnosis of *Clostridium difficile*-related enteric disease. Diagn Microbiol Infect Dis 1986;5(1):61–9.

69. Stamper PD, Alcabasa R, Aird D, et al. Comparison of a commercial real-time PCR assay for tcdB detection to a cell culture cytotoxicity assay and toxigenic culture for direct detection of toxin-producing *Clostridium difficile* in clinical samples. J Clin Microbiol 2009;47(2):373–8.

70. Stamper PD, Babiker W, Alcabasa R, et al. Evaluation of a new commercial TaqMan PCR assay for direct detection of the *Clostridium difficile* toxin B gene in clinical stool specimens. J Clin Microbiol 2009;47(12):3846–50.

71. Depitre C, Avesani V, Delmee M, et al. Detection of *Clostridium difficile* toxins in stools. Comparison between a new enzyme immunoassay for toxin A and other routine tests. Gastroenterol Clin Biol 1993;17(4):283–6.

72. Shanholtzer CJ, Willard KE, Holter JJ, et al. Comparison of the VIDAS *Clostridium difficile* toxin A immunoassay with *C. difficile* culture and cytotoxin and latex tests. J Clin Microbiol 1992;30(7):1837–40.

73. Sloan LM, Duresko BJ, Gustafson DR, et al. Comparison of real-time PCR for detection of the *tcdC* gene with four toxin immunoassays and culture in diagnosis of *Clostridium difficile* infection. J Clin Microbiol 2008;46(6):1996–2001.

74. Nemat H, Khan R, Ashraf MS, et al. Diagnostic value of repeated enzyme immunoassays in *Clostridium difficile* infection. Am J Gastroenterol 2009;104(8):2035–41.

75. Drees M, Snydman DR, O'Sullivan CE. Repeated enzyme immunoassays have limited utility in diagnosing *Clostridium difficile*. Eur J Clin Microbiol Infect Dis 2008;27(5):397–9.

76. Renshaw AA, Stelling JM, Doolittle MH. The lack of value of repeated *Clostridium difficile* cytotoxicity assays. Arch Pathol Lab Med 1996;120(1):49–52.

77. Aichinger E, Schleck CD, Harmsen WS, et al. Nonutility of repeat laboratory testing for detection of *Clostridium difficile* by use of PCR or enzyme immunoassay. J Clin Microbiol 2008;46(11):3795–7.

78. Wren MW, Kinson R, Sivapalan M, et al. Detection of *Clostridium difficile* infection: a suggested laboratory diagnostic algorithm. Br J Biomed Sci 2009;66(4): 175–9.
79. Novak-Weekley SM, Marlowe EM, Miller JM, et al. *Clostridium difficile* testing in the clinical laboratory by use of multiple testing algorithms. J Clin Microbiol 2010;48(3):889–93.
80. Goldenberg SD, Cliff PR, Smith S, et al. Two-step glutamate dehydrogenase antigen real-time polymerase chain reaction assay for detection of toxigenic *Clostridium difficile*. J Hosp Infect 2010;74(1):48–54.
81. Snell H, Ramos M, Longo S, et al. Performance of the TechLab C. DIFF CHEK-60 enzyme immunoassay (EIA) in combination with the *C. difficile* Tox A/B II EIA kit, the Triage *C. difficile* panel immunoassay, and a cytotoxin assay for diagnosis of *Clostridium difficile*-associated diarrhea. J Clin Microbiol 2004;42(10):4863–5.
82. Crobach MJ, Dekkers OM, Wilcox MH, et al. European Society of Clinical Microbiology and Infectious Diseases (ESCMID): data review and recommendations for diagnosing *Clostridium difficile*-infection (CDI). Clin Microbiol Infect 2009; 15(12):1053–66.
83. Terhes G, Urban E, Soki J, et al. Comparison of a rapid molecular method, the BD GeneOhm Cdiff assay, to the most frequently used laboratory tests for detection of toxin-producing *Clostridium difficile* in diarrheal feces. J Clin Microbiol 2009;47(11):3478–81.
84. Huang H, Weintraub A, Fang H, et al. Comparison of a commercial multiplex real-time PCR to the cell cytotoxicity neutralization assay for diagnosis of *Clostridium difficile* infections. J Clin Microbiol 2009;47(11):3729–31.
85. Eastwood K, Else P, Charlett A, et al. Comparison of nine commercially available *Clostridium difficile* toxin detection assays, a real-time PCR assay for *C. difficile* tcdB, and a glutamate dehydrogenase detection assay to cytotoxin testing and cytotoxigenic culture methods. J Clin Microbiol 2009;47(10):3211–7.
86. Peterson LR, Manson RU, Paule SM, et al. Detection of toxigenic *Clostridium difficile* in stool samples by real-time polymerase chain reaction for the diagnosis of *C. difficile*-associated diarrhea. Clin Infect Dis 2007;45(9):1152–60.
87. van den Berg RJ, Vaessen N, Endtz HP, et al. Evaluation of real-time PCR and conventional diagnostic methods for the detection of *Clostridium difficile*-associated diarrhoea in a prospective multicentre study. J Med Microbiol 2007;56(Pt 1):36–42.
88. Teasley DG, Gerding DN, Olson MM, et al. Prospective randomised trial of metronidazole versus vancomycin for *Clostridium-difficile*-associated diarrhoea and colitis. Lancet 1983;2(8358):1043–6.
89. Zar FA, Bakkanagari SR, Moorthi KM, et al. A comparison of vancomycin and metronidazole for the treatment of *Clostridium difficile*-associated diarrhea, stratified by disease severity. Clin Infect Dis 2007;45(3):302–7.
90. Herpers BL, Vlaminckx B, Burkhardt O, et al. Intravenous tigecycline as adjunctive or alternative therapy for severe refractory *Clostridium difficile* infection. Clin Infect Dis 2009;48(12):1732–5.
91. Louie TJ, Peppe J, Watt CK, et al. Tolevamer, a novel nonantibiotic polymer, compared with vancomycin in the treatment of mild to moderately severe *Clostridium difficile*-associated diarrhea. Clin Infect Dis 2006;43(4):411–20.
92. Pillai A, Nelson R. Probiotics for treatment of *Clostridium difficile*-associated colitis in adults. Cochrane Database Syst Rev 2008;(1):CD004611.
93. Aboudola S, Kotloff KL, Kyne L, et al. *Clostridium difficile* vaccine and serum immunoglobulin G antibody response to toxin A. Infect Immun 2003;71(3): 1608–10.

94. Kelly CP. Immune response to *Clostridium difficile* infection. Eur J Gastroenterol Hepatol 1996;8(11):1048–53.
95. Kyne L, Warny M, Qamar A, et al. Asymptomatic carriage of *Clostridium difficile* and serum levels of IgG antibody against toxin A. N Engl J Med 2000;342(6):390–7.
96. Kyne L, Warny M, Qamar A, et al. Association between antibody response to toxin A and protection against recurrent *Clostridium difficile* diarrhoea. Lancet 2001;357(9251):189–93.
97. Salcedo J, Keates S, Pothoulakis C, et al. Intravenous immunoglobulin therapy for severe *Clostridium difficile* colitis. Gut 1997;41(3):366–70.
98. Garey KW, Sethi S, Yadav Y, et al. Meta-analysis to assess risk factors for recurrent *Clostridium difficile* infection. J Hosp Infect 2008;70(4):298–304.
99. Sougioultzis S, Kyne L, Drudy D, et al. *Clostridium difficile* toxoid vaccine in recurrent *C. difficile*-associated diarrhea. Gastroenterology 2005;128(3):764–70.
100. McFarland LV, Elmer GW, Surawicz CM. Breaking the cycle: treatment strategies for 163 cases of recurrent *Clostridium difficile* disease. Am J Gastroenterol 2002;97(7):1769–75.
101. Johnson S, Schriever C, Galang M, et al. Interruption of recurrent *Clostridium difficile*-associated diarrhea episodes by serial therapy with vancomycin and rifaximin. Clin Infect Dis 2007;44(6):846–8.
102. Bakken JS. Fecal bacteriotherapy for recurrent *Clostridium difficile* infection. Anaerobe 2009;15(6):285–9.
103. You DM, Franzos MA, Holman RP. Successful treatment of fulminant *Clostridium difficile* infection with fecal bacteriotherapy. Ann Intern Med 2008;148(8):632–3.
104. Tvede M, Rask-Madsen J. Bacteriotherapy for chronic relapsing *Clostridium difficile* diarrhoea in six patients. Lancet 1989;1(8648):1156–60.
105. Lowy I, Molrine DC, Leav BA, et al. Treatment with monoclonal antibodies against *Clostridium difficile* toxins. N Engl J Med 2010;362(3):197–205.

Erratum

An error occurred in the article 'Developments in Immunologic Assays for Respiratory Viruses' by Marie Louise Landry, Volume 29, Issue 4, Page 638 (December 2009). The credit line for Table 1 should have been placed with Table 2, and read "*Data from* Landry ML, Ferguson D. Suboptimal detection of influenza virus in adults by the Directigen Flu A+B enzyme immunoassay and correlation of results with the number of antigen-positive cells detected by cytospin immunofluorescence. J Clin Microbiol 2003;41:3407–9." We apologize for this oversight.

Clin Lab Med 30 (2010) 343
doi:10.1016/j.cll.2009.12.002
0272-2712/10/$ – see front matter © 2010 Elsevier Inc. All rights reserved.

labmed.theclinics.com

Index

Note: Page numbers of article titles are in **boldface** type.

A

Clin Lab Med 30 (2010) 345–364
doi:10.1016/S0272-2712(10)00028-4
0272-2712/10/$ – see front matter © 2010 Elsevier Inc. All rights reserved.

labmed.theclinics.com

Moving?

Make sure your subscription moves with you!

To notify us of your new address, find your **Clinics Account Number** (located on your mailing label above your name), and contact customer service at:

Email: journalscustomerservice-usa@elsevier.com

800-654-2452 (subscribers in the U.S. & Canada)
314-447-8871 (subscribers outside of the U.S. & Canada)

Fax number: 314-447-8029

Elsevier Health Sciences Division
Subscription Customer Service
3251 Riverport Lane
Maryland Heights, MO 63043

*To ensure uninterrupted delivery of your subscription, please notify us at least 4 weeks in advance of move.

Printed and bound by CPI Group (UK) Ltd, Croydon, CR0 4YY

03/10/2024

01040450-0013